P9-EDE-819

POINT LOMA NAZARENE COLLEGE
*Ryan Library*
3900 Lomaland Drive, San Diego, CA 92106-2899

# HANDBOOK OF
# ADULT & PEDIATRIC
# RESPIRATORY HOME CARE

618,92
H236r

# HANDBOOK OF
# ADULT & PEDIATRIC
# RESPIRATORY HOME CARE

**JOAN TURNER, RN, MS**

Assistant Clinical Professor
University of California San Francisco School of Nursing
Coordinator, Pulmonary Research Unit
San Francisco General Hospital
San Francisco, CA

**GWENDOLYN J. McDONALD, RN, MS**

Clinical Assistant Professor
University of Washington School of Nursing
Respiratory Clinical Nurse Specialist
Division of Pulmonary and Critical Care Medicine
University of Washington Medical Center
Seattle, Washington

**NANCI L. LARTER, RN, MSN**

Clinical Nurse Specialist
Pediatric Pulmonary Center
University of Washington, Seattle
Community Health Liaison
Children's Hospital and Medical Center
Seattle, Washington

POINT LOMA NAZARENE COLLEGE
WITHDRAWN
RYAN LIBRARY

*With **114** illustrations*

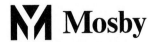 Mosby

St. Louis  Baltimore  Boston  Chicago  London  Madrid  Philadelphia  Sydney  Toronto

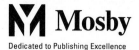

Executive Editor: N. Darlene Como
Senior Developmental Editor: Laurie Sparks
Project Manager: Patricia Tannian
Manuscript Editor: Kathy Lumpkin
Senior Book Designer: Gail Morey Hudson
Manufacturing Supervisor: Theresa Fuchs

**Copyright © 1994 by Mosby–Year Book, Inc.**

All rights reserved. No part of this publication may be reproduced,
stored in a retrieval system, or transmitted, in any form or by any
means, electronic, mechanical, photocopying, recording, or otherwise,
without prior written permission from the publisher.

Permission to photocopy or reproduce solely for internal or personal
use is permitted for libraries or other users registered with the Copyright
Clearance Center, provided that the base fee of $4.00 per chapter plus $.10
per page is paid directly to the Copyright Clearance Center, 27 Congress
Street, Salem, MA 01970. This consent does not extend to other kinds
of copying, such as copying for general distribution, for advertising or
promotional purposes, for creating new collected works, or for resale.

Printed in the United States of America
Composition by Graphic World, Inc.
Printing/binding by R.R. Donnelley & Sons Company

Mosby–Year Book, Inc.
11830 Westline Industrial Drive, St. Louis, Missouri 63146

**Library of Congress Cataloging in Publication Data**

Handbook of adult & pediatric respiratory home care  /  [edited by] Joan
  Turner, Gwendolyn J. McDonald, Nanci L. Larter.
       p.      cm.
    Includes index.
    ISBN 0-8016-5163-8
    I. Turner, Joan.      II. McDonald, Gwendolyn J.      III. Larter, Nanci
      L.     IV. Title: Handbook of adult and pediatric respiratory care.
    [DNLM:   1. Respiratory Therapy—handbooks.   2. Home Care Services—
      handbooks.   3. Respiratory Distress Syndrome—therapy—handbooks.
      4. Respiratory Distress Syndrome, Adult—therapy—handbooks.   WF 39
    H236 1993]
    RC735.H65H36      1993
    616.2′0046—dc20
    DNLM/DLC
    for Library of Congress                                    93-25213
                                                               CIP

       93  94  95  96  97  /  9  8  7  6  5  4  3  2  1

# CONTRIBUTORS

**VIRGINIA CARRIERI-KOHLMAN, RN, DNSc**

Professor and Coordinator,
Critical Care/Trauma,
Graduate Nursing Program,
University of California San Francisco School of Nursing,
San Francisco, California

**PATRICIA A. DETTENMEIER, RN, MSN(R), CCRN**

Clinical Nurse Specialist,
Division of Pulmonology and Pulmonary Occupational Medicine,
St. Louis University Medical Center,
St. Louis, Missouri

**LINDA K. FAHR, RN, MN**

Manager, Medical/Surgical Unit,
Pacific Communities Hospital,
Newport, Oregon

**MARSHA D.M. FOWLER, RN, MS, PhD, M.Div**

Professor, School of Nursing and Graduate School of Theology,
Azusa Pacific University;
Director, Parish Nurse Clinical Specialization,
Pastoral Staff, Westminster Presbyterian Church
Temple City, California

**MARGARET F. GLONINGER, RD, MS**

Formerly Assistant Professor of Nutrition,
Department of Epidemiology ESPH,
Cystic Fibrosis Clinic, Children's Hospital,
Pittsburgh, Pennsylvania

**MARGARET M. IRWIN, RN, MN**

Assistant Vice President,
Department of Nursing,
Allegheny General Hospital,
Pittsburgh, Pennsylvania

**SUSAN JANSON-BJERKLIE, RN, DNSc, FAAN**

Professor, Department of Physiological Nursing,
Adjunct Professor, Department of Medicine,
University of California San Francisco,
San Francisco, California

**JANET JONES, MPT**

Physical Therapist, Pulmonary Medicine,
Children's Hospital and Medical Center,
Seattle, Washington

**KATHRYN A. KANDAL, BA, RRT**

Respiratory Care Practitioner,
Respiratory Care Services,
California Pacific Medical Center,
San Francisco, California

**NANCI L. LARTER, RN, MSN**

Clinical Nurse Specialist,
Pediatric Pulmonary Center,
University of Washington, Seattle;
Community Health Liaison,
Children's Hospital and Medical Center,
Seattle, Washington

**SUSAN G. MARSHALL, MD**

Assistant Professor, Department of Pediatrics,
School of Medicine, University of Washington;
Attending Physician, Pulmonary Medicine,
Children's Hospital and Medical Center,
Seattle, Washington

**JUDY I. MASSONG, BSN, MS, JD**

Schroeter, Goldmark and Bender, PS,
Seattle, Washington

**GWENDOLYN J. McDONALD, RN, MS**

Clinical Assistant Professor,
University of Washington School of Nursing;
Respiratory Clinical Nurse Specialist,
Division of Pulmonary and Critical Care Medicine,
University of Washington Medical Center,
Seattle, Washington

**ANN CONDON MEYERS, RD, MS**

Formerly Chief Clinical Dietitian,
Children's Hospital,
Pittsburgh, Pennsylvania

**MARIJO MILLER-RATCLIFFE, RN, MN**

Clinical Nurse Specialist,
Pediatric Pulmonary Center,
University of Washington,
Seattle, Washington

**NANCY A. MIZUMORI, BS**

Formerly Freelance Medical Writer,
Seattle, Washington

**A. BRUCE MONTGOMERY, MD**

Assistant Clinical Professor,
University of California San Francisco,
San Francisco General Hospital,
San Francisco, California

**ELLAN J.P. NELSON, MBA, RN, RRT**

Manager, Endocrinology, Asthma, and Allergy,
Virginia Mason Medical Center,
Seattle, Washington

**LOUISE M. NETT, RN, RRT**

Research Associate,
Presbyterian–St. Luke's Center for Health Sciences Education,
Denver, Colorado

**DIANA R. OPENBRIER, RN, PhD**

Pulmonary Clinical Nurse Specialist,
Formerly Veterans Administration Medical Center,
Pittsburgh, Pennsylvania

**AMY L. PADAVICH, RN, BSN**

Yakima, Washington;
Formerly Nurse Clinician,
Asthma and Allergy Associates,
Seattle, Washington

**WILLIAM S. PRENTICE, RN, BSN**

Pulmonary Liaison Nurse,
Rancho Los Amigos Medical Center,
Downey, California

**THEDA RICKERSON-WONG, RN, MS**

Instructor/Facilitator,
Better Breather's Course and Club,
American Lung Association of San Francisco and American Red Cross,
San Francisco, California

**CAROL M. TAYLOR, RN, MN**

Oncology Services Manager,
Group Health Cooperative of Puget Sound,
Seattle, Washington

**ROBIN B. THOMAS, RN, PhD**

Individual, Couple, and Family Therapist,
Seattle, Washington

**SALLY CRIM TIBBALS, RN, MS**

Assistant Professor, Nurse Science,
Oklahoma State University,
Oklahoma City, Oklahoma

**JOAN TURNER, RN, MS**

Assistant Clinical Professor,
University of California San Francisco School
of Nursing;
Coordinator, Pulmonary Research Unit,
San Francisco General Hospital,
San Francisco, California

**MARY S. VOGT-YANTA, RN, MS**

Pulmonary Clinical Nurse Specialist,
Clinical Faculty,
Lewis and Clark Community College School
of Nursing,
St. Louis, Missouri

**KAY A. WICKS, BSN**

Administrative Director, Department of Surgery,
Children's Hospital and Medical Center,
Seattle, Washington

**LYNN M. WITHEY, RN**

Prince Nursing Service,
Ontario, California

For our patients who taught us so much . . . .

JRT, GJMcD, NLL

*This book is also dedicated to*

*my children*

**Christine, Nancy, and Michael**

whose love and encouragement sustain me

JRT

*my father*

**Howard**

who has been my lifelong academic role model

*my mother*

**Audrey**

who followed this project with great pride but
did not live to celebrate its completion

*and my husband*

**Curt**

who supported me through all
the ups and downs of its long gestation

GJMcD

*my children*

**Christopher and Elizabeth**

whose love and laughter enrich and support
the balance of work and play in my life

NLL

# PREFACE

In the face of escalating health care costs and increased pressure to limit hospital stays, patients with lung disease are being discharged much earlier and at a stage in their convalescence when they continue to require close monitoring of cardiopulmonary status. Patients are often discharged with new equipment or medications that they must learn to use safely and effectively. Thus care of the patient in the home requires professional staff with specialized knowledge and skills in cardiopulmonary assessment, respiratory rehabilitation, and the use and maintenance of a wide variety of home respiratory therapy equipment. It also requires an understanding of psychosocial and behavioral responses to chronic respiratory impairment, and of current approaches to the medical management of respiratory problems.

The home is a less expensive alternative to the institution for many types of complicated therapy such as long-term ventilatory care and intravenous therapy for cystic fibrosis. Professional support in the home enables the patient and family to cope with sophisticated medication and treatment regimens and to identify significant problems early. Having a qualified professional in the home permits evaluation of the patient's adherence and response to therapy, as well as the assessment of family and environmental factors that may influence patient progress. For a child with chronic lung disease, care in the home promotes developmental growth, better adaptation into the family, and psychosocial support in a warm, caring environment.

## PURPOSE OF THIS BOOK

In this book we address the etiology, assessment, treatment, and nursing care of physical and psychosocial problems that are encountered most frequently in the home care of adults and children with chronic lung disease. The book is written from the perspective of the home care nurse who usually cares for adults, but who occasionally sees pediatric patients. We hope that it will be a useful guide for other home care professionals as well. We believe that the problems of adults and children, and their assessment and management, have more similarities than differences. Therefore we have chosen to integrate pediatric and adult content whenever possible. Approaches to the physical assessment and psychosocial problems that are unique to the adult or child are discussed in separate chapters. Other differences between children and adults are noted within chapters. For ease of identification, content relating specifically to children is italicized throughout the book.

Recommended procedures such as cleaning of equipment and use of clean versus sterile techniques have been adapted from consensus reports whenever possible or are based on the authors' experience about accepted practice. However, the reader must recognize that care procedures vary from region to region and change with time. Thus home care nurses must know the standards of care within their own agencies and communities and must remain current through journals and continuing education programs.

## IDEAL CANDIDATES FOR HOME CARE

Generally patients with chronic lung disease are referred for home care after hospitalization for an acute exacerbation. Patients who are most likely to benefit from home care include:

1. The patient with a newly diagnosed chronic lung disease, especially if that diagnosis has an emotionally charged significance or if the treatment regimen requires technical skill
2. The patient (or caregiver) with poor coping assets, significant anxiety, confusion, or forgetfulness
3. The patient who is going home with new equipment or with any major change in therapy
4. The unstable patient with labile cardiopulmonary status who needs close supervision and frequent cardiopulmonary assessment
5. The "revolving door patient" who has developed a pattern of cycling through the emergency department or being readmitted to the hospital
6. The patient with significant disability who needs assistance to identify and access community resources so that he or she can function independently at home

## DISCHARGE PLANNING

Discharge planning is the first step toward ensuring a smooth transition from the hospital to home and is critical to the successful management of complicated home care regimens. Early in discharge planning the level of care the patient requires must be determined and a nursing agency or registry chosen if needed. Options for care include private duty nursing, intermittent visits by home health agency staff, and nonlicensed caregivers. The choice depends on the severity of the patient's disability, the complexity of nursing needs, patient and family support systems, funding, and the adequacy of support services available from community agencies and the equipment vendor.

It is important for the home care nurse to be involved in the discharge planning process. This is particularly so for patients with complex care needs such as ventilator-dependent patients. Special discharge planning needs of patients receiving mechanical ventilation are addressed in Chapter 16. A home visit to evaluate the safety and adequacy of the home may be indicated before discharge.

It is important for the home care nurse to obtain a discharge summary for all patients referred for home care following a hospitalization for an acute exacerbation. This must include a listing of all current prescribed medications, any pertinent abnormal physical findings, and results of diagnostic tests. A copy of the discharge teaching plan should be obtained, especially if the patient is a child, so that patient and family education that has been initiated in the hospital is continued at home until educational goals have been achieved.

It is also important for the home care nurse to provide feedback to the hospital-based caregivers about the patient's condition, progress toward mastery of the educational goals, and any problems or successes that may relate to hospital interventions. This establishes a cyclic pattern of ongoing communication that helps to bridge the gap between hospital and home.

## MEDICARE REIMBURSEMENT ISSUES

The vast majority of home care agencies in the United States in the 1990s are Medicare-certified agencies that must adhere to Health Care Financing Administration guidelines in order to be reimbursed for services they provide. Clear and skillful documentation that reflects adherence to these guidelines is key to ensuring reimbursement. A discussion of specific strategies for documentation would be useful in a book such as this but is generally not feasible because Medicare guidelines change often and are subject to regional interpretation. Therefore individual home care agency administrators will need to assume responsibility for educating their nurses about policies and procedures for Medicare documentation.

## ACKNOWLEDGMENTS

The editors wish to thank the many colleagues who have provided support and feedback at critical times during the development of this manuscript. These include Moira L. Aitken, MD; Kathryn Anderson, RN, PhD; MaryAnne Blake, MSLS; Soo Borson, MD; Marianne Breskind, RD; Beverly Davis, RN, MSN, OCN; Douglas Eckman, MBA, RRT; Carol Franzen, RRT; Mia Hannula, MLS; Philip Hopewell, MD; Leonard Hudson, MD; S. Lakshminarayan, MD; Sue Lareau, RN, MS; Kathryn Lee, RN, PhD; Michael Mahlmeister, MS, RRT; Tom Martin, MD; David Ralph, MD; Nancy Risser, MN, RNC, ANP; Deanna Ritchie, RN, MN; Joanne Rokosky, RN, MN; Ruth Shride, RRT; Patricia Spencer, RN; and Martha L. Tyler, RN, MN, RRT.

The editors are especially grateful for the invaluable insights and personal experiences Nancy Mizumori provided for Chapter 16. Nancy was a medical writer and a courageous, productive, and wise woman who lived for many years on full ventilatory support. Nancy died of progressive neuromuscular disease on July 6, 1989.

The editors also wish to acknowledge the core consultative contribution of Dr. Soo Borson to the discussion of depression and anxiety in Chapter 17. Dr. Borson is an Associate Professor, Department of Psychiatry and Behavioral Sciences, University of Washington Medical Center, Seattle, Washington.

## ABOUT THE AUTHORS

Gwen McDonald is a Respiratory Clinical Nurse Specialist who has worked in home care for over 10 years. While with the San Francisco Visiting Nurse Association in the 1970s, she participated in the development of the first respiratory home care program in the nation. In 1979 she moved to Seattle to develop a highly successful Respiratory Home Care Program for Seattle/King County Visiting Nurse Services. She is an experienced consultant in respiratory home care and has developed an extensive curriculum and has taught many courses and classes on this subject. She has coordinated several research studies including a major study of the safety and efficacy of treatment for depression in people with COPD, and most recently the rhDNase trials for people with cystic fibrosis. She has published several articles, has presented research findings, and has been an invited speaker at national and international meetings. She is currently coordinator of the Adult Cystic Fibrosis Center at the University of Washington Medical Center and holds a clinical faculty position with the University of Washington School of Nursing. She has served as chair of the American Thoracic Society Section on Nursing and is active in both state and national respiratory organizations.

Nanci Larter, a Pediatric Pulmonary Clinical Nurse Specialist since 1975, has provided direct patient care and coordination to children with chronic lung disease in both the inpatient and outpatient settings. She has authored several articles, chapters, and teaching booklets about chronic lung diseases including cystic fibrosis and asthma. She has given numerous presentations about pediatric lung diseases to nurses throughout the United States and has taught graduate level pediatric pulmonary nursing care at the University of Arizona and the University of Washington.

Joan Turner has been a pulmonary clinical nurse specialist since 1974. She was a home care pulmonary nurse specialist for the Visiting Nurse Association of San Francisco before becoming the coordinator of the Pulmonary Research Unit at San Francisco General Hospital in 1985. She has been the nurse coordinator for the University of California San Francisco for two major multicenter research studies sponsored and funded by the Division of Lung Diseases, National Heart, Lung and Blood Institute, and National Institutes of Health. The first was a study of the long-term effects of IPPB therapy in patients with COPD, and the second is a prospective study of the pulmonary complications of HIV infection. She has been an invited speaker at international meetings and is the author of several publications. She is a nonsalaried faculty member of the University of California San Francisco School of Nursing and has worked actively for the American Lung Association of San Francisco and the California Thoracic Society.

**Joan Turner**
**Gwendolyn J. McDonald**
**Nanci L. Larter**

# CONTENTS

# HANDBOOK OF
# ADULT & PEDIATRIC
# RESPIRATORY HOME CARE

# LUNG DISEASES COMMONLY SEEN IN HOME CARE

The chapters in this book are written from the perspective of problems that home care nurses frequently encounter when working with patients who have respiratory diseases. The following table summarizes information about the diseases affecting respiratory functioning that are frequently seen in home care, the age groups affected, respiratory manifestations, and treatment. In addition to these diseases, respiratory tract infection is discussed in Chapter 4, and sleep disorders are discussed in Chapter 12.

Most children and adults with chronic lung disease who require home care have obstructive diseases. Therefore these diseases are the main focus of the book. Obstructive diseases are primarily disorders of the airways that cause airflow reductions, air trapping, and hyperinflation with normal or impaired oxygenation. They include chronic bron-

chitis and emphysema (chronic obstructive pulmonary disease), asthma, and cystic fibrosis.

Diseases of the lung parenchyma or the chest wall may result in restrictive respiratory disorders. In these disorders lung volumes are reduced, airflow can be normal, increased, or decreased in proportion to the lung volume, and oxygenation is frequently impaired. Interstitial pulmonary fibrosis is an example of a restrictive disease that involves the lung parenchyma. It is not unusual for patients to have both obstructive and restrictive disorders. Severe kyphoscoliosis causes abnormalities in the thoracic cage that may significantly inhibit effective ventilation. Neuromuscular diseases and spinal cord injuries may cause alterations in respiratory functioning because of depression of respiratory drive, impaired neurologic functioning, or abnormalities of respiratory muscles.

| Disorder | Definition | Age group | Cause |
|---|---|---|---|
| **OBSTRUCTIVE DISORDERS** | | | |
| Asthma | Intermittent wheezing, chest tightness, and cough with bronchial hyperresponsiveness *or* a 20% reduction in $FEV_1$ with provocation challenge *or* a 20% increase in $FEV_1$ after inhaled bronchodilator; inflammatory changes in wall of airways | All ages | Etiology not clear; interaction between genetic factors (atopy and airway hyperresponsiveness) and environmental factors (allergens, viral infections, pollutants); *extrinsic asthma* usually caused by allergy and starts in childhood; *intrinsic asthma* does not have evidence of allergy and usually starts in adulthood; *occupational asthma* is caused by workplace exposures |
| Chronic bronchitis | Cough and sputum production 3 mo per yr for 2 yr in succession *or* chronic productive cough present for half the time for 2 yr without known cause | Adults | Chronic airway irritation from inhaled substances, especially cigarette smoke |
| Emphysema | "Abnormal permanent enlargement of airspaces distal to the terminal bronchioles accompanied by destruction of their walls and without fibrosis" (Snider, 1985) | Adults | Cigarette smoking; $\alpha_1$-antitrypsin deficiency |

Data from *Am Rev Respir Dis* 146:1349, 1992; Murray JF, Nadel JA, editors: *Textbook of respiratory medicine,* Philadelphia, 1988, WB Saunders; Snider GL et al: *Am Rev Respir Dis* 132:182, 1985; and Wyngaarden JB, Smith LH, Bennett JC, editors: *Cecil textbook of medicine,* ed 19, Philadelphia, 1992, WB Saunders.
*ABGs,* Arterial blood gases; *C3,* third cervical vertebra; *C8,* eighth cervical vertebra; *CNS,* central nervous system; *$FEV_1$,* forced expiratory volume in 1 second; *$FIO_2$,* fraction of inspired oxygen; *FVC,* forced vital capacity; *IgG,* immunoglobulin class G; *IV,* intravenous; *$PaCO_2$,* partial pressure arterial carbon dioxide; *$PaO_2$,* partial pressure arterial oxygen; *PEFR,* peak expiratory flow rate; *VC,* vital capacity.

| Respiratory manifestations | | Treatment |
| --- | --- | --- |
| **Signs** | **Symptoms** | **Treatment** |
| *Physical exam:* reduced airflow; wheezes; tachypnea; tachycardia; pulsus paradoxus in severe exacerbations<br>*Spirometry:* decreased $FEV_1$, PEFR, FVC<br>*ABGs:* hypoxemia, hypocapnia usually; hypercapnia seen with respiratory failure | Wheezing: chest tightness; breathlessness; cough | *Relieve airway inflammation:* inhaled corticosteroids, oral or IV preparations may be necessary<br>*Relieve bronchospasm:* inhaled bronchodilators, oral or IV preparations may be necessary; inhaled anticholinergics<br>*Prevent bronchospasm:* sodium cromoglycate may be administered to prevent early and late response to allergens; environmental strategies to control allergens and irritants |
| *Physical exam:* crackles and rhonchi; peripheral edema, jugular venous distention, $S_3$ and $S_4$ if heart failure present; increased anterior-posterior diameter and flattened diaphragms with severe obstruction<br>*Spirometry:* decreased $FEV_1$, PEFR, FVC<br>*ABGs:* may see hypoxemia, hypercapnia | Productive cough; breathlessness | Promote secretion clearance; smoking cessation; bronchodilators, usually inhaled and oral; maybe corticosteroids and anticholinergics; measures to enhance secretion clearance; antibiotics for exacerbations; low-flow oxygen for hypoxemia; diuretics for heart failure; strategies to control breathlessness |
| *Physical exam:* increased anterior-posterior diameter; flattened diaphragms; decreased air movement on chest auscultation<br>*Spirometry:* decreased $FEV_1$, PEFR, FVC<br>*Other pulmonary function tests:* decreased diffusing capacity for carbon monoxide<br>*ABGs:* hypoxemia; hypercapnia | Breathlessness | *Relieve breathlessness:* bronchodilators, inhaled and oral; low-flow oxygen for hypoxemia; strategies to control breathlessness; smoking cessation |

| Disorder | Definition | Age group | Cause |
|---|---|---|---|
| Chronic obstructive pulmonary disease (COPD); may be called chronic obstructive lung disease (COLD) or chronic airflow obstruction (CAO) | Airway obstruction that may be partially reversible with presence of emphysema or chronic bronchitis; may also include cystic fibrosis and other obstructive diseases | Adults | Same as chronic bronchitis and emphysema |
| Cystic fibrosis (CF) | Exocrine pancreatic insufficiency and/or chronic airway obstruction *Diagnostic criteria:* pulmonary manifestations and/or gastrointestinal manifestations and/or history of CF in immediate family and sweat chloride concentration >60 mEq/L | Neonate to adult | Autosomal recessive genetic disorder; incidence 1:2500 whites |
| Bronchiectasis | Abnormal dilation of bronchi more than 2 mm diameter from destruction of muscular and elastic tissue; can be localized or generalized | Childhood to adult | Associated with chronic bacterial infection, bronchial obstruction, congenital defects such as cystic fibrosis, Kartagener's syndrome, $\alpha_1$-antitrypsin deficiency |
| Bronchiolitis obliterans | Chronic obstruction of bronchioles after acute bronchiolitis | Infants and young children | Formation of bronchiolar granulation tissue and peribronchiolar fibrosis |

| Respiratory manifestations | | |
|---|---|---|
| **Signs** | **Symptoms** | **Treatment** |
| Same as chronic bronchitis and emphysema | Same as chronic bronchitis and emphysema | Same as chronic bronchitis and emphysema |
| *Pulmonary disease:* crackles; increased anterior-posterior diameter; flattened diaphragms, clubbing of digits; bronchiectasis; colonization with *Pseudomonas*<br>*Spirometry:* decreased $FEV_1$, PEFR, FVC<br>*ABGs:* hypoxemia, hypercapnia (end stage)<br>*Gastrointestinal disease:* meconium ileus in newborns and meconium ileus equivalent in adults; protein and fat malabsorption<br>*Other exocrine gland dysfunction:* sweat gland dysfunction with excessive salt loss; male infertility<br>*Associated problems:* sinusitis; nasal polyps; diabetes; pancreatitis; biliary cirrhosis; cholelithiasis; pneumothorax; frank hemoptysis; hematemesis | *Pulmonary disease:* Productive cough; breathlessness; maybe hemoptysis; recurrent infection<br>*Gastrointestinal disease:* frequent, foul-smelling, greasy stools<br>*Exocrine dysfunction:* weakness, lethargy due to hyponatremia (heat prostration) | *Promote secretion clearance:* Chest physical therapy; bronchodilators; inhaled corticosteroids as needed; regular exercise<br>*Control infection:* antibiotics, oral, inhaled, and/or IV; avoid crowds in flu season; flu vaccine<br>*Promote nutrition:* pancreatic enzyme replacement; vitamins; dietary supplements; hydration/salt replacement if necessary<br>*Psychosocial support:* promote self-care/independence; normalize life as much as possible; genetic counseling<br>*Lung transplantation* |
| *Physical exam:* crackles; rhonchi; wheezes; sometimes clubbing, cyanosis, right ventricular failure<br>*Spirometry:* decreased $FEV_1$, FVC, PEFR<br>*ABGs:* May see hypoxemia; hypercapnia | Chronic cough with purulent sputum (three layers); fever; weakness; weight loss; sometimes hemoptysis | *Promote secretion clearance:* chest physical therapy; bronchodilators; antibiotics |
| *Physical exam:* wheezing | Wheezing; cough; dyspnea | Steroids; surgical resection if localized |

| Disorder | Definition | Age group | Cause |
|----------|-----------|-----------|-------|
| Bronchopul- monary dys- plasia (BPD) | Bronchiolar metaplasia, obliteration, and cyst formation | Infants (can be seen in adults who have had adult respira- tory distress syndrome) | Long-term positive-pressure ventilation with high oxy- gen concentrations to treat infant respiratory distress syndrome (hyaline mem- brane disease or other dis- eases requiring respiratory support measures) |

**RESTRICTIVE DISORDERS**

| | | | |
|----------|-----------|-----------|-------|
| Interstitial pul- monary fibro- sis (crypto- genic fibrosing alveolitis) | Chronic inflammation of the alveolar walls leading to progressive fibrosis | Infant to adult; mean age 50- 60 yr | Unknown |
| Coal worker's pneumoconi- osis (black lung disease) | Coal macules and nodules; focal em- physema and fibrosis from deposi- tion of coal dust | Adult | Inhalation and deposition of coal dust in lung; fre- quently associated with bronchitis and emphysema from cigarette smoking; in- dividual susceptibility is a factor |
| Asbestosis (pul- monary paren- chymal fibro- sis) | Pulmonary fibrosis and pleural thick- ening from inhalation of asbestos fi- bers | Adult | Inhalation of asbestos fibers; disease dependent on amount inhaled and indi- vidual response; frequently associated with lung cancer and cigarette smoking; cig- arette smoking is added pollutant and may reduce asbestos fiber clearance |
| Kyphoscoliosis (with chronic respiratory failure) | Excessive curvature of spine (ky- phosis—posterior curvature; sco- liosis—lateral curvature) causing reduced lung volumes and pulmo- nary vascular bed, stiff chest wall, reduced respiratory muscle strength, and hypoventilation | Adults more than 35 yr; cause of <1% of chronic respi- ratory failure in adults | Defect in vertebrae, connec- tive tissue, or neuromuscu- lar support of spinal col- umn; one third of patients also have emphysema and bronchitis; two thirds have atelectasis |

| Respiratory manifestations | | |
| --- | --- | --- |
| **Signs** | **Symptoms** | **Treatment** |
| *Physical exam:* retractions; expiratory grunting; nasal flaring; crackles; wheezing<br>*ABGs:* hypoxemia; hypercapnia | Cough; irritability; lethargy | *Correct hypoxemia:* mechanical ventilation; oxygen therapy (gradual withdrawal of both as tolerated); chest physical therapy<br>*Relieve bronchospasm:* bronchodilators; steroids<br>*Treat infection:* antibiotics<br>*Supportive care:* nutritional support; developmental support |
| *Physical exam:* finger clubbing in 40%-80% of patients; fine end inspiratory crackles (Velcro rales); tachypnea<br>*Spirometry:* normal PEFR and $FEV_1$; decreased VC<br>*ABGs:* Severe hypoxemia; normal or low $Paco_2$; hypercapnia when end stage | Breathlessness; cough (may be dry or productive of scant mucoid sputum) | *Control breathlessness:* corticosteroids; immunosuppressant therapy; nursing strategies<br>*Relieve hypoxemia:* oxygen therapy |
| *Physical exam:* crackles; signs of right ventricular failure<br>*Spirometry:* decreased VC; decreased $FEV_1$ and PEFR if associated bronchitis and emphysema<br>*ABGs:* maybe hypoxemia, hypercapnia | Productive cough (may see black sputum); breathlessness | *Control breathlessness:* nursing strategies; control exposures to coal dust; bronchodilators if obstruction present; oxygen for hypoxemia; diuretics for heart failure<br>*Smoking cessation strategies*<br>*Surveillance for tuberculosis* |
| *Physical exam:* basilar crackles; coarse rhonchi; sometimes finger clubbing<br>*Spirometry:* not diagnostic<br>*ABGs:* sometimes hypoxemia and hypercapnia | Breathlessness; productive cough; chest tightness; chest pain | *Relieve breathlessness:* bronchodilators may be helpful; nursing strategies; oxygen for hypoxemia<br>*Smoking cessation strategies* |
| *Physical exam:* abnormal thoracic cage, reduced breath sounds, heart failure (end stage)<br>*Spirometry:* decreased VC ($FEV_1$ decreased in proportion to VC in patients with scoliosis curves greater than 90-100 degrees<br>*ABGs:* hypoxemia, hypercapnia | Breathlessness; reduced activity tolerance; repeated respiratory infections | Surgery usually does not correct lung complication in adults<br>*Supportive care:* avoidance of infection; treatment of infection; avoidance of sedatives; oxygen for hypoxemia; mechanical ventilation for respiratory failure if necessary |

| Disorder | Definition | Age group | Cause |
|---|---|---|---|
| **NEUROMUSCULAR DISORDERS** | | | |
| Myasthenia gravis | Motor end-plate disease causing muscle weakness aggravated by muscle contraction | Adult | IgG autoantibody affecting skeletal muscle acetylcholine receptors |
| Amyotrophic lateral sclerosis (Lou Gehrig's disease) | Upper and lower motor neuron deficits causing muscle atrophy | Adult | Progressive degeneration of cortico-spinal tract neurons, brainstem, and spinal cord motor cells |
| Poliomyelitis | Destruction of motor neurons in anterior horn cells of spinal cord causing muscle paralysis | Any age; rare now because of vaccination; now see late denervation of muscles that were reinnervated earlier | Viral infection |
| Myopathy | Muscle weakness | Child to adult | Congenital defects; infection; diabetes mellitus; steroids; alcohol; impaired nutrition; inflammatory autoimmune disease |

| Respiratory manifestations | | |
|---|---|---|
| **Signs** | **Symptoms** | **Treatment** |
| *Physical exam:* tachypnea; muscle wasting<br>*Spirometry:* decreased VC<br>*ABGs:* hypoxemia and hypercapnia in respiratory failure | Progressive weakness; breathlessness; decreased cough: dysphagia; difficult speech; decreased gag reflex | *Treat cause:* anticholinesterase drugs; corticosteroids; plasmapheresis to remove IgG autoantibody<br>*Supportive care:* prevention of infection; respiratory support as required; promote secretion clearance |
| *Physical exam:* peripheral muscle weakness; tachypnea; decreased diaphragmatic movement; sometimes heart failure<br>*Spirometry:* decreased VC<br>*ABGs:* hypoxemia and hypercapnia in respiratory failure | Limb and respiratory muscle weakness; may have muscle cramps and fasciculations: fatigue and breathlessness with exertion progressing to breathlessness at rest; decreased cough, speaking and swallowing ability, and gag reflex: may have morning headache, disturbed sleep, daytime somnolence | *Supportive care:* intermittent to continuous ventilatory support (negative-pressure body respirators); postural drainage; chest physical therapy with abdominal assist coughing; tracheal suctioning |
| *Physical exam:* decreased chest expansion; decreased reflexes; muscle atrophy<br>*Spirometry:* decreased VC<br>*ABGs:* hypoxemia, hypercapnia dependent on degree of respiratory failure | Muscle paralysis; breathlessness | *Promote ventilation:* ventilatory assistance dependent on degree of paralysis; glossopharyngeal breathing<br>*Promote secretion clearance:* same as spinal cord injuries |
| *Physical exam:* may see muscle atrophy and fasciculation. tachypnea; if advanced may see impaired gag reflex, decreased diaphragmatic excursion, and heart failure<br>*Spirometry:* decreased VC<br>*ABGs:* hypoxemia, hypercapnia if severe | Limb and respiratory muscle weakness; breathlessness; if extreme, difficulty speaking, coughing, swallowing; may also have morning headache, difficulty sleeping, and daytime sleepiness | *Treat cause*<br>*Supportive care:* speech and cough techniques; phrenic nerve pacing; mechanical ventilation |

| Disorder | Definition | Age group | Cause |
|---|---|---|---|
| Spinal cord injuries | | | |
| High cervical injury | Injury above C3 leading to respiratory muscle paralysis | Any age | Usually traumatic; may be tumors, epidural abscess, vascular accident |
| Mid and low cervical injury | *Quadriplegia:* C3-C8 lesion with paralysis of all four limbs; usually some respiratory function | Any age | Same as high cervical injury |
| Thoracic cord injury | Paraplegia | Any age | Same as high cervical injury |
| **OTHER DISORDERS** | | | |
| Pulmonary embolism | Partial or complete obstruction of pulmonary arteries and vasoconstriction causing increased pulmonary vascular resistance and increased right ventricular work | Adult | 95% of occurrence from venous thrombosis of legs, rarely from arms, hepatic or renal veins, right atrium or ventricle (more likely with right heart failure or indwelling catheter); venous thrombosis is associated with venous stasis from immobility, right ventricular failure, and peripheral edema; thrombosis is result of internal injury and coagulation defects |

| Respiratory manifestations | | |
| --- | --- | --- |
| **Signs** | **Symptoms** | **Treatment** |
| *Physical exam:* apnea; decreased breath sounds; sometimes basilar rhonchi; sometimes hypertrophy of sternocleidomastoid and trapezius muscles; flaccid abdominal muscles; no diaphragmatic excursion with respiration | Inability to breathe, talk, or cough; asphyxia; dyspnea; difficulty clearing secretions | *Promote ventilation:* glossopharyngeal breathing, speech, and cough techniques; phrenic nerve pacing and/or mechanical ventilation<br>*Promote secretion clearance:* turn every 2 hr; suctioning as necessary; bronchodilators for retained secretions; antibiotics for infection |
| *Physical exam:* paradoxic movement of rib cage; crackles and rhonchi with retained secretions and infection<br>*Spirometry:* decreased VC (increased VC in supine position)<br>*ABGs:* normal awake $Paco_2$ to mild hypercapnia and hypoxemia | Breathlessness with retention of secretions and infection | *Promote secretion clearance:* change position every 2 hr; deep breathing exercises and incentive spirometry every 4 hr; chest physical therapy; assisted coughing; bronchodilators and bronchoscopy for retained secretions; antibiotics for infection<br>*Increase ventilatory muscle strength:* inspiratory and expiratory muscle resistance training |
| May be same as mid and low cervical injury or less severe depending on level of injury | Same as high cervical injury | *Enhance cough effectiveness*<br>*Enhance expiratory muscle strength* |
| *Physical exam:* tachypnea; tachycardia, cyanosis; right ventricular failure; sometimes hemoptysis; crackles, dullness<br>*Spirometry:* nondiagnostic<br>*ABGs:* hypoxemia | Sudden onset of chest pain, breathlessness, palpitations, and sense of impending doom | *Relieve obstruction of pulmonary arteries:* anticoagulant therapy; rarely thrombolytic agents, surgical embolectomy, and inferior vena cava interruption to prevent recurrences<br>*Supportive care:* oxygen therapy for hypoxemia; treatment of heart failure<br>*Prevention of venous thrombosis:* Low-dose anticoagulants and leg compressive devices for patients at significant risk |

| Disorder | Definition | Age group | Cause |
|---|---|---|---|
| Spontaneous pneumothorax | Air in pleural space | Infant to adult | Can be primary from rupture of subpleural bleb of unknown cause or secondary to underlying lung disease, when it can be life threatening; associated with chronic obstructive pulmonary disease, cystic fibrosis, *Pneumocystis carinii* pneumonia, bronchogenic carcinoma, tuberculosis, neonatal respiratory distress syndrome; may occur with positive-pressure mechanical ventilation |
| Lung cancer (bronchogenic carcinoma 90% of lung cancer) | Carcinoma arising from basal cells of bronchial mucosa; includes squamous cell, adenocarcinoma, large cell, and adenosquamous cell carcinoma (small cell and non–small cell) | Adult | 80%-85% of cases from cigarette smoking; other associated factors are inhalation of asbestos and other carcinogens, low dietary vitamin A, familial tendency, immunocompromise, and chronic obstructive pulmonary disease |

| Respiratory manifestations | | |
|---|---|---|
| **Signs** | **Symptoms** | **Treatment** |
| *Physical exam:* tachycardia; cyanosis; hypotension; mediastinal shift toward opposite side; hyperresonance, distant breath sounds, decreased tactile fremitus on affected side<br>*Spirometry* (if performed): decreased VC<br>*ABGs:* hypoxemia; hypercapnia; tension pneumothorax may cause acute respiratory failure | Sudden onset of breathlessness, chest pain on affected side | *Removal of pleural air:* tube thoracostomy<br>*Prevention of recurrence:* pleural instillation of sclerosing agent; thoracotomy to oversew or remove bullae<br>*Supportive care:* oxygen, pain control |
| *Physical exam:* may be normal; stridor or absent breath sounds if partial or complete obstruction of bronchus; pneumonitis or pleural effusion; may see clubbing<br>*Spirometry:* not diagnostic<br>*ABGs:* depend on degree of pulmonary disease | Dependent on location and whether primary or metastatic<br>*Primary lung:* cough; sputum; hemoptysis; breathlessness; chest pain; fever<br>*Intrathoracic extrapulmonary:* breathlessness; wheezing; chest pain; hoarseness; dysphagia; superior vena cava obstruction; cardiac symptoms<br>*Metastases:* lymph node enlargement, central nervous system symptoms; liver enlargement and pain; bone pain; cutaneous or subcutaneous masses<br>*Systemic symptoms:* anorexia; weight loss; weakness; neurologic symptoms | *Surgical resection if possible*<br>*Pain control*<br>*Radiation/chemotherapy*<br>*Psychosocial support*<br>*Nutritional support*<br>*Palliative control of symptoms* |

| Disorder | Definition | Age group | Cause |
|---|---|---|---|
| Respiratory failure | Abnormal gas exchange resulting in ventilatory failure with $Paco_2$ >45 mm Hg and/or impaired oxygenation with $Pao_2$ <60 mm Hg while breathing room air; can be acute or chronic; many home care patients have chronic respiratory failure | Infant to adult | *Ventilatory failure:* impaired central control (Ondine's curse, cerebrovascular accident, head trauma, encephalitis, drug overdose, central apnea); impaired respiratory muscle function (neuromuscular disease, spinal cord injury); mechanical problems of lungs and chest wall (airway obstruction, obesity, kyphoscoliosis)<br>*Impaired oxygenation:* alveolar hypoventilation (see ventilatory failure); impaired diffusion; emphysema; ventilation-perfusion mismatching; pulmonary embolism; airway obstruction; right to left shunting of blood; pneumonia; atelectasis; pulmonary edema (intracardiac shunt, arteriovenous failure); reduced $Fio_2$; fire exposure |
| Acute respiratory failure in patient with chronic respiratory failure | Inability to maintain $Pao_2$ of approximately 60 mm Hg with variable $Paco_2$ on maximal therapy | Infant to adult | *Infection:* inflammation; excessive secretions<br>*Acute bronchoconstriction:* allergen exposure; noxious gas inhalation<br>*Pneumothorax*<br>*Pulmonary embolism*<br>*Reduction in maintenance doses of medications* |

| Respiratory manifestations | | |
| --- | --- | --- |
| **Signs** | **Symptoms** | **Treatment** |
| *Physical exam:* rapid, shallow breathing or decreased ineffective respirations or apnea; sometimes coma and cardiovascular collapse (see also acute respiratory failure in patient with chronic respiratory failure, below) | Breathlessness; orthopnea (see also acute respiratory failure in patient with chronic respiratory failure, below) | *Hospitalization*<br>*Treat cause if known:* antibiotics for infection; chest tube for pneumothorax; anticoagulants for pulmonary embolus; adjust maintenance medications; bronchodilators; corticosteroids for acute airway obstruction<br>*Maintain oxygenation:* increase $FIo_2$; intubation and mechanical ventilation if necessary<br>*Maintain secretion clearance:* chest physical therapy; suctioning if necessary |
| Must know what is usual for patient<br>*Physical exam:* may see increased use of accessory muscles, grunting, nasal flaring; pulsus paradoxus 15 mm Hg or more; reduced breath sounds; tachycardia (more than 130 beats/min); inability to cooperate; restlessness; increased signs of heart failure; fever<br>*Spirometry:* patient may be unable to perform; decreased FVC, $FEV_1$, PEFR<br>*ABGs:* worsening $Pao_2$ on usual flow rate of supplemental oxygen; variable $Paco_2$ | Must know what is usual for patient; may see increased breathlessness, increased cough, increase or decrease in sputum production, more tenacious sputum | See respiratory failure (above) |

# ASSESSMENT OF THE CHILD AND ADULT IN THE HOME ENVIRONMENT

# CHAPTER 1

# HISTORY AND SYMPTOM EVALUATION

MARY S. VOGT-YANTA • PATRICIA A. DETTENMEIER

The patient history and symptom assessment serves as a guide for the physical examination, establishes a baseline from which to assess changes over time, and helps to determine priorities for the plan of care. A detailed history is rarely provided with the home care referral; therefore it must be obtained by the nurse during the initial visits.

The patient is the primary source of information for the history; however, valuable information may also be obtained from family members and caregivers. Parents or caregivers can provide the history for the young child and for adults who are unable to relate it themselves because they are confused or otherwise incapacitated. The history and assessment of the child are presented in Chapter 3.

Effective questioning and careful listening are important so that the patient is at ease and the necessary information is gathered. Specific questions are organized by problem or physiologic system. Frequently two or three home visits are required before all of the historical data can be gathered. Whenever possible, a history, treatment plan, and hospital discharge summary should be obtained from the referring physician. Techniques for interviewing patients with chronic lung disease are summarized in Table 1-1.

The format for history and symptom assessment is as follows:

- Precipitating events
- Chronologic development of illness
- Cardiopulmonary symptoms
- Review of physiologic systems
- Medications and treatments
- Allergies
- Smoking history
- Use of alcohol and recreational drugs
- Personal and social history

**Table 1-1**  Interviewing techniques

| Technique | Rationale |
|---|---|
| Keep unnecessary conversation to a minimum | Conserves patient energy and interviewer's time |
| Ask questions that can be generally answered by few words | Protects patient from unnecessary breathlessness |
| Be aware of the patient's vocal tone and fluctuations, facial expressions, and body position and movements | Provides important information about degree of breathlessness or discomfort |
| Focus on important issues | Ensures brief interview, which may be limited by the status of the patient (i.e., by physical distractions, ability to communicate, memory, control of speech, level of consciousness) or time constraints of home care nurse |

## PRECIPITATING EVENTS

Initially it is important to determine why the home care referral was made and the events that precipitated the current episode or exacerbation.

## DIAGNOSIS AND CHRONOLOGIC DEVELOPMENT OF ILLNESS

The patient is asked to state the diagnosis and chief complaint in his or her own words. This provides information on the patient's level of knowledge about the illness and the problems the patient considers to have the highest priority. Sometimes the chief complaint does not appear to be related to the diagnosis or to the problems observed. However, this may reveal an area of particular importance to the patient. Any differences between patient and nursing priorities must be considered in the plan of care.

The patient is asked to give a chronologic history of the illness, describing the date of onset of each incident, the duration, the treatment, and the relation to other occurrences. The dates of previous hospitalizations, surgical procedures, and injuries should be obtained. Dates of pneumococcal vaccines and flu vaccines should also be noted. It is important to note any past episodes requiring intubation and ventilatory assistance. This information also sets the stage for later discussions of the patient's desires regarding invasive interventions.

## CARDIOPULMONARY SYMPTOMS

Commonly occurring cardiopulmonary symptoms are cough, sputum, nasal symptoms (rhinitis, postnasal drip, and nasal stuffiness), dyspnea, wheezing, chest pain, palpitations, syncope, symptoms of right and left ventricular failure, and generalized fatigue and weakness. The patient is asked about each symptom during the initial assessment. This symptom profile then becomes the baseline for comparison during follow-up visits and exacerbations of chronic lung disease. There are seven characteristics to evaluate for each symptom:

1. Chronology—onset (sudden or gradual), pattern (variable or constant), and duration
2. Quality—what it feels like (sharp, dull, or burning), intensity (mild, moderate, or severe, or graded on a scale of 1 to 10)
3. Location—area of the body affected; radiating or localized
4. Setting—what the patient was doing when the symptom occurred
5. Associated manifestations—other symptoms that occur at the same time
6. Aggravating factors—factors that make the symptom worse
7. Alleviating factors—factors that make the symptom better

### Cough

A cough may be described as dry or wet; productive (associated with sputum production) or nonproductive; and hacking, coarse, or barking. Coughing may be more prevalent at certain times of the day, such as morning or evening, or may occur throughout the day or night. It is important to determine what factors improve or worsen coughing. Effective coughing clears secretions, whereas episodes of uncontrollable coughing can be exhausting. Coughing may be relieved by avoiding irritants, by using medications such as bronchodilators, antibiotics, corticosteroids, and expectorants that facilitate secretion clearance, and by using cough suppressants or decongestants. Patients should be taught breathing techniques and effective cough methods to facilitate the removal of excessive respiratory secretions. Effective cough techniques are discussed in Chapter 7.

A new cough or a change from usual coughing habits may be associated with an acute infectious process, such as bronchitis or pneumonia, whereas a chronic cough is usually a symptom of diseases such as chronic bronchitis, bronchiectasis, and asthma. Coughing may also be caused by exposure to allergens and irritants, postnasal drip, aspiration, bronchogenic carcinoma, pulmonary fibrosis, congestive heart failure, and anxiety. It may be associated with sputum production, dyspnea, wheezing, chest pain or tightness, palpitations, syncope, sleep disturbances, fatigue, or weakness. Some people, particularly children and young adults with cystic fibrosis, vomit with excessive coughing. Violent coughing may cause hemoptysis, rib fractures, and rupture of the rectus abdominis muscles.

## Sputum Production

Mucus production in the normal respiratory tract is thought to be less than 100 ml daily. Because this amount is swallowed, it is rarely noticed. Secretions in excess of this amount are usually expectorated and referred to as sputum.

Sputum is described by its color, consistency, quantity, and odor. A history of usual sputum production is important to assess changes over time. Patients are asked to describe the characteristics of the sputum on a normal day and during an exacerbation. Patterns of sputum production may then become apparent. Patients are taught to observe their sputum so exacerbations can be treated early.

### Color

Sputum is usually clear, although some patients with chronic bronchitis often produce sputum that is white, tan, or gray. A change from the usual color of the sputum to green, yellow, or rust often indicates a respiratory tract infection. Patients with cystic fibrosis and bronchiectasis usually expectorate green purulent sputum. Discoloration of early morning expectoration that clears later in the day is due to the effects of an enzyme, verdoperoxidase, on retained nocturnal secretions and does not indicate infection. Patients should be encouraged to use white rather than colored tissues for expectoration so that the color of the sputum may be evaluated more accurately.

### Consistency

Normal sputum is thin or watery. Thicker secretions often indicate the presence of a respiratory tract infection, especially when associated with an increase in cough, dyspnea, fever, chills, or loss of appetite. Patients with cystic fibrosis and bronchiectasis usually produce thick, tenacious, purulent sputum, whereas asthmatics produce tenacious mucous plugs that are difficult to expectorate. The sputum of patients with bronchiectasis typically settles into three layers: a purulent bottom layer, a thin clear or grayish middle layer, and a frothy top layer. Frothy, bubbly, pink-tinged secretions are associated with pulmonary edema.

### Quantity

The patient is asked to estimate the volume of sputum (in teaspoons, tablespoons, or cups) that is produced during a 24-hour period. Such measurements are preferable to estimates such as small, moderate, or large because these determinations vary from person to person. Accurate measurements of expectorated sputum volume are possible if the patient expectorates all sputum into a container. Sputum containers should be kept covered and should be cleaned or changed daily. A small amount of water in the bottom of reusable containers facilitates cleaning and should be deducted from the sputum volume.

The patient may produce sputum daily or infrequently, in the early morning or throughout the day. Children or self-conscious patients sometimes deny sputum production or swallow rather than expectorate it, making the assessment of volume difficult. The volume of sputum that is expectorated depends on the volume that is produced and the ease with which it can be expectorated. Thus sputum volume may be increased or decreased with respiratory tract infection. Any change in the quantity of sputum must be interpreted in the context of other symptoms.

### Odor

An unusual odor of the sputum may be caused by organisms such as *Pseudomonas aeruginosa*, which tends to colonize the airways in cystic fibrosis and bronchiectasis. The purulent secretions of the patient with chronic bronchitis usually do not have an odor, whereas those associated with a lung abscess can be extremely foul smelling.

## Hemoptysis

The patient should be asked if he or she ever coughs up blood in the form of blood-streaked sputum or frank blood. Blood streaking is often seen with infection or excessive coughing. Massive pulmonary hemorrhage (200 to 600 ml of blood in a 24-hour period) is caused by inflammation or erosion of the bronchial arteries and may be seen in active pulmonary tuberculosis, bronchiectasis, and chronic necrotizing pneumonia. The following conditions are associated with hemoptysis:

- Infections such as bronchitis, tuberculosis, and pneumonia
- Severe cystic fibrosis
- Bronchiectasis
- Pulmonary edema or emboli
- Lung cancer
- Recent chest trauma, rib fractures, vigorous coughing, or chest physical therapy
- Anticoagulant therapy
- Smoke inhalation

Efforts must be made to differentiate true hemoptysis from blood in oral, nasal and gastric secretions. The following characteristics of hemoptysis must be described:

- Color—fresh blood is bright red, whereas old blood appears dark brown or dark red; pink-tinged sputum may contain blood or simply be caused by inhalation of the bronchodilator, isoetharine (Bronkosol)
- Frequency
- Amount—the amount of blood produced in a 24-hour period; because there is a tendency for patients or family members to exaggerate the volume expectorated, it is helpful to have the patient save all expectorated blood or blood-tinged sputum
- Duration

Hemoptysis should always be evaluated by the physician, especially if there are recurring episodes. The larger and fresher the bleed, the more urgent it is for the patient to go to the emergency room for evaluation.

## Excessive Nasal Secretions

The patient should be asked to describe the color, consistency, and quantity of nasal secretions. Nasal or postnasal secretions are described as serous, mucoid, purulent, and sanguineous. Frankly bloody nasal secretions are called epistaxis. It is important to differentiate an increase in nasal secretions from an increase in sputum because the nursing interventions differ. Purulent sinus drainage may be a source of infection for the lower respiratory tract.

Nasal secretions are often associated with a head cold, allergy, rhinitis, or sinusitis. Patients with cystic fibrosis have a high incidence of chronic sinusitis with complaints of rhinorrhea and nasal stuffiness. Symptoms of sinus infection include low-grade fevers, purulent postnasal drip, headaches, and pressure and discomfort over the sinuses on palpation. The patient is asked if nasal secretions occur during any particular season or time of the day. Occasionally the patient is aware that sinus drainage or obstruction occurs in certain positions, such as when reclining. Coughing may be precipitated by the drainage of nasal secretions into the posterior pharynx. Sometimes the only clue to increased pharyngeal drainage is frequent clearing of the throat. This may not even be noticeable to the patient, but it is often observed by others. Associated symptoms may include anorexia and a diminished sense of smell or taste.

Fluid in the middle ear drains into the posterior pharynx through the eustachian tubes. A history of earaches or hearing loss may be associated with excessive nasal secretions, especially in infants and young children, and should be thoroughly evaluated. Infections of the middle ear are frequently associated with sinusitis, colds, and flu.

## Dyspnea

Dyspnea is a symptom of both cardiac and lung disease. The patient may be asked to describe the degree of dyspnea as mild, moderate, or severe or to indicate the intensity of the symptom on a numeric or visual analog scale. Dyspnea is fully discussed in Chapter 8.

The onset of shortness of breath is usually gradual when it is caused by a chronic disease, such as chronic obstructive pulmonary disease (COPD), and sudden with an acute problem, such as pulmonary edema or infection. It is important to determine when the dyspnea occurs and to recognize

**Table 1-2**    Etiology of chest pain

| Type of chest pain | Cause | Signs and symptoms |
|---|---|---|
| Musculoskeletal | Rib fracture, muscle strain from coughing | Aggravated by deep inspiration, pressure, coughing, and specific movement; "point tenderness" present over site of rib fracture; crepitus may be present |
| Cardiac | Angina | May be located substernally or to left of sternum; may be referred to shoulder, arm, or jaw, especially on left; relieved with rest or nitrite therapy; often precipitated by activity or excitement; described as heavy, stabbing, or viselike |
| | Acute myocardial infarction | May occur in same location as angina with similar descriptives; sustained pain that is usually not relieved by rest or nitrite therapy; may be no apparent precipitant |
| Esophageal | Heartburn, esophagitis | Typically not associated with activity; usually described as burning pain that is relieved by food or antacids; may be similar to angina |
| Pleuritic | Inflammation of pleura often due to pneumonia | Severe, sharp, or stabbing pain aggravated by coughing and deep breathing; may be confused with musculoskeletal chest pain; may persist for days to weeks after inflammation resolved |
| Other | Acute tracheobronchitis | Raw, burning substernal pain associated with coughing |
| | Pneumothorax | Sharp, knifelike chest pain associated with marked increase in dyspnea |
| | Pneumonia | Dull, aching parenchymal pain or soreness |

any precipitating factor, such as talking, coughing, anxiety, or exercise. Strategies the patient uses to obtain relief from the dyspnea are important, as is the time it usually takes to recover.

## Wheezing

The patient is asked to describe how and when the wheezing begins and whether it is always present or occurs intermittently. It is important to clarify what the patient means by "wheezing," because many use the term incorrectly to describe respiratory sensations such as chest congestion. Wheezing is often associated with the complaint of tightness in the chest. An associated productive or nonproductive cough may indicate the presence of mucous plugs or a respiratory tract infection. *Coughing may be the equivalent of wheezing in children* and in some adults with asthma. Precipitating factors should be noted. Examples include respiratory tract infection, exercise, or exposure to

cold air, strong scents, irritants such as cigarette smoke, or allergens such as animal dander.

## Chest Pain

Chest pain is a common complaint of the patient with chronic lung disease. The intensity of the pain is best quantified using a scale of 0 (no pain at all) to 10 (extreme pain). A numeric score is usually more accurate than descriptive statements such as mild, moderate, or severe. Complaints of chest pain should always be thoroughly evaluated by a physician. Types of chest pain, causes, and associated signs and symptoms are presented in Table 1-2.

## Palpitations

Patients often describe palpitations as a sensation of "fluttering" in the chest or a feeling that the heart is "jumping around." Palpitations may be caused by excitement, exertion, excessive intake of caffeine or nicotine, or many types of medications, including bronchodilators, especially at toxic levels. Palpitations may be related to minor arrhythmias, such as premature systoles and paroxysmal tachycardia, or more serious disturbances, such as organic heart disease and thyrotoxicosis.

Palpitations often occur paroxysmally and resolve spontaneously. Most palpitations do not interfere with the patient's ability to function. However, if prolonged, they can be debilitating, especially when associated with excessive anxiety.

### Syncope

Syncope, or temporary loss of consciousness, may be described by the patient as "fainting" or "blacking out." Some patients are more prone to syncope than others. Syncopal episodes may occur at a variable frequency and usually last only a few seconds, although they may last for several hours. Some patients report that syncope is accompanied by light-headedness, a spinning sensation, or dizziness. Other patients describe seeing spots or colored lights just before they lose consciousness. Syncope has little medical significance when it is associated with an emotional upset, but it is significant in aortic stenosis, complete heart block, transient ischemic attacks, cerebrovascular accidents, or head trauma. Valsalva maneuvers during toileting or strenuous exercise and coughing are known to induce syncope. Syncope associated with coughing is termed *cough syncope*. Light-headedness or syncope may occur with a sudden change in position in people with postural hypotension, a common problem for older people receiving diuretic and antihypertensive medications. *In children, severe temper tantrums may cause syncope.* People who have syncopal episodes are at risk of falling and should use care when operating machinery.

### Symptoms of Right and Left Ventricular Failure

Patients with chronic lung disease are at increased risk for right ventricular failure caused by pulmonary heart disease and for left ventricular failure caused by coexisting cardiovascular prob-

lems such as systemic hypertension and myocardial infarction. Thus the initial history must include questions about the symptoms of heart failure. Although there are differences in the causes and the signs and symptoms of right and left ventricular failure, most patients exhibit features of both.

Right ventricular failure is associated with peripheral edema and passive congestion of abdominal organs with symptoms that include the following:

- Weight gain not associated with increased food intake
- Peripheral edema (shoes may be tight)
- Abdominal tenderness and fullness; anorexia
- Constipation

Left ventricular failure causes increased backward pressure within the pulmonary capillary bed and is therefore associated with symptoms of pulmonary edema, as well as reduced cardiac output. These symptoms include the following:

- Unusual fatigue or weakness; exertional dyspnea
- Angina
- Orthopnea and paroxysmal nocturnal dyspnea
- Wheezing; chest congestion; frothy, pink-tinged sputum
- Impaired cognition; anxiety

The assessment and management of right and left ventricular failure are discussed in depth in Chapter 10.

### Generalized Fatigue and Weakness

Patients with chronic lung disease frequently complain of generalized fatigue and weakness associated with repeating cycles of shortness of breath and decreased exercise tolerance. Patients often complain of increased fatigue just before an infection, and it may persist days to weeks after resolution of the infection. Patients with chronic lung disease often complain of greater fatigue when they raise their arms above their shoulders, an activity that is frequently necessary for personal hygiene. Sometimes fatigue is more severe with weather changes or in seasons when allergen levels are high. Other factors associated with an increase in fatigue and weakness include worsening left ventricular failure; low levels of body protein stores and minerals such as calcium, phosphorus, potassium, and magnesium; systemic corticosteroid therapy; and neuromuscular diseases.

## REVIEW OF PHYSIOLOGIC SYSTEMS

Patients with chronic lung disease are at risk for a variety of problems involving other organ systems. Information about associated problems is essential in formulating the home care plan, yet is rarely provided in the home care referral. Therefore the baseline history must include a brief review of physiologic systems.

## Cardiovascular System

A history of cardiovascular disease is significant because of the close relation between the cardiac and respiratory systems. Symptoms of cardiovascular disease include cardiac irregularities, chest pain, peripheral edema, orthopnea, and paroxysmal noctural dyspnea. Headaches, blurred vision, seeing "spots," and feeling light headed when assuming a sitting or standing position may indicate blood pressure abnormalities or arrhythmias. Intermittent claudication, complaints of coldness or numbness in the extremities, and changes in the color of the skin with sores that do not heal may indicate arterial insufficiency or venous stasis.

## Neurologic System

A history of neurologic disease is significant because of its potential impact on respiratory muscle function. Examples of neurologic and neuromuscular diseases include myasthenia gravis, muscular dystrophy, spinal cord injury, and the long-term effects of poliomyelitis. Symptoms that may reflect an impact on respiratory function include muscle weakness and difficulty swallowing, coughing, and clearing secretions.

## Musculoskeletal System

A history of musculoskeletal disorders that affect the chest wall or respiratory muscles is important. Muscle weakness and fractures of the ribs and vertebrae are more common in patients who have been receiving long-term corticosteroid therapy. Post-

menopausal women are predisposed to osteoporosis and are at risk for fractures.

## Gastrointestinal System

Gastrointestinal problems are relatively common in patients with chronic lung disease. There may be problems with the purchase and preparation of food and with adequate nutritional intake. The home care patient often complains of anorexia, gastrointestinal pain, heartburn, bloating, gas, indigestion, nausea, and vomiting. Gastroesophageal reflux (GER) is a possible cause of recurrent middle or lower lobe pneumonia and wheezing in adults. These problems are discussed in Chapter 13.

Fungal and viral infections in the mucosa of the mouth and esophagus are common in patients who are immunocompromised because of organ transplantation, HIV infection, or chemotherapy, and such infections may cause a sore mouth, difficulty swallowing, and a bad taste.

### Bowel Habits

Bowel habits are an important component of the gastrointestinal history. The decreased activity associated with chronic lung disease predisposes the patient to constipation. This may increase the work of breathing by causing abdominal distension and excessive straining to evacuate the stool. The history should include the use of laxatives, stool bulkers, and softeners.

A liquid or diarrheal stool may be associated with drug toxicity or gastrointestinal infection. Frequent liquid stools may cause dehydration and electrolyte deficiencies, *particularly in young children*. A chronically debilitated patient also may not be able to increase his or her nutritional intake enough to compensate for the electrolyte losses from significant diarrhea.

Frequent floating, malodorous stools with a high fat content are seen in pancreatic insufficiency associated with cystic fibrosis. Black stools may be seen with iron supplementation, medications containing bismuth (Pepto-Bismol), and old gastrointestinal bleeding. Maroon or red bowel movements may be caused by the ingestion of red vegetables, such as beets, and by active gastrointestinal bleeding.

## Genitourinary System

A history of frequent urination may be associated with urinary tract infection, diabetes, anxiety, and the use of medications such as diuretics, cardiotonics, and theophylline. Nocturia may be associated with congestive heart failure, renal or bladder infection, drinking too much liquid, or taking diuretics at bedtime.

## Fluid Balance

Dehydration and fluid retention are potential problems for the patient with chronic lung disease. Symptoms of light-headedness when arising from a sitting or lying position and rapid weight loss, particularly when it is associated with an acute febrile illness and vomiting or diarrhea, may be indications of dehydration.

Rapid weight gain, dependent or periorbital edema, and increased dyspnea may be associated with fluid retention. A complaint of tight-fitting rings and shoes may be an early indication of peripheral edema.

## Psychiatric History

Mood or cognitive problems such as anxiety, depression, or organic brain syndrome can significantly affect the implementation of a plan of care. Anxiety and depression are common in patients with COPD. Cognitive impairment is frequently seen in patients who are elderly, depressed, or severely hypoxemic and in alcoholics.

## MEDICATIONS AND TREATMENTS

Chronically ill and elderly patients often take multiple prescription and over-the-counter medications, often without the knowledge of a physician. This significantly increases the likelihood of adverse drug interactions and toxicities. Patients frequently do not understand their medication therapy. It is extremely important to review with the patient the purpose of each drug, the frequency and dosage, any special instructions for use, and any side effects that may have been experienced.

It is also important to review and observe the patient's or caregiver's technique with treatments such as inhaled medications and chest physical therapy to assess the need for additional instruction.

## ALLERGIES

Allergies and reactions to irritant substances should be noted in the patient's record. Common allergens include animal danders, dust mites, seasonal pollens, molds, and certain foods or medications. It is particularly important to identify an allergy to eggs because many vaccines, including flu vaccines, are egg based. Allergic reactions include hives, urticaria, joint pain and swelling, bronchospasm, laryngospasm, and anaphylaxis.

Skin rashes (as distinguished from hives) may be caused by medications, foods, infection, and environmental agents. Many physicians do not consider rashes to be a true indication of allergy or a contraindication to drug use. Some patients may be premedicated with antihistamines.

Common irritants include dust, smog, smoke, solvents, perfumes, laundry detergents, and scented antistatic preparations used in the clothes dryer. Symptomatic responses to irritants are not considered to be allergies and should not be described as such.

## SMOKING HISTORY

A past and current smoking history should be obtained from the patient. Because of the known harmful effects of secondhand smoke, the parents (if the patient is a child) and other household members must also be asked if they smoke.

The smoking history should include the pack year history, the current smoking pattern (including the brand of cigarettes smoked; if they are filtered or unfiltered, with low or high tar and nicotine content), information about current desire to quit smoking, and if there were previous attempts to quit. The pack year history is calculated by multiplying the number of packs per day (ppd) by the number of years smoked. For example, someone who has smoked 2 ppd for 10 years has a 20 pack year history. The pack year history for periodic smoking is determined by calculating the pack years for each period of time and adding them together (e.g., 2 ppd × 5 years = 10 pack years + 1 ppd × 3 years [or 3 pack years] = 13 pack years). Strategies for smoking cessation are presented in Chapter 20.

## USE OF ALCOHOL AND RECREATIONAL DRUGS

The history of alcohol use includes the amount and type of alcohol ingested and the usual pattern of consumption such as social drinking or binges. The patient with addictive behavior often uses a combination of substances such as nicotine and alcohol. Excessive alcohol ingestion in the patient with chronic lung disease may be associated with the following:
- Impaired clearance of medications, such as theophylline, that are metabolized by the liver, predisposing the patient to drug toxicity
- Psychosocial problems, including marked enhancement of depression, anxiety, and cognitive dysfunction
- Reduced compliance with medication therapies, treatments, and cleaning and maintenance of respiratory equipment
- Aspiration pneumonia secondary to respiratory depression and an inhibited gag reflex

It is also important to note whether the patient or caregiver uses "recreational" drugs such as marijuana, amphetamines, cocaine, or heroin. Occasionally patients or caregivers abuse prescription narcotics and other medications.

## PERSONAL AND SOCIAL HISTORY

The personal and social history includes information about the patient's residence, work or school, finances, family relationships, health habits, and medication compliance. Usually pertinent information is obtained over several home visits.

### Places of Residence

Current and past places of residence are significant because of possible exposures to endemic diseases. For example, histoplasmosis is endemic to the midwestern regions of the United States and coccidioidomycosis is endemic to the desert Southwest. Urban dwellers may be exposed to excessive air pollution, whereas rural dwellers may be at risk for water-borne infections from contaminated well water or occupational diseases such as farmer's lung.

### Education

Effective home care plans include teaching strategies that are geared to the level of education of the patient or caregiver. Some patients and caregivers try to conceal the fact that they lack a formal education or are illiterate. The home care nurse must be alert for clues to such problems when planning patient education. Strategies for teaching in the home are presented in Chapter 21.

### Occupation

Occupational exposures may predispose the patient to respiratory diseases such as black lung and asbestosis. Important occupational exposures include toxic fumes, dusts, chemicals, tobacco smoke, asbestos, and other pollutants. Occupations that are known to cause lung disease include mining, welding, foundry work, glass and insecticide manufacturing, stone cutting, sandblasting, construction, and shipbuilding.

### Use of Community Resources

It is important to determine whether the patient has health insurance for the proposed plan of care. Many patients need help to find coverage for hourly nursing services, personal care, light housekeeping, meal preparation, and the delivery of medications. It is also important to know whether other agencies are involved in the care of the patient to prevent duplication and to facilitate coordination of services. Finally, community resources can vary greatly from one community to another. The home care nurse must be familiar with local services and the procedures for referral. A referral to a social worker may be indicated.

### Personal Relationships

Chronic lung disease often causes changes in traditional roles that may make the patient feel diminished as a person. Loss of the ability to earn a wage, carry out usual family responsibilities, and engage in sexual activity may be particularly significant for the patient and may affect his or her personal relationships. It is important to assess how the patient and others in the household interact with each other. The home care nurse must be alert to clues suggesting problems, such as unrealistic expectations, inadequate support, and physical abuse or neglect. Counseling may be indicated to help resolve family conflicts. Psychosocial aspects of chronic lung disease are presented in Chapters 17 and 18.

## Compliance

Compliance with medications and treatments has important implications for successful therapy. An essential part of the history is to assess the level of compliance as accurately as possible. Such information may also be obtained from family members and referral sources. The plan of care can then include strategies to help improve patient compliance if necessary. These issues are discussed in Chapter 21.

**SUGGESTED READINGS**

Billings JA, Stoeckel JD: *The clinical encounter: a guide to the medical interview and case presentation,* St Louis, 1989, Mosby.

Cohen-Cole SA: *The medical interview: a functional and operational approach,* St Louis, 1990, Mosby.

Dettenmeier PA: *Pulmonary nursing care,* St Louis, 1992, Mosby.

Hodgkin JE, editor: Chronic obstructive pulmonary disease. In *Clinics in chest medicine,* vol 11, no 3, Philadelphia, 1990, WB Saunders.

Kersten LD: *Comprehensive respiratory nursing,* Philadelphia, 1989, WB Saunders.

Sackner MA: Cough. In Murray JF, Nadel JA, editors: *Textbook of respiratory medicine,* Philadelphia, 1988, WB Saunders.

Thompson JM: Respiratory system. In Thompson JM et al: *Mosby's manual of clinical nursing,* ed 2, St Louis, 1989, Mosby.

West JB: Respiration. In *Best and Taylor's physiological basis of medical practice,* sec 5, Baltimore, 1990, Williams & Wilkins.

Wilkins RL: *Clinical assessment in respiratory care,* ed 2, St Louis, 1990, Mosby.

# CHAPTER 2

# PHYSICAL ASSESSMENT OF THE PATIENT AND THE ENVIRONMENT

PATRICIA A. DETTENMEIER • MARY S. VOGT-YANTA

## GENERAL OBSERVATIONS

Important information about the patient's respiratory, cardiac, cognitive, and emotional status can be obtained by astute observations made during home care visits. General appearance, body habitus (obese or thin), apparent comfort, grooming, posture, and speech patterns should be noted. In addition, the nurse should assess whether the patient appears to be in respiratory distress or in pain and whether the patient is relaxed or tense.

### Communication

The patient's facial expression, vocal tone, body language, and specific responses to questions provide a variety of verbal and nonverbal clues to the patient's physical status. The inability to complete a full sentence and the use of very brief answers to questions are important indicators of breathlessness and should be documented.

### Mental Status

Inappropriate responses to questions suggest confusion, disorientation, and impaired mental status, which may reflect coexisting cognitive disorder, drug toxicity, or blood gas abnormalities. Mental dullness, monotone speech, lack of facial expression, and irritability may reflect either cognitive or affective problems and require further evaluation. Any limitation in intellectual or emo-

---

**Components of the Assessment**

**GENERAL OBSERVATION**

Communication
Mental status
Grooming
Posture

**PULMONARY ASSESSMENT**

Inspection
Palpation
Percussion
Auscultation

**CARDIAC ASSESSMENT**

Pulse
Blood pressure
Heart sounds
Jugular venous pressure
Hepatojugular reflux
Edema

**ASSESSMENT OF THE ENVIRONMENT**

Safety
Cleanliness
Allergens and irritants
Personal hygiene
Cooking facilities
Location

tional functioning must be considered in the development of an appropriate plan for patient care or education.

## Grooming

Grooming may be affected by financial limitations, shortness of breath, dyspnea on exertion, and mental status. Dental caries and gum infections may predispose the patient to pulmonary infections. Male patients may be unshaven because they are too short of breath to lift their arms to shave or too depressed to care. If the patient is wearing nightclothes during the day, he or she may be depressed or too short of breath to change clothes.

## Posture

The patient's posture may provide important clues to problems. Patients will assume postures and positions that enhance their ability to breathe more easily. Patients with severe emphysema often lean forward with their elbows on a table (the tripod position) to improve breathing; sometimes they practice this so often their elbows are heavily calloused. An inability to recline suggests worsening congestive heart failure; a slumped or "caved-in" posture may reflect depression.

## PULMONARY ASSESSMENT

The health history and symptom evaluation serve as background data and as a guide for the pulmonary examination. The physical assessment of the chest includes four components: inspection, palpation, percussion, and auscultation.

Whenever possible, the chest examination is performed in a warm, private room with good lighting. The patient is positioned comfortably in a chair or on a bed. The patient's clothes should be removed above the waist, exposing the chest. A shirt or loose robe may be used as a drape. The examination is performed in a systematic manner from top to bottom, comparing right with left, evaluating the anterior, posterior, and lateral aspects of the chest.

The assessment findings are described in relation to imaginary lines of reference drawn on the chest. These lines refer to landmarks and are named accordingly (Fig. 2-1).

## Inspection

Inspection of skin, muscle, and body development, thoracic shape and movement, and respiratory pattern is the first component of the chest examination.

### Skin

It is important to inspect the skin for color, rashes, bruises, or lesions. The skin should be assessed with natural lighting because artificial light often imparts a bluish color distortion. Cuts or scars are often clues to past conditions the patient may not have thought to mention in the history. Bruises may be caused by physical abuse, falls, excessively vigorous chest physical therapy, steroid therapy, or blood clotting abnormalities. Rashes may be caused by systemic diseases; local infections from bacterial, viral, or fungal organisms; and drug or hypersensitivity reactions. Yellow stains on the fingers and nails indicate heavy cigarette smoking.

The visibility of cyanosis depends on tissue perfusion, cardiac output, the rate of blood flow, the skin thickness and color, the amount of hemoglobin present, adequacy of lighting, and the assessment skills of the examiner. Because cyanosis depends on the amount of reduced hemoglobin, it may not be detected in anemic patients. Conversely, patients who are polycythemic are often cyanotic with only mild hypoxemia. Therefore cyanosis is considered a late and unreliable sign of hypoxemia. Other signs of poor oxygenation, such as tachycardia, tachypnea, or increased systemic blood pressure, are usually noted sooner.

Cyanosis can be central or peripheral. Central cyanosis is caused by low blood oxygen content associated with cardiac or respiratory failure. It is most easily observed on the mucous membranes of the mouth, the sclera and conjunctiva, the ear lobes, and the nail beds. Because the hemoglobin is not fully saturated, arterial oxygen saturation values will be abnormally low. Peripheral cyanosis is observed in the extremities when perfusion is decreased. This may be caused by very cold temperatures and vasoconstriction or cessation of blood

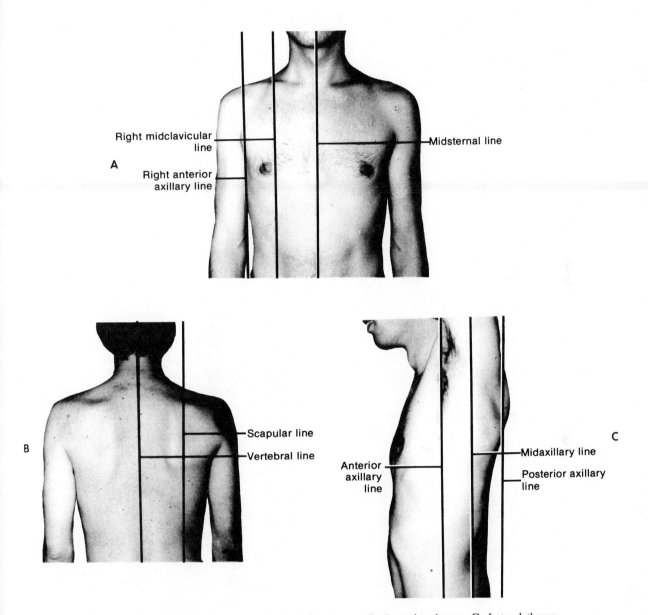

**Fig. 2-1** Topographic landmarks. **A,** Anterior thorax. **B,** Posterior thorax. **C,** Lateral thorax. (From Bowers AC, Thompson JM: *Clinical manual of health assessment,* ed 3, St Louis, 1988, Mosby.)

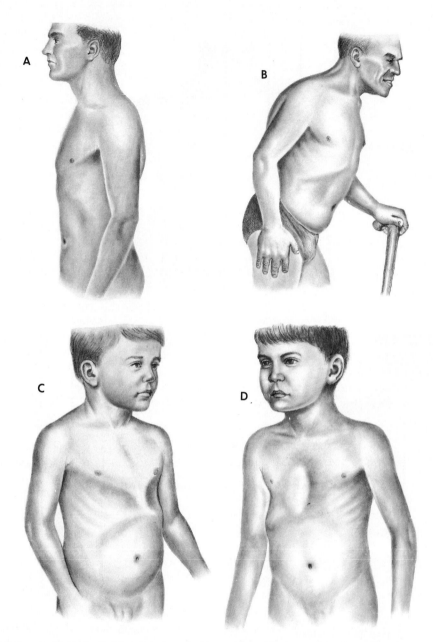

**Fig. 2-2** **A,** Thoracic diameter of normal healthy adult. **B,** Increased anterior-posterior diameter, or barrel chest. **C,** Pectus carinatum, or pigeon chest. **D,** Pectus excavatum, or funnel chest. (From Seidel H et al: *Mosby's guide to physical examination,* ed 2, St Louis, 1991, Mosby.)

flow from obstruction or obliteration of a blood vessel. Arterial oxygen saturation is often normal in peripheral cyanosis.

### Muscle and Body Development

The patient's general body development is noted. Patients with some forms of chronic lung disease, such as cystic fibrosis and emphysema, are often thin and emaciated with hypertrophy of accessory muscles of respiration.

### Thoracic Shape and Movement

■ *Anterior-Posterior Diameter.* The anterior (A) to posterior (P) dimensions of the chest are compared with the lateral chest dimensions (Fig. 2-2). In the normal adult chest, this AP/lateral ratio is 1:2, increasing slightly with normal aging and increasing markedly with obstructive diseases such as emphysema or cystic fibrosis. Patients with significant obstructive disease have a rounded or "barrel" chest with an AP/lateral ratio close to 1:1.

Deformities of the thorax and spine are noted. The term "pigeon chest" refers to the deformity pectus carinatum, or protruding sternum. Conversely, when the sternum angles inward, the deformity is termed funnel chest, or pectus excavatum. An exaggerated outward posterior curvature of the thoracic spine is termed kyphosis, or commonly hunchback. Kyphosis is common in postmenopausal women with vertebral decalcification. When kyphosis is combined with scoliosis, an abnormal lateral curvature of the spine, the resultant chest deformity is called kyphoscoliosis. An abnormally straight spine is known as poker spine. Severe deformities of the chest and spine can markedly impair pulmonary and cardiac functioning.

■ *Symmetry.* Symmetry of the chest is best assessed with the patient in the sitting position. If the patient is unable to sit, the nurse should stand at the foot of the bed to observe the patient in the reclining position. Normally both sides of the chest expand equally. Asymmetric movement may be caused by trauma, pneumothorax, pleural disease, effusions, severe atelectasis, or a surgically induced abnormality. A flail chest is the paradoxic inward movement of part of the chest on inspiration and outward movement on expiration. Flail chest is caused by rib fractures in two or more places and is rarely seen in the home care setting unless the patient has recently fallen and fractured ribs. Flail chest is associated with a marked increase in dyspnea and requires immediate medical evaluation.

■ *Accessory Muscles.* Patients with obstructive or restrictive lung disease frequently use accessory muscles of the neck, shoulders, and abdomen with quiet breathing. This accessory muscle use becomes more pronounced with exercise.

■ *Retractions.* Retractions on inspiration are often seen in the substernal, suprasternal, or intercostal spaces in patients whose work of breathing is increased. Bulging of the interspaces may occasionally be seen on expiration in patients with severe airflow obstruction.

■ *Clubbing.* The fingers and toes are inspected for clubbing of the distal phalanges. Clubbing is characterized by enlargement of the distal phalanges with softening of the nail bed and an increase in the angle between the base of the nail and the skin from approximately 160 to 180 degrees or more (Fig. 2-3). For evaluation, a straight edge may be laid over the distal phalanx parallel to the finger, or the patient can be asked to position the index fingers of the right and left hands with the nails and the distal joints approximated. In clubbed fingers the space that is normally visible at the base of the nail is absent, and in advanced clubbing the fingers appear spoon shaped.

The etiology and significance of clubbing are unknown, and it generally does not cause symptoms. It may occur in patients with pulmonary neoplasms, bronchiectasis, cystic fibrosis, and interstitial fibrosis, and rarely as a familial tendency. Some patients, particularly adolescents and young adults, may be self-conscious about the appearance of clubbing.

### Respiratory Pattern

Normally the respiratory rate of the adult varies from 12 to 20 breaths per minute at rest (Fig. 2-

Clubbing—early        almost 180°

Clubbing—middle        180°

Clubbing—severe        > 180°

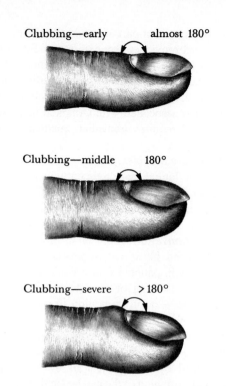

**Fig. 2-3**  Stages of clubbing in fingers from infectious and noninfectious causes. (From Seidel H et al: *Mosby's guide to physical examination*, ed 2, St Louis, 1991, Mosby.)

4). Tachypnea or an increase in the respiratory rate often occurs with fever, anxiety, and interstitial pulmonary fibrosis and after exercise. Bradypnea or a decrease in the respiratory rate may occur with neurologic diseases. Hypopnea is abnormally slow, shallow respirations, whereas hyperpnea is deep, abnormally rapid respirations. In most cases, however, respirations are in proportion to metabolic demand. These terms are not to be confused with hyperventilation and hypoventilation. Hyperventilation is increased ventilation in excess of metabolic demands, and in the normal person it results in a low arterial carbon dioxide tension. Hypoventilation is a decrease in ventilation that results in high arterial carbon dioxide tension. The diagnosis is based on arterial blood gas findings and cannot be determined by inspection alone.

Kussmaul breathing is a deep and rapid pattern of breathing that may be seen in diabetic ketoacidosis. Cheyne-Stokes respiration, characterized by periods of increasing and decreasing respiratory rate and depth with episodes of apnea, may be seen with severe congestive heart failure, uremia, cerebrovascular accidents, and terminal disease conditions. Biot's breathing, characterized by unpredictable irregularities in the rhythm, rate, and depth of respiration, including periods of apnea, is most often seen in central nervous system disorders that affect the medulla oblongata. Apneic episodes that occur during sleep may be indicative of sleep apnea syndrome and are discussed in Chapter 12.

## Palpation

Palpation techniques are used to assess the skin, chest wall, trachea, chest excursion, and voice vibrations (tactile fremitus).

### Skin Turgor

Skin turgor is an indication of body fluid status and is assessed by pinching or tenting the skin over a bony prominence, usually the forearm. The length of time it takes for the skin to return to its original state is then noted. In well-hydrated patients with normal skin turgor, the tented skin promptly returns to normal. In poorly hydrated patients with poor skin turgor, the skin remains tented or pinched for several seconds before returning to normal. Elderly patients tend to have thin, dry, less elastic skin, and in these patients it is more accurate to assess turgor over the forehead or sternum rather than the forearm.

### Temperature

Decreased skin temperature may be due to a cool environment or to circulatory impairment. Excessively warm skin, which is often evidenced by flushing or diaphoresis, may be caused by an overly warm environment, fever, hypercapnia, anxiety, or embarrassment. Local areas of warm or hot skin may be caused by cellulitis or abscesses.

| Type/Pattern | Rate (breaths per minute) | Clinical Significance |
|---|---|---|
| Eupnea | 12-20 | Normal |
| Tachypnea | >35 | Respiratory failure<br>Response to fever<br>Anxiety<br>Shortness of breath<br>Respiratory infection |
| Bradypnea | <10 | Sleep<br>Respiratory depression<br>Drug overdose<br>Central nervous system<br>(CNS) lesion |
| Apnea | Periods of no respiration lasting >15 seconds | May be intermittent such as in sleep apnea<br>Respiratory arrest |
| Hyperpnea | 16-20 | Can result from anxiety or response to pain<br>Can cause marked respiratory alkalosis, paresthesia, tetany, confusion |
| Kussmaul's | Usually >35, may be slow or normal | Tachypnea pattern associated with diabetic ketoacidosis, metabolic acidosis, or renal failure |
| Biot's | Variable | Periods of apnea and shallow breathing caused by CNS disorder: found in some healthy clients |
| Apneustic | Increased | Increased respiratory time with short grunting expiratory time: seen in CNS lesions of the respiratory center |

**Fig. 2-4**    Breathing patterns. (From Weilitz P: *Pocket guide to respiratory care*, St Louis, 1991, Mosby.)

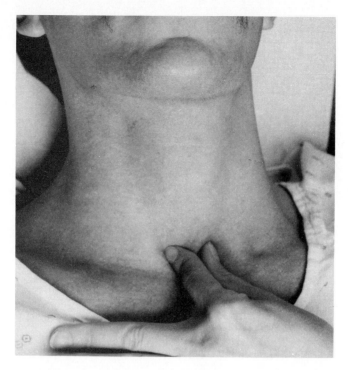

**Fig. 2-5** Tracheal position is assessed in suprasternal notch with thumbs or second and third fingers. (From Potter P, Perry A: *Fundamentals of nursing,* ed 2, St Louis, 1989, Mosby.)

### Chest Wall

The chest wall is gently palpated with the fleshy balls of three fingers to assess for bulges, masses, or subcutaneous emphysema. Bulges or masses may be associated with strained muscles, rib fractures, abscesses, or tumors. Subcutaneous emphysema is often described as the sound of bubbles popping or cellophane crackling beneath the skin. It is harmless but can be painful and frightening for the patient. Subcutaneous emphysema may be caused by a pneumothorax, a rib fracture, tracheostomy, or a transcutaneous oxygen catheter. During a severe exacerbation of asthma, it may occur because of extreme hyperinflation and the movement of air into the subcutaneous tissue. It generally is symptomatic of a medical problem, which must be evaluated and treated by the physician.

### Trachea

The trachea is palpated to determine if it is in the midline and moveable (Fig. 2-5). One or two fingers are placed between the trachea and the suprasternal notch, comparing the peritracheal space on each side. The trachea is displaced toward the affected side with problems such as atelectasis that decrease lung volume. By contrast, space-occupying lesions, such as tension pneumothorax, pleural effusion, tumor, or enlargement of the thyroid gland or lymph nodes, push the trachea toward the opposite side. Significant tracheal displacement may indicate mediastinal shift with compression of the great vessels.

### Chest Excursion

Chest excursion is assessed by placing each hand on one side of the lower chest wall with the thumbs

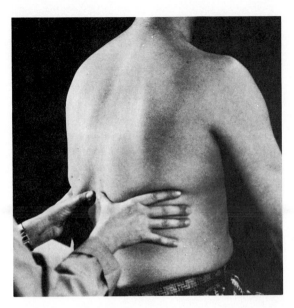

**Fig. 2-6** Thumbs are placed at level of tenth rib for palpating thoracic expansion. (From Malasanos L et al: *Health assessment,* ed 4, St Louis, 1990, Mosby.)

in the midline and the fingers spread over the lateral chest wall (Fig. 2-6). The maneuver is usually performed on the posterior chest, although the same technique is useful on the anterior chest. The fingers are pressed firmly against the chest wall, while the thumbs rest lightly on the skin so that they can move freely as the patient's chest expands. As the patient exhales fully, the thumbs are positioned so they barely touch. The patient then inhales deeply while the degree and symmetry of chest expansion are noted. The normal chest expands symmetrically, 2 to 5 cm from the midline bilaterally. Asymmetric movement or splinting may occur when one side of the chest is affected by atelectasis, pneumonia, pleuritic pain, pleural disease, pneumothorax, or other chest trauma.

### Tactile Fremitus

Tactile fremitus is the vibration caused by speaking that is palpable on the chest wall. It may be assessed with the ulnar aspect of the hands or fist or the palmar aspect of the fingers or hands while

the patient is asked to repeat a phrase such as "ninety-nine," or "blue moon." Both sides of the chest wall may be palpated simultaneously, or one hand can be moved from one side to the other. Normally the vibrations are more intense where large airways are close to the chest wall, if the voice is more resonant, and if the chest wall is very thin. Vibrations are decreased over bones, if the patient is obese or has large muscles, and if the voice is very soft. Abnormal increases in vibration are noted over areas of consolidation from pneumonia or tumor and with extensive pulmonary fibrosis. Abnormal decreases in vibration are noted when there is air trapping, when fluid or air fills the pleural space, or when airway obstruction inhibits the transmission of voice vibrations.

### Percussion

Percussion is a technique that may be used to determine the boundaries of organs and to assess the density of lung tissue. It is usually performed by placing the distal portion of the middle finger of the nondominant hand on the chest wall and striking it with the tip of the middle finger of the dominant hand just above the nail bed with a sharp, quick motion that originates from the wrist (Fig. 2-7). Care is taken not to dampen the sound by placing other fingers or parts of the hand on the chest wall. Some clinicians use the ulnar aspect of the fist, especially in the patient with a thick chest wall.

The percussion note can be described as resonant, hyperresonant, dull, flat, or tympanic. The normal lung produces a resonant percussion note; the air trapping characteristic of emphysema or a pneumothorax produces a hyperresonant percussion note; and organs such as the liver, as well as lung tissue that is consolidated or atelectactic, produce a dull percussion note. The extreme of dullness is called flatness and is similar to the sound produced when percussing over the thigh. A flat percussion note may be heard over a large pleural effusion. A tympanic note is normally heard over a gastric air bubble. It may also be heard when percussing the lung over a large pneumothorax. The percussion note is dampened if the patient is

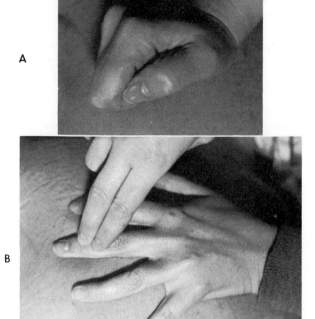

**Fig. 2-7   A,** Direct percussion using ulnar aspect of fist. **B,** Indirect percussion using fingers. (From Dettenmeier P: *Pulmonary nursing care,* St Louis, 1992, Mosby.)

obese or well muscled and increased if the patient is thin with poorly developed muscles.

### Diaphragmatic Excursion

Diaphragmatic excursion may be determined with percussion. The position of each hemidiaphragm is assessed at expiration and again at full inspiration. The distance between these two points is the diaphragmatic excursion and is usually 3 to 6 cm. Diaphragmatic excursion is assessed on the posterior chest wall with percussion beginning at about the eighth rib on the midscapular line. While the patient is breathing quietly or when the patient

has exhaled completely, the nurse percusses down the chest until the percussion note changes from resonant to dull. The patient is then instructed to take a deep breath and hold it. The nurse then quickly percusses from that point downward until the second point of dullness is reached. The distance between the two points of dullness represents the diaphragmatic excursion. The excursion of the right and left hemidiaphragms should be nearly equal, although the right hemidiaphragm may be positioned slightly higher because of displacement by the liver. Diaphragmatic excursion is usually decreased in emphysema because the diaphragms are flattened from hyperinflation. Other conditions that limit diaphragmatic excursion include ascites, hepatomegaly, and pregnancy. Paralysis of one hemidiaphragm may be noted by asymmetric excursion.

## Auscultation

Auscultation is the final component of the physical assessment of the chest. Information obtained from the history, inspection, palpation, and percussion guides the nurse in auscultation of the chest. The patient is asked to breathe in slowly and slightly deeper than normal through the mouth to enhance the intensity of the breath sounds. The diaphragm of the stethoscope is positioned firmly on the bare skin of the chest to minimize movement of the stethoscope on the skin or body hair. This precaution minimizes confusing and distracting noises. The stethoscope is moved from side to side and top to bottom as sounds from the anterior, lateral, and posterior aspects of the chest are compared.

### Normal Breath Sounds

■ *Bronchial Breath Sounds.* Bronchial sounds are normally heard over the trachea and mainstem bronchi. It is not normal to hear them over the lung parenchyma. They are described as having a high-pitched tubular quality. A similar sound can be produced by blowing air through a hollow tube. The expiratory phase is usually longer and louder than the inspiratory phase with a short pause between the two.

**Table 2-1**  Adventitious sounds

| Recommended term | Characteristics | Associated disorders | Other terminology |
|---|---|---|---|
| **DISCONTINUOUS SOUNDS** | | | |
| Coarse crackles | Interrupted, explosive sounds; loud, low pitched, and of long duration | Pulmonary edema; resolving pneumonia; secretions in medium-sized airways | Coarse bubbling rales; coarse crepitations |
| Fine crackles | Interrupted, explosive sounds; quieter, higher pitched, and of shorter duration than coarse crackles | Interstitial fibrosis; popping open of underventilated alveoli (often disappear with deep breaths) | Rales; fine crepitations |
| **CONTINUOUS SOUNDS** | | | |
| Wheezes | High-pitched sounds with musical quality | Airway narrowing or partial obstruction | Musical rales; sibilant rhonchi; high-pitched wheeze |
| Rhonchi | Low-pitched snoring sound | Secretions in large airways (often clear with cough) | Sonorous rhonchi; low-pitched wheezes |

Modified from Report of ATS Ad Hoc Committee on Pulmonary Nomenclature, 1981.

■ *Vesicular Breath Sounds.* Vesicular breath sounds are normally heard over the lung parenchyma as air moves in and out of the bronchioles and alveoli. Vesicular breath sounds are described as quiet and similar to the gentle rustling of air through the leaves on a tree. The inspiratory phase is louder and higher in pitch than the expiratory phase and audible longer by a ratio of approximately 5:2.

## Adventitious Breath Sounds

Adventitious breath sounds include crackles, wheezes, rhonchi, pleural friction rubs, and stridor. The American Thoracic Society (ATS) recommends standard terminology to describe these abnormal sounds (Table 2-1) (Mikams, 1987). Adventitious sounds can be divided into two major groups: discontinuous and continuous.

■ *Discontinuous Breath Sounds*

■ CRACKLES. Crackles (formerly called rales) are short, discontinuous crackling or bubbling sounds that are most often heard on inspiration, although they can be heard on expiration and after coughing (posttussive crackles). There are two postulated causes for crackles. One is that they result from bubbles of secretions that explode or pop as air moves into the airways. A second possible cause is the snapping open of small airways on inspiration. The latter theory is supported by the observation that fine basilar crackles often disappear after the patient takes several deep breaths.

Crackles may be coarse (low pitched) or fine

(high pitched). Low-pitched crackles are simulated by blowing through a straw into a glass of heavy syrup. High-pitched crackles are simulated by rubbing a lock of hair between the thumb and forefinger in front of the ear. Generally the pitch of the crackle depends on the size of the airway in which it is located. Crackles are often heard in bronchitis, atelectasis, consolidation, pneumonia, congestive heart failure, pulmonary edema, and pulmonary fibrosis. Those heard early in inspiration are often associated with airflow obstruction, whereas those heard late in inspiration (end-inspiratory crackles) suggest a restrictive problem. The crackles that are heard in the patient with pulmonary fibrosis occur toward the end of inspiration, sound like they are just below the diaphragm of the stethoscope, and have a dry quality resembling the sound made by pulling apart pieces of Velcro—hence, the name "Velcro crackles."

■ PLEURAL FRICTION RUB. A pleural friction rub is produced by two inflamed pleural surfaces rubbing against each other. A rub is most noticeable over the lower anterolateral chest where the movement of the chest wall is greatest. Pleural friction rubs have been described as coarse discontinuous grating, scratching, or creaking noises, often like the sound of two pieces of leather rubbing together. Some clinicians believe that pleural friction rubs resemble crackles or a pericardial rub. However, a pleural friction rub ceases with breath holding, whereas a pericardial rub does not. Pleural friction rubs may occur with pneumonia, tuberculosis, cancer, and pulmonary infarction.

■ *Continuous Breath Sounds*

■ WHEEZES. Wheezes are high-pitched, continuous, musical, whistling, or squeaking sounds that occur most often on expiration, although they can also occur on inspiration. They are produced as air moves turbulently through narrowed airways. They may be caused by bronchospasm, inflammation, encroachment of a tumor or foreign body into the airway, bronchial stenosis, or thick secretions.

■ RHONCHI. Rhonchi (low-pitched wheezes) or gurgles resemble continuous moaning or snoring sounds. They may be the result of air movement through a narrowed airway. They are usually related to the presence of secretions and decrease or disappear after coughing or suctioning the airway.

■ STRIDOR. Stridor is a crowing sound that is heard when there is laryngeal obstruction. It is generally detectable without a stethoscope and is usually heard on inspiration. It is often confused with wheezing; however, wheezing generally occurs on expiration. Stridor is usually caused by croup but can be a sign of foreign body aspiration, tracheitis, or smoke inhalation. Stridor that is heard on expiration is usually caused by an intrathoracic obstruction such as a foreign body or vascular ring. Very often stridor is a medical emergency.

### Voice Sounds

The transmission of voice sounds through the chest wall may also be assessed by auscultation. Normally, voice sounds are muffled and unclear when heard through the stethoscope. However, when there is tissue consolidation from intraalveolar fluid accumulation and inflammation, the transmission of sound waves is increased and voice sounds are enhanced.

■ *Bronchophony*. Bronchophony is the sound of the spoken voice heard through the stethoscope. The patient is instructed to repeat the phrase "ninety-nine" or "how now brown cow," while the nurse listens over the lung parenchyma with the diaphragm of the stethoscope. The words are clearly distinguishable over areas of consolidation and not over normal lung tissue.

■ *Whispered Pectoriloquy*. Whispered pectoriloquy is a finding similar to bronchophony, in which a whispered "ninety-nine" or "how now brown cow" is heard clearly over an area of consolidation and not over normal lung tissue.

■ *Egophony*. Egophony refers to the distortion of the voice sound *"ee"* so that it is heard as *"aa"* over lung tissue consolidation. Some describe egophony as similar to the bleating of a goat.

Abnormal chest examination findings are summarized in Table 2-2.

**Table 2-2**   Physical findings in some common pulmonary disorders

| Disorder | Inspection | Palpation | Percussion | Auscultation |
|---|---|---|---|---|
| Bronchial asthma (acute attack) | Hyperinflation; use of accessory muscles | Impaired expansion; decreased fremitus | Hyperresonance; low diaphragm | Prolonged expiration; inspiratory and expiratory wheezes |
| Pneumothorax (complete) | Lag on affected side | Absent fremitus | Hyperresonant or tympanitic | Absent breath sounds |
| Pleural effusion (large) | Lag on affected side | Decreased fremitus; trachea and heart shifted away from affected side | Dullness or flatness | Absent breath sounds |
| Atelectasis (lobar obstruction) | Lag on affected side | Decreased fremitus; trachea and heart shifted toward affected side | Dullness or flatness | Absent breath sounds |
| Consolidation (pneumonia) | Possible lag or splinting on affected side | Increased fremitus | Dullness | Bronchial breath sounds; bronchophony; pectoriloquy; crackles |

From Murray JF, Nadel JA: *Textbook of respiratory medicine,* Philadelphia, 1988, WB Saunders.

## CARDIAC ASSESSMENT

The examination of the patient with pulmonary disease must always include an assessment of cardiac functioning because the pulmonary and cardiac systems are closely related. Pulse rates, blood pressure readings, and body weight measurements should be obtained for all patients referred for home care at the initial visit and on follow-up visits as indicated. The chest examination should include careful auscultation of the heart for abnormalities in the rate or rhythm, the presence of murmurs, extra heart sounds, and abnormal placement of the point of maximal impulse.

### Pulse

The rate, rhythm, and strength of the peripheral pulse are usually assessed over the radial artery. If the radial artery pulse is absent or difficult to palpate, the apical, brachial, carotid, or temporal pulses may be assessed. The nurse also assesses the posterior tibial and dorsalis pedis pulses for peripheral vascular disease.

### Rate

Generally the normal resting pulse rate ranges between 60 and 100 beats per minute. Patients with severe chronic lung disease often have tachycardia in excess of 100 beats per minute. Factors associated with an increased heart rate include decreased cardiac output, poor muscle conditioning, medications such as bronchodilators, fluid overload or deficit, hypoxemia, and fever or other hypermetabolic states. Heart block causes a decreased heart rate. The heart rate for each patient should be determined at rest and with exercise.

### Rhythm

An irregular pulse indicates that there are alterations in the electromechanical functioning of the heart. If the peripheral pulse is irregular, it should be evaluated simultaneously with the apical pulse for a full minute. Ectopic beats may occur at regular or irregular intervals. Alterations in the rhythm of the heart are associated with many disorders, including electrolyte abnormalities, drug toxicity, fever, hypoxia, exercise, congestive heart failure, and myocardial ischemia or infarction.

### Pulse Deficit

A pulse deficit, in which the peripheral pulse rate is lower than the apical heart rate, may be seen with premature ventricular contractions when ventricular systole occurs before the ventricle has time to fill with blood.

### Pulse Pressure

The pulse pressure, or the difference between systolic and diastolic blood pressure, is determined by cardiac stroke volume and ejection velocity and by the systemic vascular resistance. The strength of the pulse is sometimes used to determine fluid status, but it is not always a reliable indicator. A strong, bounding pulse (pulsus magnus) is associated with fluid overload, as well as with any condition that increases pulse pressure, such as patent ductus arteriosus, essential hypertension, thyroid storm, aortic insufficiency, and arteriovenous fistula. A small, weak pulse (pulsus parvus) is found in any condition in which the pulse pressure is reduced, such as decreased cardiac output from aortic and mitral stenosis, fluid deficit, or cardiomyopathy. A pulse pressure of less than 30 mm Hg should be evaluated because it may mean that tissue perfusion is compromised. A strong pulse beat followed by a weaker pulse beat (pulsus alternans) may be noted in patients with left ventricular failure and severe arterial hypertension.

## Blood Pressure

Several factors affect blood pressure, including the cardiac output, peripheral vascular resistance, arterial elasticity, blood volume, exercise, emotions, weight, and age. The body adapts to mild or acute hypoxemia with hypertension, whereas severe or prolonged hypoxemia may be associated with hypotension. The blood pressure is measured on the right and left extremities during the initial assessment. Thereafter the extremity with the higher reading is used for measurement.

### Factors Affecting Blood Pressure

■ *Orthostatic Hypotension.* The blood pressure and heart rate should be measured after the patient has been in the supine position for 10 minutes, after 1 minute of sitting, and after 1 minute of standing. Standing from a lying position causes a 10% to 12% decrease in systolic pressure and a similar drop or increase in the diastolic pressure. The patient is considered to be orthostatic when the change is greater than 15% and is accompanied by an increased heart rate of more than 15 beats per minute. Postural hypotension may be caused by reduced intravascular volume, sodium deficit, impaired peripheral vasomotor tone, or autonomic insufficiency that prevents the heart rate from increasing in response to a decreased cardiac output. The autonomic insufficiency is commonly caused by β-adrenergic blocking agents or calcium antagonists. Orthostatic hypotension is significant in the home care patient because many are treated with diuretics.

■ *Pulsus Paradoxus.* Pulsus paradoxus is an abnormal fall in systemic blood pressure during inspiration. It develops when the intrathoracic pressure becomes so high that blood flow from the right to the left side of the heart is impaired. Pulsus paradoxus may be seen with severe bronchospasm and cardiac tamponade. It may also be "normally" present in some patients with severe chronic obstructive pulmonary disease (COPD). To evaluate a pulsus paradoxus the blood pressure cuff should be inflated from 5 to 10 mm Hg above the patient's systolic blood pressure; the air should then be *very slowly* released from the cuff (slowly enough to hear three or more beats with each 10 mm Hg drop in pressure) until the first Korotkoff sound is heard

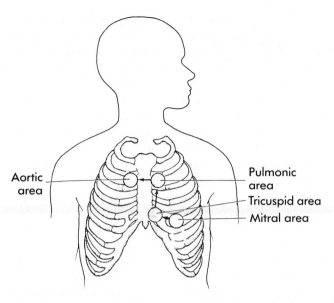

**Fig. 2-8**   Cardiac auscultation. (From Phipps WJ et al: *Shafer's medical-surgical nursing,* ed 7, St Louis, 1980, Mosby.)

only during expiration. Air should continue to be released until Korotkoff sounds are heard throughout inspiration and expiration. A difference of 10 mm Hg or less between these two points is normal. If the difference is greater than 10 mm Hg, the patient is said to have a pulsus paradoxus of *"x"* mm Hg.

## Heart Sounds

Heart sounds are caused by the opening and closing of the heart valves in conjunction with cardiac muscle contraction and the resultant blood flow. Heart sounds are louder in patients who are slender because they have a thin chest wall and are softer in those who are obese or well muscled. Heart sounds in the patient with severe COPD may be heard best just below the xiphoid process because the retrosternal airspace is increased and the heart is displaced because of hyperinflation.

### First Heart Sound

The first heart sound ($S_1$) is produced by closure of the mitral and tricuspid valves at the onset of ventricular systole. The $S_1$ is best heard with the diaphragm of the stethoscope positioned left of the sternum at the midclavicular line in the fifth intercostal space and left of the sternum in the fourth intercostal space (Fig. 2-8).

### Second Heart Sound

The second heart sound ($S_2$) is produced when the aortic and pulmonic valves close at the end of the ventricular systole. The $S_2$ is best heard with the diaphragm of the stethoscope positioned on the second intercostal space at the right and left sternal borders. In some patients, especially children, the $S_2$ is physiologically split on inspiration when the pulmonic valve closure is delayed by increased venous return to the right ventricle and slower right ventricular contraction. Persistent splitting of the $S_2$ in inspiration and expiration is abnormal and may occur in atrial septal defects, pulmonary stenosis, pulmonary hypertension, severe mitral insufficiency, aortic stenosis, and bundle branch block.

### Third Heart Sound

A third heart sound ($S_3$) is normal during diastole in young adults and in children. The $S_3$ is best heard with the bell of the stethoscope in the mitral or apical area to the left of the sternum at the mid-clavicular line in the fourth and fifth intercostal spaces. An abnormal $S_3$ (ventricular gallop) occurs during the rapid early phase of ventricular filling because of increased volume load or decreased compliance of the ventricle. A right ventricular gallop is best heard with the bell of the stethoscope on the third and fourth intercostal spaces at the left sternal border. A left ventricular gallop is best heard at the apex of the heart with the patient in the left lateral decubitus position. $S_3$ gallops sound similar to the word "Ken-tuc-ky" and are commonly associated with advanced congestive heart failure, pulmonary hypertension and cor pulmonale, tricuspid insufficiency, mitral insufficiency, and left-to-right shunts.

### Fourth Heart Sound

The fourth heart sound ($S_4$), or atrial gallop, occurs after atrial contraction and just before the $S_1$ during the late phase of ventricular filling (presystole). It may be difficult to distinguish from a widely split $S_1$. Similar to the $S_3$, a left-sided $S_4$ is best heard with the bell of the stethoscope at the apex of the heart, whereas a right-sided $S_4$ is best heard along the left sternal border. $S_4$ gallops sound similar to "Ten-nes-see." The presence of an $S_4$ is consistent with reduced ventricular compliance and is fairly common in older people. The $S_4$ does not necessarily indicate heart failure, although it may be present in patients with ventricular overload, cardiomyopathy, elevated diastolic pressure, pulmonary hypertension, aortic or pulmonary stenosis, coronary artery disease, and hyperthyroidism. It is heard in many patients with angina and in *most* patients with an acute myocardial infarction. A summation gallop may be heard in patients with an $S_3$ and $S_4$. In a summation gallop, the $S_3$ and $S_4$ are heard as one sound because the heart rate is increased and ventricular diastole is shortened.

It is very important to identify and document heart sounds at the initial assessment of the patient so that changes can be noted in follow-up assessments. For instance, an $S_4$ that is assessed at baseline and in the absence of other clinical signs of cardiac dysfunction would probably be considered "normal" for a given patient. However, if an $S_4$ was not noted at the baseline visit and was detected on a follow-up visit, it would be an abnormal finding and the physician should be notified.

### Jugular Venous Pressure

Jugular venous pressure is often used as an indicator of fluid status. Normally, people have full jugular veins in the supine position, but the veins become barely visible as the head is elevated. Right ventricular failure or volume overload is suggested if jugular venous distention (JVD) is present when the head is elevated 45 degrees. JVD is best assessed by observing the right internal jugular vein rather than the external jugular vein, because the former is more proximal to the right atrium and does not have valves to interfere with venous pulsations.

JVD is assessed by observing the vertical distance between the sternal angle and the jugular distention (Fig. 2-9). Most measurements are taken with the head of the bed elevated 30 to 45 degrees. The height of the distention is recorded in centimeters and the position of the patient in degrees relative to supine—for instance, "the jugular venous pressure is 4 cm with the head of the bed elevated 30 degrees." Future measurements must be made with the patient in the same position so that they are comparable. An alternative and perhaps more simple measure of JVD may be obtained by noting the height of the neck vein distention in relation to other anatomic landmarks in the neck with the patient positioned as before. Such a reading is recorded as follows: "The jugular veins are distended to the angle of the jaw with the patient at a 45-degree angle."

### Hepatojugular Reflux

The hepatojugular reflux is evaluated by applying firm pressure over the liver for 30 to 60 seconds

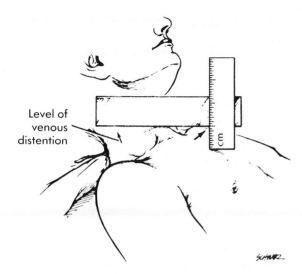

**Fig. 2-9**   Measurement of jugular venous pressure. Arrows indicate height of jugular venous distention in centimeters. (From Malasanos L et al: *Health assessment,* St Louis, 1986, Mosby.)

with the patient sitting at a 30- to 45-degree angle and observing the jugular veins for distention. If there is passive congestion from right ventricular failure, this maneuver will create back pressure in the vena cava and jugular veins. An increase of more than 1 cm of jugular distention is considered significant.

## Edema

Edema is an indicator of total body fluid accumulation and does not necessarily correlate with intravascular water. Edema occurs as a result of poor venous circulation or heart failure and is typically observed in dependent areas such as the extremities, sacrum, and periorbital area. Patients with respiratory disorders and compromised cardiac functioning commonly develop edema as a result of increasing their dietary intake of sodium. Edema may also result from phlebitis, or from hypoproteinemia (low serum albumin) that reduces plasma oncotic pressure and allows fluid to move into the interstitial spaces. Patients with chronic lung disease are at risk for phlebitis because of impaired mobility and hypoproteinemia because of poor nutrition. Chronic edema is also associated with impaired lymphatic drainage or lymphatic obstruction. Edema itself is usually only a cosmetic problem unless it is so severe that it compresses blood vessels and impairs circulation.

Edema is assessed in several ways. The most common technique is to firmly compress the tissue over a bony prominence, such as the dorsum of the foot or the anterior tibia, for 5 seconds and to note the resultant degree of pitting. Most clinicians grade the edema with "1" plus for each millimeter of pitting. Edema typically varies from "trace to 4 plus." When it is most severe, the skin may be too tight to pit and the edema is recorded as "severe, nonpitting edema." It is also important to record the location of the edema—for example, "2 plus pitting to the ankle with trace to the knee" or "1 to 2 plus pitting above the ankle." A second technique to assess edema is to measure the circumference of the extremity at a standard given point, such as 3 inches above the ankle. Subsequent measurements must always be taken at the same place. The latter technique is useful for unilateral edema that may result from deep vein thrombosis and to measure the degree of abdominal ascites.

### Weight Change

When edema is present, daily weight measurements are an adjunctive measurement of volume status. The ideal time to record weight is the early morning before breakfast with the patient clad only in nightclothes and without shoes. The scale must be placed on a firm surface rather than carpeting and should be located in an area with bright lighting, especially if the patient is visually impaired. Home care staff should carry their own scales if the patient does not have one because the patient must be weighed on the same scale each time. Agencies should purchase scales for staff to use in the home. An increase in weight in excess of 1 lb each day in the adult is an indication of increased fluid volume.

## ASSESSMENT OF THE ENVIRONMENT

The home care staff have a unique opportunity to assess the physical environment inside and outside the home, as well as the community in which the patient lives. Assessment of the environment is a basic component of all home care visits. Environmental factors that should be evaluated for the patient with chronic lung disease include:

- *Safety*—hallways free of clutter; oxygen supply tubing long enough to allow for movement from room to room and placed to minimize risk of tripping; space heaters placed away from oxygen equipment, walls, and furniture to minimize risk of fire; adequate electrical outlets for respiratory equipment with extension cords of appropriate quality; extension cords placed out of traffic areas
- *Cleanliness*—respiratory equipment properly maintained; nebulizer medications and aerosol solutions properly stored to reduce risk of infection
- *Allergens and irritants*—allergens and irritants in home reduced or eliminated to minimize risk of bronchospasm in susceptible patients
- *Personal hygiene*—adequate bathroom facilities, with a place for the patient to sit while bathing
- *Cooking facilities*—safe water supply; functioning stove and refrigerator
- *Location*—convenient access to medical facilities

## DIAGNOSTIC EVALUATIONS THAT MAY BE PERFORMED IN THE HOME

For some patients, it may be extremely difficult and expensive to find transportation to a physician's office or clinic. Several simple diagnostic tests can be performed in the home with ease and accuracy, and they can provide valuable information to guide the plan of care. These are described briefly; detailed instructions for each test are be-

---

### Home Diagnostic Evaluations

Spirometry
Oxygenation
Home sleep studies
Radiographs
Biochemical samples
Electrocardiograms
Apnea monitoring
Esophageal pH monitoring

---

yond the scope of this book and depend on the type of equipment that is used and the manufacturer's recommendations.

### Spirometry

Spirometry is one of the most important diagnostic tests that can be carried out in the home. Although a portable spirometer may be relatively expensive, it is a recommended and worthwhile investment for the home care agency. Spirometry consists of timed measurements of relaxed and forced inspiratory and expiratory flow (e.g., vital

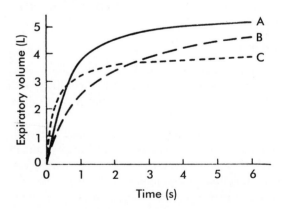

**Fig. 2-10**   Spirograms. *A*, Normal; *B*, obstructive; *C*, restrictive patterns. (From Schroeder S et al: *Current medical diagnosis and treament*, San Mateo, Calif, 1992, Appleton & Lange.)

**Table 2-3**   Spirometry

| Test | Definition | Values |
|------|-----------|--------|
| Forced expiratory volume in 1 second ($FEV_1$) | Amount of air that can be forcefully exhaled in 1 second; valid measurement requires patient effort | Normal = 80% of predicted; decreased in airflow obstruction: mild = 65%-79%, moderate = 50%-64%, severe = <50%; normal or decreased in restrictive disease |
| Forced vital capacity (FVC) | Amount of air that can be exhaled as rapidly and forcefully as possible after maximal inspiration | More than 80% of predicted; normal or decreased in obstructive disease; decreased in restrictive disease |
| $FEV_1$/FVC | Forced expiratory volume in 1 second expressed as a percentage of forced vital capacity | Normal = 75%; decreased in airflow obstruction: mild = 60%-74%, moderate = 40%-59%, severe = <40%; normal or increased in restrictive disease |
| Vital capacity (VC) | Amount of air that can be exhaled slowly after a full inspiration | Normal = 80% of predicted; normal or decreased in obstruction; decreased in restrictive disease; may be higher than forced maneuver in patient with irritable airways (e.g., asthma) |
| Peak expiratory flow rate (PEFR) (L/min) | Measurement of maximal airflow during forced exhalation after full inspiration; valid measurement requires patient effort | Decreased in obstruction; normal or increased in restrictive disease |
| Tidal volume ($V_T$) | Amount of air that is inhaled and exhaled with each breath during quiet breathing | Normal = approximately 400 ml |

capacity [VC], forced expiratory volume [FEV], forced vital capacity [FVC]). The results are displayed as a spirogram (Fig. 2-10) or as a digital reading. Normal values are calculated according to sex, height, and age and are obtained from nomograms. Spirometry is most useful in home care to assess changes in airflow obstruction. Such changes are important in assessing the significance of acute exacerbations and monitoring patient responses to therapy. The measurements that may be made with a spirometer are presented in Table 2-

3. Instructions for obtaining a spirogram are as follows:
   1. Follow the manufacturer's instructions for cleaning, calibrating, and transporting the spirometer to the home.
   2. The patient should be seated in front of spirometer with nose clip in place and mouth placed firmly around the mouthpiece.
   3. The patient is instructed to breathe quietly in and out with the mouth firmly around the mouthpiece for several breaths to record the

tidal volume, then to breathe in as deeply as possible, and finally to blow all of the air out as quickly and forcefully as possible.* With this maneuver the $FEV_1$, FVC, and $FEV_1$/FVC can be determined. If the patient does not inhale through the spirometer mouthpiece, he or she should be instructed to take several breaths of room air through the mouth, take in as deep a breath as possible, hold the breath while placing the lips around the mouthpiece, and blow out as hard and as fast as possible. Enthusiastic coaching often helps patients to perform better. The VC is obtained in the same manner but with a relaxed maximal exhalation.

4. Calculations are made from the spirogram tracing according to the manufacturer's instructions or the results are obtained from the digital recording.

## Peak Flow

The maximum rate of expiratory flow can readily be measured in the home with a peak flow meter. Peak expiratory flow primarily reflects the resistance of large airways and is an effort-dependent maneuver. It has been shown to correlate with wheezing and is an objective measurement of obstruction in patients with asthma (Clark, 1992). The hand-held meter can be used by patients who are over 4 years of age. Patients are instructed to breathe in as much air as possible, place their mouth on the mouthpiece, and blow out as hard and fast as they can. Nose clips can be used but are not necessary.

## Oxygenation
### Arterial Blood Gases

The effectiveness of the delivery of oxygen to the blood and the removal of carbon dioxide can be assessed by the measurement of arterial blood gases (ABGs). Home care staff require training to perform arterial puncture. For accurate results the blood specimen must be packed in ice water and transported to the laboratory within 1 hour from the time it is obtained.

### Oxygen Saturation

Oxygen saturation can be measured noninvasively in the home using pulse oximeters. Transcutaneous electrodes may be fastened to the ear lobe or clipped over the finger and determine the oxygen saturation by measuring the light absorption of hemoglobin. Oximeters can be used in the home to determine oxygen desaturation during exercise and sleep and to assess the effectiveness of oxygen and home ventilator therapy. They are also very useful for monitoring oxygen saturation in infants and small children from whom it is difficult to obtain arterial blood. Portable oximeters are expensive but extremely important pieces of equipment for use in the home. Grants from local philanthropic organizations may be sought to purchase spirometers and oximeters for nonprofit home care agencies. Oxygenation is discussed in Chapter 15.

## Home Sleep Studies

Home sleep studies have been advocated by some investigators because of the high cost of laboratory polysomnograms. They may be useful as a screening test for a suspected sleep disorder and to assess the efficacy of treatment. However, they do not provide as much information as laboratory studies (Romaker, 1987). Portable oximeters with printout capabilities may be useful to document desaturation during sleep. Probes must be attached carefully so that they are not dislodged during sleep. It is possible that the spouse or caregiver can monitor the patient during sleep. Sleep is discussed in Chapter 12.

## Radiographs

It is possible to take radiographs in the home if the local radiology service has portable facilities. In most instances, however, it is more cost effective to arrange for transportation to a hospital or radiology office when radiographs are required.

---

*If more than one patient breathes from the spirometer, filters must be used and changed after each use to prevent the spread of infection.

## Biochemical Samples

Sputum, blood, urine, and stool samples may readily be obtained from home care patients and analyzed in the home or transported to a laboratory. It is important to follow universal precautions and agency procedures for obtaining and transporting body fluids. Usually the laboratory provides the specimen containers or collection tubes and specifies if the sample needs to be obtained under any special circumstances, such as with fasting, after a special kind of meal, or within a certain number of hours after the prescribed dose of a medication. Home care agencies often stock blood collection tubes. The home care nurse must be certain that the tubes are appropriate for the laboratory to which the samples will be taken or they may not be properly processed. Biochemical samples usually can be transported in plastic foam containers that protect them from extremes of temperature and breakage. Ideally, they should reach the laboratory within 1 to 2 hours after they have been obtained. Some laboratories provide a centrifuge if blood samples need to be spun down promptly. Samples obtained for drug level analysis should also be labeled with the name of the drug to be analyzed, the time and amount of the last dose, and the time the blood was drawn.

## Electrocardiograms

Twelve-lead electrocardiograms and rhythm strips can readily be obtained in the home with a portable electrocardiograph device. Holter monitors can also be used for extended monitoring of arrhythmias that may not be assessed on a routine electrocardiogram.

## Apnea Monitoring

Apnea monitors are frequently used in the home to monitor high-risk infants. Apnea monitoring is briefly discussed in Chapter 12.

## Esophageal pH Monitoring

It may be useful to record the pH of the esophagus to rule out problems caused by gastroesophageal reflux. These studies are carried out with a portable monitor similar to the Holter monitor.

**REFERENCES**

Clark NM, Evans D, Mellins RB: Pulmonary perspective: patient use of peak flow monitoring, *Am Rev Respir Dis* 145:722, 1992.

Mikams R et al: International symposium on lung sounds: synopsis of proceedings, *Chest* 92:342, 1987.

Romaker AM, Ancoli-Israel S: The diagnosis of sleep-related breathing disorders, *Clin Chest Med* 8:1, 1987.

**SUGGESTED READINGS**

Dettenmeier PA: *Pulmonary nursing care,* St Louis, 1992, Mosby.

Hill NS: The cardiac exam in lung disease, *Clin Chest Med* 8:2, 1987.

Kersten LD: *Comprehensive respiratory nursing,* Philadelphia, 1989, WB Saunders.

Potter PA: *Pocket guide to physical assessment,* ed 2, St Louis, 1990, Mosby.

# CHAPTER 3

# SPECIAL CONSIDERATIONS FOR CHILDREN

NANCI L. LARTER • MARIJO MILLER-RATCLIFFE

Caring for children with chronic lung disease and their families is in many ways similar to caring for adults. The purpose of this chapter is to focus on differences in the child, with an emphasis on issues unique to children and their families.

## GROWTH AND DEVELOPMENT OF THE LUNG

As in the adult, the purpose of the upper airway in a child is to protect and humidify the lower airways. The nasal passages provide approximately 50% of the total resistance to inspiration, a significant proportion because many infants are obligate nose breathers. The adenoids are proportionally larger in babies and decrease in size in late childhood (Murray, 1986). Any factors such as inflammation or secretions that decrease the caliber of the nasal passage further increase resistance to airflow and may compromise the infant's breathing. This can result in an overall increase in the work of breathing or difficulty in the infant's ability to coordinate sucking, swallowing, and breathing.

The nasal passages are linked with the middle ear via the eustachian tubes. The angle of the eustachian tube in an infant is relatively horizontal and may not drain fluid that enters from the nasopharynx. The resulting fluid stasis predisposes the infant to middle ear infections (e.g., otitis media). Young children should not be put to bed with a propped bottle because this increases the likelihood of ear problems in addition to promoting dental caries. As the child grows, the angle of the eustachian tube increases, facilitating drainage and preventing fluid movement from the nasopharynx into the eustachian tube.

Within the lower respiratory tract the formation and number of airways are completed by 16 weeks of gestation; no further generation of airways occurs after birth. The infant's airways grow in length and diameter and become more stable with the development of cartilage, muscle, and connective tissue (Boyden, 1984). The number of mucus-producing glands is the same in the infant and the adult. Therefore the density of mucous glands is proportionately higher in the infant with shorter, more narrow airways in comparison with the adult. The infant's lessened ability to tolerate the increased amount of secretions produced with respiratory disease further compromises the narrow airways, thus increasing the work of breathing.

In young children, alveoli are fewer in number and less complex in anatomic structure than those found in adults; however, capillaries surround the alveoli and gas exchange occurs as it does in the adult. Babies are born with approximately 20 to 25 million alveoli. With lung growth, mainly through alveolar multiplication, the number of alveoli progresses to the adult number (between 300 and 600 million) during the first several years of life (Murray, 1986). After this, alveoli increase in size until the chest wall stops growing.

The number of arteries leading to the lung and airways is completely formed at birth. At the time of birth, however, there are relatively fewer arterioles and capillaries near the incompletely developed alveoli. Over the next few years arterioles, capillaries, and veins increase significantly in number and size as they develop in conjunction with alveolar development. Of significant importance is the linear relationship between increases in body surface area and lung growth, particularly growth in height. Therefore adequate nutrition to promote growth is crucial.

Alveolar stability also changes with age. The elastic tissue in the septa of alveoli provides stability, enabling airways to remain open. Because babies have relatively few alveoli, the alveoli collapse more readily. With alveolar growth there is greater support for the airway (as well as the alveoli) and less airway instability with age. The pores of Kohn (which channel between alveoli) and canals of Lambert (which channel between bronchioles) are thought to be nonfunctional at birth but develop over time. These collateral channels permit ventilation of alveoli and bronchioles when there is airway obstruction above the level of the small bronchioles. Because of this absence, the alveoli and small bronchioles may collapse more readily, leading to atelectatic regions in the lung of an infant.

The thoracic cage affects the efficiency of ventilation, and in young children its developing structure can have a large impact on its subsequent function. The sternum is cartilaginous at birth and even in a young child is soft and provides an unstable base for the ribs. The ribs themselves are highly compliant and do not provide the basic support found in the adult. Mechanically, the "bucket-handle motion" (on which adult thoracic respiration depends for greatest efficiency) is not present in children. The normal diaphragmatic contribution of increasing lung volume on inspiration when contracting downward from a domed position is lost or diminished over time in the presence of disease. As in the adult, any process that results in a distended abdomen or hyperinflated lungs in young children can increase the work of breathing. Intercostal and accessory suprasternal muscles attempt to elevate the thorax to compensate for this loss.

Because of the relative underdevelopment (immaturity) of these muscles, the child experiences increased work of breathing as the respiratory efforts become less efficient. Ultimately, gas exchange is compromised as capillary perfusion and alveolar ventilation become progressively mismatched. Because of these anatomic and physiologic differences, infants and children have more difficulties with respiratory diseases than do adults. However, young children have the advantage of growth in airway size, length, and stability and growth in the number of gas exchange units, which allows them to overcome some lung damage from respiratory deficiencies and diseases occurring early in life.

## HISTORY

Parents or usual caregivers should provide the historical information. Children between 8 and 12 years of age can provide some information; by 15 or 16 years of age, teenagers should be able to provide much of the pertinent information. Important information to include in the history for children with respiratory problems is similar to that for adults and is discussed in Chapter 1.

Other information pertinent to the care of a child includes the following:

Well child care
    Primary care provider
    Nutrition: method of feeding; type of formula; food intolerance
    Allergies
    Immunizations
    Developmental milestones
Chronic illness history and continuing management
    Origin of problem
    Initial treatment
    Ongoing treatment
    Ultimate goals of treatment
    Parental (and child's) understanding of illness and problems
    Physicians, nurses, therapists, nutritionists, and social workers involved
    Medications, side effects
    Community resources assisting in care provisions

Social history
Family constellation
Relationship with parents and peers
Sources for income; medical insurance coverage
Social supports
School attendance
Grades or other assessment of achievement

## ASSESSMENT
### General Appearance

The child's general appearance is assessed by looking at the child's interactions and activity level (e.g., sitting; smiling; playing as opposed to lying down; no protest to a stranger's approach) and the physical appearance (e.g., thin; frail; pale as opposed to robust; healthy looking). This quickly gives information about the child's level of illness. In assessing the child, attention should be directed to any unusual bruises, burns, or obvious injuries that might indicate child neglect or abuse.

### Growth

Children with chronic lung disease may use many calories because of their increased work of breathing. Growth is important to monitor on a continuous basis. The child's weight, height, and (for children under 2 years of age) head circumference need to be assessed and charted on an appropriate growth grid. Weight for all children under 2 years of age should be on a baby scale without clothes or diapers and is charted on the growth grid for children from birth to 36 months of age. Heights for children in this age group should be measured on a height statiometer board with the child lying supine. When the child is weighed on a stand-up scale or height is taken standing, the measurements should be charted on a growth grid for 2- to 18-year-olds. There are four pediatric growth grids: two for girls (birth to 36 months and 2 to 18 years of age) and two for boys (birth to 36 months and 2 to 18 years of age), and it is important to use the correct grid to chart and monitor growth (Figs. 3-1 to 3-4). Even if the child is at less than the 5th percentile (meaning that he or she is smaller than

95% of children the same age) on the growth grid, he or she should follow the growth grid curve. A trend or deviation away from the usual growth curve, or "falling off" the growth curve, is cause for concern and signals the need for nutritional intervention. Infants should gain between 10 and 30 g per day when weight gain is calculated on a weekly basis. If the infant gains less than 70 g in a week and this trend continues or worsens, referral for nutritional intervention is necessary. Height and head circumference are usually measured weekly, whereas weights are assessed daily in moderately ill children under 2 years of age.

Fluid retention is partially assessed by daily weights (e.g., weight gain of more than 30 g per day as assessed by cumulative weight gain over several days). Frequent liquid stools may cause dehydration and electrolyte deficiencies. In dehydrated infants the fontanelle is depressed, the eyes appear sunken, and there are few wet diapers or tears. Infants who are breast fed have more and softer stools, whereas those on cow's milk formulas or iron supplements may have problems with constipation.

Gastroesophageal reflux is often a problem for children with chronic lung disease (Orenstein, 1988). With expiration, abdominal muscles are used to push air out of obstructed lungs and also push against the stomach, resulting in reflux of gastric contents. When the gastric contents are refluxed into the back of the upper airway in a child, aspiration into the lungs is a constant concern. Many infants reflux or spit up after feedings. Therefore upright positioning or side-lying positions are preferable for sleeping, especially if the infant is put to bed immediately following a feeding.

### Development

To evaluate the child's psychosocial and developmental growth, a developmental assessment also needs to be completed. A formal developmental assessment through a developmental clinic or by a pediatric physical or occupational therapist should be completed for any child suspected of having developmental delay. Children with chronic lung

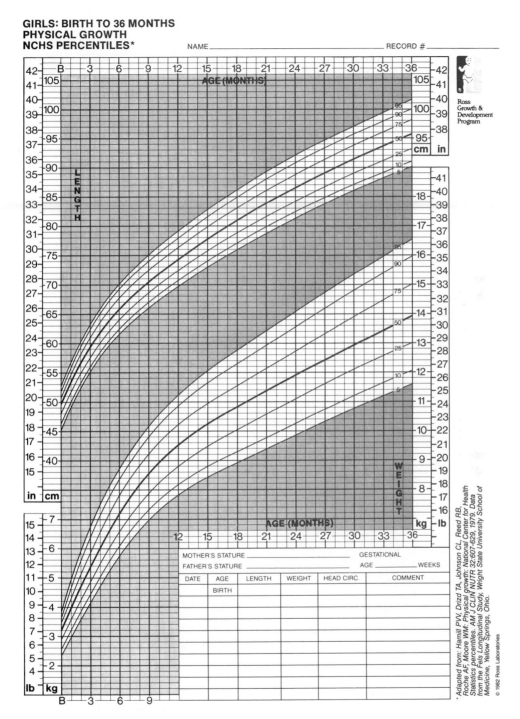

**Fig. 3-1** Girls' growth grid, birth to 36 months. (From Ross Laboratories, Columbus, Ohio.)

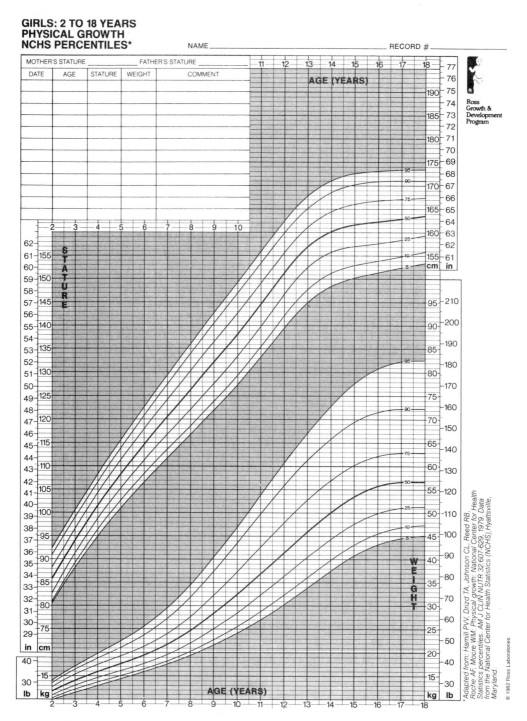

**Fig. 3-2** Girls' growth grid, 2 to 18 years. (From Ross Laboratories, Columbus, Ohio.)

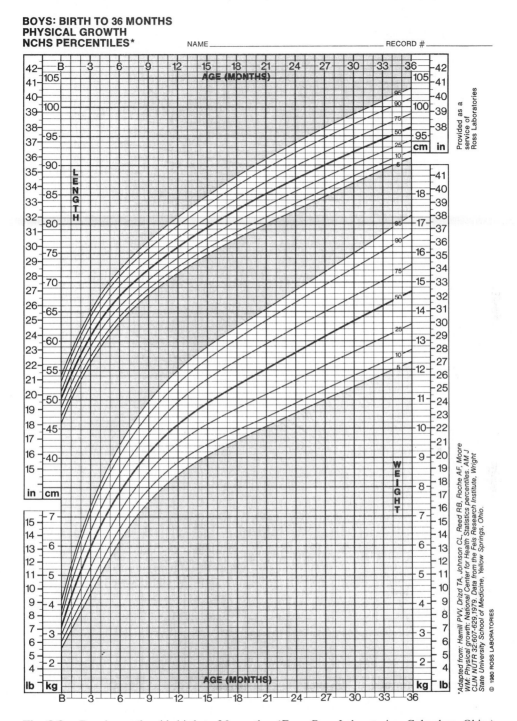

**BOYS: BIRTH TO 36 MONTHS**
**PHYSICAL GROWTH**
**NCHS PERCENTILES***

**Fig. 3-3** Boys' growth grid, birth to 36 months. (From Ross Laboratories, Columbus, Ohio.)

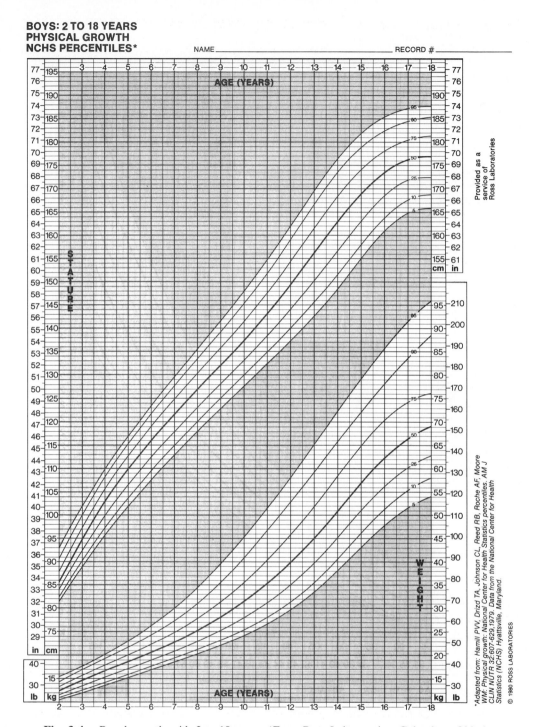

**Fig. 3-4** Boys' growth grid, 2 to 18 years. (From Ross Laboratories, Columbus, Ohio.)

---

## Age-Appropriate Developmental Tasks for Normal Infants and Preschool Children

**BIRTH TO 3 MONTHS**

Lifts head and chest while prone
Turns head to follow objects
Startles at loud noises
Coos
Smiles

**3 TO 6 MONTHS**

Head held upright without support
Roll from stomach to back; back to stomach
Reach for a toy
Plays with feet when supine
Turns head toward sounds

**6 TO 12 MONTHS**

Sits without support
Pulls self to stand with support
Feeds self finger foods
Waves "bye-bye"
Imitates sounds

**12 TO 18 MONTHS**

Walks without support
Drinks from a cup
Says several words
Picks up small objects
Knows parents from strangers

**18 MONTHS TO 2 YEARS**

Walks up and down stairs with help
Uses two-word sentences
Takes off clothes
Plays next to (but not with) other children
Feeds self

**2 TO 3 YEARS**

Stacks more than two objects
Names familiar objects
Runs
Names body parts (e.g., eyes, nose)

**3 TO 4 YEARS**

Jumps, runs, and throws
Understands the concepts "under," "over," "behind," and "up"
Plays with other children
Uses toys to create things

**4 TO 5 YEARS**

Hops on one foot
Draws a recognizable face
Understands the concepts "many," "big," "small"
Speech is clear except for *s, z, th,* and *r*
Asks "why" questions

Modified from Siegel M: *The developmental wheel,* Washington Birth to Six State Planning Project, Olympia, Wash, 1987, Washington State Department of Social and Health Services.

disease are often delayed in some aspects of their development. Many of these children have social skills that are age appropriate, although this depends on the severity of respiratory disease, neurologic involvement, and treatment modalities. When infants are attached to a ventilator, are positioned on a wedge for gastroesophageal reflux precautions, or have a tracheostomy or gastrostomy, they are often delayed in developing normal skills. The box above lists the age-appropriate skills attained in the first 5 years of life.

All children with chronic lung disease need a developmental assessment before their initial hospital discharge to define their individual developmental level or the need for referral to an occupational, speech, or physical therapy program. A child with a tracheostomy should have a communication or speech pattern evaluation and be referred to a therapy program. The home care nurse and parents will be given therapy exercises to assist the infant's development. These exercises are done daily or with feedings or may involve positioning during sleep, depending on the type of therapy.

## Respiratory System

When the caregiver is examining a child, particularly between 7 months and 3 years of age, it is helpful to begin by taking a history from the parents while the child plays in the room. At the beginning of the physical assessment the parents should remove the child's clothing. The child will be somewhat less resistant if held on a parent's lap during the physical examination. Watching the chest movement can yield a respiratory rate in most children. Chest shape, anterior-posterior diameter, and deformities can also be assessed at this time. A barrel-shaped chest appearance may occur with chronic or acute air trapping. Pectus excavatum (sometimes called funnel chest), pectus carinatum (commonly known as pigeon chest), or Harrison's grooves (flaring out of lower frontal ribs) may be noted in a child with chronic respiratory disease. Because breathing patterns vary, the respiratory rate should be counted for at least 30 seconds and doubled, or counted for 1 full minute if possible. Table 3-1 lists normal respiratory rates for children. Respiratory rates vary greatly with feedings, activity, or emotional expression. A respiratory rate during sleep provides a steady state for ongoing respiratory rate monitoring.

An increasing respiratory rate may indicate a problem, but it is nonspecific for problem identification (e.g., fever and pneumonia both cause increased respiratory rates). Signs and symptoms to evaluate increased work of breathing include:

- Tachypnea
- Nasal flaring
- Retractions
- Head bobbing
- Irritability
- Grunting
- Cyanosis
- Decreased activity level
- Poor feeding; prolonged feeding time
- Poor-quality sleep

**Table 3-1** Normal respiratory rates in children

| Age | Asleep | Awake |
|---|---|---|
| 6-12 mo | 22-31 | 58-75 |
| 1-2 yr | 17-23 | 30-40 |
| 3-6 yr | 14-25 | 19-36 |
| 7-10 yr | 13-23 | 15-31 |
| 11-14 yr | 13-19 | 15-26 |

From Kendig E, Cherniak V: *Disorders of the respiratory tract in children,* ed 4, Philadelphia, 1983, WB Saunders.

The ratio of inspiratory time to expiratory time in the infant and young child is fairly equal. Airway obstruction causes difficulty in exhalation, prolonging the expiratory phase and necessitating use of abdominal muscles to facilitate expiration. Accessory muscle use in the child consists of retractions (supraclavicular, suprasternal, substernal, subcostal, or intercostal), nasal flaring, grunting, and head bobbing. As the work of breathing increases, activity may decrease and feedings may be difficult.

Coughing frequently occurs with respiratory disease and is the most common sign of asthma in children. When young children produce excess mucus, they swallow it. Swallowing of mucus may lead to loss of appetite or feelings of nausea but otherwise is harmless. Most children will not expectorate until the school-age years; however, children as young as 3 years of age who have constant increased mucus production (e.g., in cystic fibrosis) may be able to expectorate. Often young children cough to the point of vomiting, and large amounts of sputum may be seen in the emesis.

Auscultation of breath sounds elicits sounds similar to those heard in adults (e.g., wheezes, rhonchi, crackles); however, breath sounds are easily transmitted from the upper airway or across lung fields in children, making interpretation of findings somewhat more difficult. Most young children will not or cannot cooperate with instructions to breathe deeply on command. Listening to inspiration between crying provides the opportunity to hear sounds during maximum inspiration. Whether the child's color appears normal, pale, or cyanotic is important to note; however, cyanosis is a late sign of hypoxemia. Signs of decreased oxygenation in growing children may be reflected by poor feeding, irritability, or decreased activity level. These are nonspecific but may assist in the total evaluation of the child with respiratory disease.

## Cardiac System

When the caregiver is listening to heart sounds a quiet background is helpful, and listening while the young child is held on the parent's lap may assist the examination. In children the $S_2$ is physiologically split and an $S_3$ is normal during diastole.

## Health Care Maintenance

Although children with chronic lung disease are not more susceptible to viral infections, they may have increased respiratory problems with respiratory infections and thus may require hospitalization. Reducing the child's exposure to those with obvious upper respiratory infections (URIs) and frequent hand washing by caregivers (Marcy, 1985) may help prevent some respiratory illnesses. Parents, however, should be aware that the child is likely to become infected with respiratory viruses, and they should not feel guilty when this occurs. As the child grows and becomes better able to tolerate secretions and infections, protection against exposure by restricting out of home activities is reduced to promote normal development.

Respiratory equipment should be treated in the same manner as medications. Dangers such as aspiration of small parts, contamination with viruses or bacteria, and inadvertently altered respiratory support (e.g., oxygen flow rates) are some of the concerns. Therefore extra precautions regarding safety are necessary when respiratory equipment is used in the care of a child in the home setting. A list of factors to consider in evaluating or in making a home "childproof" is provided in the box at right.

If both parents work outside the home, day care

---

### Childproofing a Home

Place all medications with MR. YUK stickers in locked cabinets or on shelves that cannot be reached. MR. YUK stickers can be obtained from poison control centers and some pharmacies.

Keep the poison control center phone number available, and have syrup of ipecac available in the home.

Keep household cleaning products, also labeled with MR. YUK, on out-of-reach shelves or behind childproof door latches.

Set water heater temperature gauge at 120° F to minimize chance of scalding burns.

Keep small toys and objects (e.g., buttons, coins, pins) out of reach of children less than 3 years of age to prevent aspiration. There may be small pieces with respiratory home care equipment.

Discard or secure drapery and blind cords, strings, necklaces, plastic bags, and other objects that can lead to suffocation. Many pieces of respiratory equipment come in a plastic bag with small twist ties.

Cover electrical outlets with safety caps or plugs (found in safety sections in some hardware, toy, and children's stores).

Use toilet lid locks, which are available for bathrooms.

Tape oxygen tubing on floor.

Keep air or oxygen tanks in containers, and store upright to prevent falling or tipping.

Prohibit smoking in the home, especially when oxygen is in use.

Secure knobs or dials on respiratory equipment with tape or cover to prevent accidental setting changes.

Do not use bed cushions filled with polystyrene beads for young infants (Kemp, 1991).

**Table 3-2** Recommended immunizations for children

| Vaccine | Route of administration* | Volume (ml) |
|---|---|---|
| Diphtheria, tetanus, pertussis (DTP) | Intramuscular | 0.5 |
| Tetanus, diphtheria (Td) | Intramuscular | 0.5 |
| Inactivated poliovaccine (IPV) | Subcutaneous | 1.0 |
| Oral poliovaccine (OPV) | Oral | |
| Measles, mumps, rubella (MMR) | Subcutaneous | 0.5 |
| *Haemophilus* b conjugate vaccine (HbCV) | Intramuscular | 0.5 |

From Peter G, editor: *The red book: report of the Committee on Infectious Disease,* ed 22, Elk Grove Village, Ill, 1991, American Academy of Pediatrics.
*For infants and children less than 18 months of age, the preferred site for injections is the anterolateral thigh muscle. For children 18 months of age or older, depending on muscle mass, the deltoid muscle in the upper arm should be used. These areas should ordinarily be used whether injection is intramuscular or subcutaneous. If multiple vaccines are administered, a different site should be used for each injection.

**Table 3-3** Immunization schedule

| Age | Vaccine |
|---|---|
| 2 mo | DTP, HbCV, and No. 1 OPV or IPV |
| 4 mo | DTP, HbCV, and No. 2 OPV or IPV |
| 6 mo | DTP and HbCV |
| 15 mo | MMR No. 1 and any HbCV |
| 15 or 18 mo | DTP and No. 3 OPV or IPV |
| 4-6 yr | DTP and No. 4 OPV or IPV |
| 11-12 yr | MMR No. 2 |
| 14-16 yr | Td |

From Peter G, editor: *The red book: report of the Committee on Infectious Disease,* ed 22, Elk Grove Village, Ill, 1991, American Academy of Pediatrics.
*DTP,* Diphtheria, tetanus, pertussis; *HbCV, Haemophilus* b conjugate vaccine; *OPV,* oral poliovaccine; *IPV,* inactivated poliovaccine; *MMR,* measles, mumps, rubella; *Td,* tetanus, diphtheria.

may be necessary for the child. Children who are cared for in day care have more URIs (Denny, 1986). High-density day care should be avoided. However, the parents' financial ability will influence day care placement for the child. Children exposed to passive smoking also have a higher incidence of respiratory infection. Smoking in the home and in enclosed areas (e.g., cars) by parents, friends, or caregivers should be prohibited.

All children with chronic respiratory disease need to receive the usual childhood immunizations listed in Table 3-2. Table 3-3 lists the schedule recommended by the American Academy of Pediatrics. Premature babies should receive their immunizations based on their chronologic age (age from birth). Children on high-dose corticosteroid therapy or those who are immunocompromised should not receive live-virus vaccines (e.g., oral polio vaccine). Flu shots are available in late fall for chronically ill children who are not allergic to eggs and who are over 6 months of age.

## COMPLICATIONS OF CHRONIC LUNG DISEASE

Complications often develop in children with chronic pulmonary disease because of their basic disease process or their need for certain treatment modalities. Nurses in the home can assist in early identification of these problems, provide continuous assessment to monitor the problem and efficacy of treatment, and promote treatment regimens prescribed by other health care professionals (e.g., implementing a schedule for developmental therapies as directed by physical therapists). Complications and contributing factors are summarized in Table 3-4.

**Table 3-4** Complications and contributing factors in chronic lung disease

| Problem | Contributing factors | Nursing interventions |
|---|---|---|
| Developmental delay | Prolonged ventilation, tracheostomy, gastrostomy, prematurity | Provide physical therapy exercises as directed; provide oral stimulation or oral feedings while giving gastrostomy feedings |
| Retinopathy of prematurity | High oxygen concentrations | Monitor oxygen saturations |
| Hearing loss | Noise level, aminoglycosides, furosemide (Lasix) | Reduce noise levels; monitor drug levels per physician orders |
| Vocal cord or airway abnormalities | Endotracheal intubation, tracheostomy | Ensure speech therapy per physican order; assist with other forms of communication (e.g., signing) |
| Systemic hypertension | Corticosteroid therapy | Monitor blood pressure |
| Gastroesophageal reflux | Increased work of breathing, poor cardiac sphincter function | Upright positioning after feeding |
| Oral hypersensitivity | Noxious oral stimuli such as endotracheal intubation or suctioning; lack of oral feeding; lack of stimulation | Provide oral stimulation program per feeding consultant; reduce trauma when suctioning; suction as infrequently as possible |

## DISCHARGE PLANNING

Discharge from hospital to home should become an option for the pediatric patient only when the home care regimen is feasible and the child's health remains stable. Parents or other caregivers should be trained during the child's hospitalization so that they feel comfortable caring for the child at home. Parents may become so overwhelmed on discharge that they forget some details of care. A checklist (Fig. 3-5) should be sent to the home care nurse to document teaching provided in the hospital and to help plan necessary instruction in the home.

It is important to know whether the parents are living together and whether one or both work. Also, it is important to ask about the anticipated impact the child's care will have on siblings, the family unit, and the family's life-style. Discussions with the entire family will provide important insight into family dynamics.

A treatment plan that takes into account the normal family routines and the way treatments will be managed at home should be established before discharge. A written schedule or plan of care can be invaluable to a parent who must juggle the child's care with other responsibilities. In addition, an emergency plan should be written that includes the phone numbers and locations of the nearest emergency room, the primary physician or clinic, family or neighbors who can be called for immediate assistance, paramedics in the area, and services for the restoration of electrical power or telephone services should a power failure occur.

Ongoing communication between the hospital discharge team and community-based providers will assist in promoting a smooth transition. Home care nurses, equipment vendors, case managers, and the primary physician should have a written summary of the care plan, medications, usual vital

Check yes if taught; no if not taught

Cardiopulmonary resuscitation   yes _____ no _____ (date) _____

Medications (write in information)

| Name | Schedule | Dose | Side effects | How to give |
|------|----------|------|--------------|-------------|
| _____ | _____ | _____ | _____ | _____ |
| _____ | _____ | _____ | _____ | _____ |
| _____ | _____ | _____ | _____ | _____ |

Respiratory

Respiratory rate (count)   yes _____ no _____          Trach tube change   yes _____ no _____

Heart rate (count)          yes _____ no _____          Trach care          yes _____ no _____

Retractions (recognize)    yes _____ no _____          Suctioning          yes _____ no _____

Cyanosis (recognize)       yes _____ no _____          Oxygen use          yes _____ no _____

Temperature (normal ranges; method [axillary]:   yes _____ no _____

Cleaning respiratory equipment   yes _____ no _____

Chest physiotherapy   yes _____ no _____

Nutrition:

| | | |
|---|---|---|
| Formula: mixing concentrations | yes _____ | no _____ |
| Schedule for feeds | yes _____ | no _____ |
| Restrictions | yes _____ | no _____ |
| Supplements | yes _____ | no _____ |
| Gastrostomy care | yes _____ | no _____ |
| Central line | yes _____ | no _____ |

**Fig. 3-5**   Pediatric discharge teaching checklist.

Preventive care

| | | |
|---|---|---|
| Hand washing | yes_____ | no _____ |
| Flu vaccine | yes_____ | no _____ |
| Flu season precautions | yes_____ | no _____ |
| Day care | yes_____ | no _____ |
| Smoking | yes_____ | no _____ |

Developmental

| | | |
|---|---|---|
| Feeding | yes_____ | no _____ |
| Positioning | yes_____ | no _____ |
| Motor | yes_____ | no _____ |
| Social | yes_____ | no _____ |

Copies sent to:

PHN/VNS nursing agency _____

_____

Private physician _____

Equipment vendor _____

Other _____

Attending physician _____ Phone no. _____

Emergency contacts _____

Additional
comments _____

**Fig. 3-5, cont'd.**

signs, equipment settings, and recent examination findings. All follow-up appointments should be made before the child is discharged from the hospital. Fig. 3-6 is an example of a discharge referral summary form.

Children who grow up with chronic disease adjust to their level of disease amazingly well. Although the children may have signs of significant increased work of breathing, they may be playful and smiling. Their ability to tolerate this abnormal

**Identifying data**

Name _____ Discharge date _____

Birthdate _____ Admission date _____

Medical diagnosis _____

Parents _____ Address _____ Phone _____

**Social history**

Mother's age _____ Father's age _____ Marital status _____

Primary caretaker(s) _____

Significant support(s) _____

Sibling(s) name _____ (age) _____ name _____ (age) _____

Home nursing care: yes _____ no _____ No. of hours _____ Agency _____

Primary language _____  _____

**Health status**

A.  Respiratory status

   Respiratory rate (resting) _____

   Lung sounds _____

   Retractions at rest: yes _____ no _____  History of apnea: yes _____ no _____

   $SaO_2$ _____ On room air _____ Oxygen _____ Amount _____

B.  Cardiac status

   Heart rate (resting) _____ beats/min

   ECG date _____ ECHO date _____

**Fig. 3-6**  Discharge referral summary for infants and children with chronic lung disease.

C. Health maintenance

    1. Immunizations

        DTP: Date _____ No. _____    OPV: Date _____ No. _____

    2. Development

        OT/PT referral: yes _____ no _____;   Agency _____

    3. Nutrition

        Name of formula _____ Concentration (cal/oz) _____

    4. ROP (retinopathy of prematurity) screen: Date _____

    5. Hearing screen: Date _____

**Technical care needs**

A. Oxygen: yes _____ no _____;   L/min or FiO$_2$ _____

    Use _____

    24 hours _____ Nighttime _____ Meals _____ Naps _____

    Oxygen delivery: Nasal cannula _____;   Oxyhood _____

B. Tracheostomy: yes _____ no _____;   Size _____ Brand name _____

C. Nebulizer: yes _____ no _____;   Treatments per day _____

D. Ventilator: yes _____ no _____;   Rate _____ PEEP _____ Volume _____ Pressure _____

E. Suction machine: yes _____ no _____;   Portable: yes _____ no _____

    Catheter size _____

F. Monitor: yes _____ no _____;   Settings: Heart rates (high/low) _____

    Apnea: delay _____

**Fig. 3-6, cont'd.**

state may challenge the home care nurse's ability to observe changes and assess the respiratory status. The family can be particularly helpful in assessing changes in the child's status and assisting the home care nurse in learning about the child. In addition to astute observation and assessment skills, knowledge of normal growth and development will assist in the total evaluation of the physical and psychosocial needs of the child and family.

## REFERENCES

Boyden EA: Development of the human lung. In Kelly E, editor: *Practice of pediatrics,* vol 2, Philadelphia, 1984, Harper & Row.

Denny F, Clyde W: Lower respiratory tract infections in non-hospitalized children, *J Pediatr* 108:635, 1986.

Kemp J, Thach BT: Sudden infant death in infants sleeping on polystyrene filled cushions, *N Engl J Med* 324:1858, 1991.

Kendig E, Cherniak V: *Disorders of the respiratory tract in children,* ed 4, Philadelphia, 1983, WB Saunders.

Marcy S: Prevention of respiratory infections, *Pediatr Infect Dis* 4:442, 1985.

Murray JF: *The normal lung,* ed 2, Philadelphia, 1986, WB Saunders.

Orenstein S, Orenstein D: Gastroesophagel reflux and respiratory disease in children, *J Pediatr* 112:847, 1988.

Peter G, editor: *The red book: report of the committee on infectious disease,* ed 22, Elk Grove Village, Ill, 1991, American Academy of Pediatrics.

Siegel M: *The developmental wheel,* Washington Birth to Six State Planning Project, Olympia, Wash, 1987, Washington State Department of Social and Health Services.

## SUGGESTED READINGS

Chernick V, Kendig E: *Disorders of the respiratory tract in children,* ed 5, Philadelphia, 1990, WB Saunders.

Fireman P, editor: Pediatric allergic disease, *Pediatr Clin North Am* 35:953, 1988.

Nelson J, McCracken G, editors: Respiratory tract infections in children, *Pediatr Infect Dis J* 7:441, 1988.

# MANAGEMENT OF PHYSICAL PROBLEMS

# CHAPTER 4

# RESPIRATORY TRACT INFECTION

A. BRUCE MONTGOMERY • JOAN TURNER

Respiratory tract infection is a serious problem for the adult and child with chronic lung disease. The most commonly occurring infections are upper respiratory tract infections (colds or URIs), bronchitis, and pneumonia. It is important for the home care nurse to understand the etiology of respiratory tract infection, to recognize early signs and symptoms of respiratory tract infection, to contact the physician about initiation of antibiotic therapy when appropriate, and to supervise patients in the prevention, recognition, and treatment of infection.

## ETIOLOGY
### Compromise of Respiratory Tract Defense Mechanisms

Factors that compromise the respiratory tract defense mechanisms predispose the patient to respiratory tract infections and allow chronic colonization of the usually sterile lower airways. Impairment of the mucociliary defense mechanism from chronic cigarette smoking or recurrent localized infection, such as that seen in chronic bronchitis and cystic fibrosis, creates a self-perpetuating cycle of damage from infection. This prevents the effective clearance of sputum and the regeneration of a functioning mucociliary epithelium. Patients with cystic fibrosis generally have repeated respiratory tract infections from *Haemophilus influenzae* and *Staphylococcus aureus* that interfere with normal defense mechanisms and allow subsequent mucosal adherence and colonization of *Pseudomonas* organisms (*P. aeruginosa, cepacia*, and *malto-*

*phila*) (Geppert, 1990). Eventually their airways become colonized with the organisms that multiply and readily become resistant to antibiotics (Levy, 1988). Respiratory tract defense mechanisms and the agents that compromise them are summarized in Table 4-1.

## Mechanisms of Transmission of Respiratory Tract Infection

Mechanisms of transmission of respiratory tract infection differ between viral, bacterial, mycobacterial, and opportunistic infections.

### Transmission of Viral Infections

Respiratory tract infections can be caused by more than 200 serologically distinct viruses belonging to six major virus families. Respiratory viruses can be transmitted from person to person by small-particle aerosols, large droplets, and hand-to-hand contact (Douglas, 1986).

Small-particle aerosols (less than 10 μm in diameter) are produced by coughing and sneezing and are so light that they do not settle by gravity. The epidemic spread of influenza viruses in susceptible populations is an example of small-particle aerosol transmission. In contrast, large droplets (greater than 10 μm in diameter), also produced by sneezing or coughing, may result in transmission but require close person-to-person contact because such droplets seldom travel more than 3 feet. Direct contact of viral particles to mucous membranes of the nose and conjunctiva from fomites

**Table 4-1**  Factors that compromise respiratory tract defenses

| Defense mechanism | Function | Agent of compromise |
| --- | --- | --- |
| **MECHANICAL** | | |
| Filtration | Nasopharynx filters out microorganisms, dust, and irritants | Intubation, tracheostomy, mechanical ventilation |
| Gag reflex | Prevents aspiration | Same as above; sedatives, narcotics, paralysis |
| Cough reflex | Ejection of organisms, dust, irritants, and mucus | Same as filtration and gag reflex |
| **MUCOSAL** | | |
| Mucociliary clearance | Microorganisms, dust, and irritants deposited on mucous blanket, cilia move mucus to oropharynx where swallowed or removed by coughing | Smoking, recurrent infection, high inspired oxygen concentration |
| **IMMUNE INFLAMMATORY** | | |
| B lymphocytes | Effect cellular synthesis and secretion of specific antibodies | Malnutrition, infant X-linked agammaglobulinemia |
| T lymphocytes | Regulate immune response, express delayed hypersensitivity, mediate cellular cytotoxic reactions | Corticosteroids, chemotherapy, human immunodeficiency virus infection |
| Macrophages | Engulf cells and debris; process antigen | Malnutrition |
| Killer lymphocytes | Kill neoplastic cells and cells infected by virus | |
| Neutrophils | Engulf, devitalize, and remove particulates | Suppression of bone marrow reduces production |

or hand-to-hand contact are an important vector of rhinoviruses, the viral group responsible for the common cold.

## Transmission of Bacterial Infections

The transmission of bacterial organisms is usually nonepidemic. Most bacteria responsible for bacterial bronchitis are commonly found in many individuals; however, the occurrence rate increases seasonally and in patients with chronic lung disease whose normal respiratory tract defense mechanisms have been compromised. *Pseudomonas aeruginosa* infection can be spread by contaminated respiratory therapy equipment; however, pro- longed intimate contact is thought to be required for cross-colonization with other patients (Hoiby, 1988). The most common acute alteration of host defenses occurs in viral infections. Viral infection decreases mucociliary clearance and the functioning of all types of inflammatory cells involved in host defenses and usually precedes acute episodes of bacterial bronchitis.

## Transmission of Tuberculosis

Tuberculosis is a contagious infection that is transmitted by inhalation of aerosolized droplets containing the organism. When the organisms reach the lungs, they may be ingested by macrophages and not cause disease, or they may multiply and cause symptomatic disease in susceptible persons. Infection may occur only in the lungs or may disseminate throughout the body.

## Opportunistic Infection

Opportunistic infection occurs in individuals who have previously been infected with an organism and are no longer able to maintain resistance to disease caused by the organism. There are defects in the synthesis and release of antibodies (humoral immunity), as well as in the regulation of cells (cell-mediated immunity) that confer protec-

tion against infection. T lymphocytes are responsible for cell-mediated immunity and B lymphocytes for humoral immunity. *Many immune deficiencies are genetically determined and therefore occur in children,* whereas others are acquired and occur in adults.

## Common Infections of the Patient with Chronic Respiratory Disease

Infections commonly seen in the patient with chronic lung disease are summarized in Table 4-2. Types of pneumonia that may occur in home care patients are summarized in Table 4-3.

**Table 4-2**    Common acute respiratory tract infections

| Infection | Occurrence/ signs and symptoms | Pathogen | Treatment |
|---|---|---|---|
| Upper respiratory tract infection (URI, cold) | Occurs in all ages; *children under 5 yr average six to nine URIs per yr, school age children average less than five per yr,* and adults average three to four per yr. Symptoms include nasal obstruction and discharge, sneezing, moderate sore throat, cough, mild constitutional symptoms, headache, and no fever. | Over 200 viral serotypes; common viruses include respiratory syncytial virus (RSV), parainfluenza virus, influenza virus, and adenovirus; occasionally caused by *Mycoplasma pneumoniae* | No specific therapy; supportive care as needed; may need decongestants |
| Otitis media | Occurs in all ages; *more common in infants and children; occurs in approximately 25% of children with URI.* Symptoms include fever, irritability, earache, and pain on side of face or neck. Eardrum appears pale or red and may bulge. | *Streptococcus pneumoniae, Streptococcus pyogenes, Haemophilus influenzae,* and occasionally *Mycoplasma pneumoniae* | Specific antibiotic therapy—amoxicillin 20-40 mg/kg/day or erythromycin 50 mg/kg/day plus sulfonamide 150 mg/kg/day; may need decongestants |

*Continued.*

**Table 4-2**   Common acute respiratory tract infections—cont'd

| Infection | Occurrence/ signs and symptoms | Pathogen | Treatment |
|---|---|---|---|
| Croup | *Generally occurs in children 6 mo to 3 yr of age. Signs and symptoms include hoarseness, cough, expiratory stridor, and suprasternal retractions.* | Parainfluenza virus | Cool humidity in a mist tent; hydration; dexamethasone, 0.6 to 1 mg/kg IM or IV if necessary; monitor oxygenation; intubation if necessary; exclude foreign body aspiration |
| Epiglottitis | *Usually occurs in children 3 to 6 yr of age;* can occur in adults. Signs and symptoms include inspiratory stridor, fever, difficult and painful swallowing. | *Haemophilus influenzae* | Emergent care; humidified oxygen; intubation; hydration; cefuroxime, ceftizoxime, or ampicillin and chloramphenicol; dexamethasone 0.6 to 1 mg/kg IV; adults need intubation less often |
| Influenza | Usually occurs in epidemics. Signs and symptoms include sudden onset of fever, chills, malaise, cough, myalgia, and runny nose. | Orthomyxovirus; respiratory route of transmission | Supportive care; bed rest; analgesics; antipyretics *(use Tylenol in children instead of acetylsalicylic acid [aspirin] to prevent Reye's syndrome);* severely ill patients may benefit from ribavirin. |
| Tracheobronchitis | All ages. Symptoms include cough, rhonchi, purulent sputum, malaise, dyspnea, anorexia, and weight loss; usually occurs in airways previously damaged by URIs, chronic bronchitis, or cystic fibrosis. | Influenza viruses, adenoviruses, *Mycoplasma pneumoniae;* secondary bacterial infection from *S. pneumoniae* and *H. influenzae,* especially | Supportive care; bronchodilators; chest physiotherapy; corticosteroids; usually broad-spectrum antibiotics, such as ampicillin, Septra, erythromycin, and tetracycline |
| Bronchiolitis | *Infants and children under 2 years of age. Signs and symptoms include tachypnea, expiratory wheezing, and substernal retractions.* | RSV, adenovirus | Supportive care |
| Pneumonia | See Table 4-3. | | |

**Table 4-3** Pneumonias that may occur in the patient with chronic lung disease

| Type of pneumonia | Occurrence/signs and symptoms | Treatment |
| --- | --- | --- |
| **VIRAL PNEUMONIA** | | |
| Influenza | Usually starts approximately 1 week after onset of influenza; severe dyspnea and cyanosis, scant and bloody sputum, and reduction in white blood cell count; usually see perihilar infiltrates on chest x-ray examination; rapid progression with high fatality rates | High-dose oral amantadine (400-550 mg/day in adults for influenza A only); bed rest; fluids; oxygen for hypoxemia; supportive care |
| Respiratory syncytial virus (RSV) | *Occurs in preschool and school age children; see consolidation on x-ray examination* | Supportive care; ribavirin aerosol for moderate to severe cases |
| **BACTERIAL PNEUMONIA** | | |
| *Streptococcus pneumoniae* (pneumococcal pneumonia) | Increased prevalence in chronic obstructive pulmonary disease (COPD), alcoholics, renal failure, cirrhosis, myeloma, splenectomy, sickle cell anemia; seasonal incidence common in winter and early spring; sudden onset of fever, myalgias, weakness; vomiting, cough, dyspnea, productive sputum, and pleuritic chest pain common; may mimic acute abdomen if lower lobe pneumonia with abdominal distention; may see only confusion from hypoxia in elderly; may see focal consolidation and pleural friction rub | Usually requires hospitalization; antibiotic therapy (especially penicillin); oxygen; IV fluids; chest physiotherapy; postural drainage; nasotracheal suctioning may be necessary to clear secretions |
| *Staphylococcus aureus* | Generally rare and usually occurs after influenza; more common in patients with colonized wound or skin infections; early diagnosis important because of high morbidity and mortality; usually rapid onset with productive cough, fever, rigor, and pleuritic chest pain; increased white blood cell count (usually); usually see abundant neutrophils in sputum with gram-positive cocci in clumps; often bilateral infiltrates on radiograph with cavitation and pleural effusion | Same as pneumococcal pneumonia; treat with penicillinase-resistant penicillin or vancomycin |
| *Haemophilus influenzae* | Occurs frequently in patients with COPD who are over 50 yr of age; onset may be abrupt as in *S. pneumoniae* but is usually insidious; usually see fever, productive cough, chills, dyspnea and pleuritic chest pain; see elevated white blood cell counts; sputum shows pleomorphic slender gram-negative organisms and abundant neutrophils; usually see diffuse infiltrates on chest radiograph and may see alveolar consolidation | Treat with general supportive care as with pneumococcal pneumonia; ampicillin is antibiotic of choice, unless allergy or known resistant strains present; need intensive bronchodilator therapy if patient has COPD |

*Continued.*

**Table 4-3**   Pneumonias that may occur in the patient with chronic lung disease—cont'd

| Type of pneumonia | Occurrence/signs and symptoms | Treatment |
| --- | --- | --- |
| *Klebsiella pneumoniae* | Often seen in alcoholics and patients with diabetes mellitus; fever, increased white blood cell count, cough, and purulent sputum with new or progressive infiltrates on chest x-ray examination | Supportive measures as needed; usually treat with combination of an aminoglycoside and a third-generation penicillin or cephalosporin |
| *Pseudomonas aeruginosa* | Patients with cystic fibrosis commonly are colonized with a mucoid *Pseudomonas* organism, which often causes pneumonia; same symptoms as *K. pneumoniae* | Same as *K. pneumoniae* with addition of broad-spectrum quinolone |
| *Serratia marcescens* | Rare; usually occurs when tracheobronchial tree colonized with the organism; same symptoms as *K. pneumoniae* | Same as *K. pneumoniae* |
| *Escherichia coli* | Same as *S. marcescens* | Same as *K. pneumoniae* |
| **ATYPICAL PNEUMONIA** | | |
| Pneumonias from common bacterial and viral pathogens that present differently from usual bacterial pneumonia | Incidence in patients with chronic lung disease unknown | — |
| *Mycoplasma pneumoniae* (causes most common clinical syndrome) | Insidious onset with prominent cough that is nonproductive or yields scant mucoid sputum; neutrophils or mononuclear cells seen in sputum without many organisms; low-grade fever usually and may have severe headache; rigors and pleuritic chest pain uncommon; culture of sputum not helpful; diagnosis based on serologic tests; white blood cell count normal or minimally elevated; chest x-ray examination shows segmental pneumonia or interstitial pattern | Supportive care as needed; erythromycin usual treatment |
| *Legionella* | May occur in general outbreaks or sporadically; organism grows in water, and outbreaks have been associated with contaminated air conditioners or other collectors of stagnant water; myalgia and headache followed by fever, chills, and a nonproductive or minimally productive cough, mimicking an influenza infection; organism does not show on Gram stain of sputum and few leukocytes are seen; chest x-ray examination shows airspace consolidation in poorly marginated, rounded opacities that can be unilateral or bilateral; diagnosis made by analysis of bronchoalveolar lavage | General supportive measures; treat with erythromycin |

**Table 4-3** Pneumonias that may occur in the patient with chronic lung disease—cont'd

| Type of pneumonia | Occurrence/signs and symptoms | Treatment |
| --- | --- | --- |
| **ASPIRATION PNEUMONIA** | More likely to be seen in patients with neurologic or muscular disease, the very young and very old patient, and the patient with gastroesophageal reflux; presents initially as acid injury to airways with bronchospasm, wheezing, and occasional consolidation on chest x-ray examination; *right upper lobe most affected in infants who are bottle fed;* may progress to bacterial pneumonia with purulent sputum, infiltrates on radiographs, fever, and increased white blood cell counts | General supportive care very important; antibiotics prescribed if bacterial pneumonia; nursing care includes nutritious food, frequent turning, and airway protection |
| *MYCOBACTERIUM TUBERCULOSIS* (TB) | HIV infection important risk factor; relatively rare in patients with chronic lung disease; presents as primary infection or as reactivation of earlier infection; many elderly patients lived in era when TB was common and have had prior infections; risks for reactivation include advanced age, poor nutrition, debility, steroid use; many physicians recommend isoniazid (INH) prophylaxis for patients who require steroid therapy, if they have positive skin test results for TB; symptoms include persistent cough, fever, night sweats, fatigue, weight loss, infiltrates on chest x-ray examination that do not clear with antibiotic therapy; in anergic patients, negative skin test finding does not rule out TB | Prolonged therapy with at least two drugs such as isoniazid, rifampin, ethambutol, pyrazinamide, or streptomycin |
| *PNEUMOCYSTIS CARINII* PNEUMONIA (PCP) | Opportunistic infection seen in immunocompromised patients; symptoms include cough, fever, chest tightness, shortness of breath; generally patient has diffuse interstitial infiltrates on chest x-ray examination, hypoxemia, and reduced diffusing capacity on pulmonary function test | Supportive care; IV trimethoprim/sulfamethoxazole or pentamidine for severe disease: oral trimethoprim/sulfamethoxazole or trimethoprim/dapsone for mild disease: clindamycin/primaquine, atovaquone, and aerosol pentamidine if cannot tolerate other therapy; oxygen therapy as necessary; may require intubation and mechanical ventilation; corticosteroids for moderate to severe disease if treated early in course |

## ASSESSMENT

The diagnosis of respiratory tract infection involves the history, physical examination, and appropriate diagnostic tests. A history of previous chest illnesses, travel, a previous residence near or exposure to other infected persons, and life-style and habits help to determine the type of acute process that may be present. Cardinal signs and symptoms of acute respiratory tract infection include the following:

- Increased cough
- Purulent sputum
- Increased breathlessness
- Increased fatigue
- Weight loss
- Decreased lung volumes and flow rates on pulmonary function tests
- Tachypnea

*Irritability, decreased activity, and poor feeding may be the only signs of respiratory infection in the young child. Children generally swallow sputum when they are younger than 5 or 6 years of age, making it difficult to determine whether the sputum is purulent. It is not unusual for children to vomit with coughing, and the color of the sputum may then be identifiable.*

Often the patient with chronic lung disease who has an acute infection does not have fever, increased white blood cell counts, or infiltrates on chest x-ray examination. An acute process may be difficult to differentiate from the chronic complaints of the respiratory home care patient. Therefore it is important to know what signs and symptoms are normal or usual for a given patient. Changes from these usual signs and symptoms may indicate that an acute infectious process is present. Signs and symptoms of specific respiratory tract infections are summarized in Tables 4-2 and 4-3.

The home care nurse should contact the physician when an acute respiratory tract infection is suspected. Tests that may be appropriate to confirm the diagnosis of acute respiratory tract infection are summarized in Table 4-4.

## NURSING INTERVENTIONS
### Care of the Patient with Acute Infection

Treatment of acute respiratory tract infections is summarized in Tables 4-2 and 4-3. Most physicians treat acute bronchitis empirically with broad-spectrum antibiotics because there is a low risk of therapy. Patients with chronic obstructive pulmonary disease (COPD) may also experience faster resolution of bronchospasm and fewer treatment failures when antibiotics are used to treat acute bronchitis (Anthonisen, 1987). Some physicians allow patients to start a course of antibiotic therapy based on subjective symptoms, whereas others prefer to evaluate the symptoms with each exacerbation and then decide on a course of treatment. To prevent treatment failure caused by the resistance of the organisms to a given antibiotic, some physicians rotate antibiotics between courses, whereas others rely on sputum cultures and antibiotic sensitivities with each exacerbation.

The administration of antibiotics directly to the respiratory tract via aerosol is common in Europe (Hodson, 1988), but not in the United States. Aerosol delivery of pentamidine has been successful in the treatment of acute *Pneumocystis carinii* pneumonia (Montgomery, 1987), but it is expensive and generally reserved for patients who cannot tolerate conventional systemic therapy.

### Cystic Fibrosis

In patients with cystic fibrosis, some physicians advocate prophylatic use of continuous antibiotics, whereas others reserve them for acute exacerbations. The initiation of treatment for an exacerbation is based primarily on a subjective increase in symptoms noted earlier (see the section on Assessment). Objective indicators—such as fever, elevated white blood cell count, and changes on x-ray examination or chest auscultation—may or may not be present. Oral antibiotics may suffice for patients with less severe pulmonary involvement, but eventually intravenous (IV) drugs will be required. Because of enhanced drug clearance and aminoglycoside binding to mucin, IV dose re-

**Table 4-4**  Tests to diagnose acute respiratory tract infection

| Test | Purpose | Finding |
|------|---------|---------|
| Chest x-ray examination | Determines presence of acute process | Normal if acute bronchitis; infiltrate if pneumonia; see Tables 4-2 and 4-3 |
| Sputum Gram's stain, culture, and sensitivity studies | Determine type of infection and sensitivity to antibiotics; less useful in patients with chronic bronchitis and cystic fibrosis who have chronic colonization of airways; symptoms such as change in color or amount of sputum, increased cough and breathlessness, and decreased activity and appetite may be more useful; sputum culture and sensitivity studies useful to assess resistance of organism to antibiotic | Presence of abnormal organisms on Gram's stain; specific organism determined by culture; appropriate antimicrobial therapy determined by sensitivity studies; abnormal predominance of neutrophils; see Tables 4-2 and 4-3 |
| Blood counts | Help determine diagnosis and patient response to infection | See Tables 4-2 and 4-3 |
| Pulmonary function test | Helps determine diagnosis and patient response to infection | Reduced lung volumes in pneumonia; reduced flow rates in bronchitis; reduced diffusing capacity of the lung for carbon monoxide ($DL_{CO}$) in *Pneumocystis carinii* pneumonia |
| Skin tests | Determine if patient has antibodies to infectious agents; determine if patient is anergic (common in HIV infection and debilitated patients) | 10 mm induration to purified protein derivative (PPD) if patient infected with TB (5 mm induration considered positive finding in HIV-infected patient) |

quirements tend to be higher and courses of therapy longer than for patients with COPD. Patients with cystic fibrosis may also require vitamin K supplements because they have a high incidence of cholestatic liver disease and antibiotics cause a reduction in gastrointestinal tract flora (a major source of vitamin K). Antibiotics that are frequently prescribed for exacerbations of cystic fibrosis are presented in Table 4-5.

Home IV therapy permits the continuation of usual daily activities and is less expensive than hospitalization (Kuzemko, 1988). Patients who are required to undergo several courses of IV therapy every year and who have lost peripheral access may be candidates for an implanted venous access line. The kinds of lines that are used and the procedures for maintaining them are presented in Table 4-6.

**Table 4-5**   Antibiotics used frequently for exacerbations of cystic fibrosis

| Drug | Usual dosage | Side and toxic effects | Comments |
|------|--------------|------------------------|----------|
| **BROAD-SPECTRUM QUINOLONES** | | | |
| Ciprofloxacin | 500-750 mg q 12 hr, po | Nausea, vomiting, diarrhea; *arthropathies in children; fetal wasting* | Effective against *Pseudomonas aeruginosa;* contraindicated for children and pregnant women; drug interactions: decreased theophylline clearance, antacids decrease ciprofloxacin availability |
| Ofloxacin | 200-400 mg q 12 hr | Same as ciprofloxacin | Same as ciprofloxacin |
| **THIRD-GENERATION CEPHALOSPORINS** | | | |
| Ceftazidime (Tazidime; Fortaz) | 1-2 g q 8 hr to maximum of 6 g daily, IV | Side effects rare and usually minor; occasionally rash or anaphylaxis | When prescribed for *Pseudomonas* infection, used with an aminoglycoside; possibly effective against *Pseudomonas cepacia* and gram-negative rods; important to maintain serum concentration; expensive |
| **AMINOGLYCOSIDES** | | | |
| Tobramycin | Inhalation: up to 600 mg tid IV: titered to the individual; range 50-200 mg q 8 hr | Renal damage; ototoxicity; hypomagnesemia | Effective against some mycobacteria; narrow therapeutic/toxic ratio, therefore requires peak and trough levels on day 2 and weekly, goal: peak level >6, trough level <2; good hydration decreases risk of renal damage; if toxic levels, monitor renal and auditory function; aerosol administration expensive (up to $3000/mo), but less toxicity, and may be prescribed for continuous use (i.e., prophylaxis) |
| **FOURTH-GENERATION PENICILLIN DERIVATIVE** | | | |
| Imipenem | 750 mg to 1 g q 8 hr IV | Risk of peripheral venous damage/thrombosis with repeated use; potential for allergic reaction, sodium overload | Very broad-spectrum drug effective against most organisms; expensive; short stability; must monitor hepatic and hematologic function |

**Table 4-6**  Intravenous access options

| Type of access line | Indications | Access and care* | Advantages | Disadvantages |
|---|---|---|---|---|
| **TEMPORARY PE-RIPHERAL VENOUS LINES** | Good veins; infre-quent need for IVs | | | |
| Angiocath | | Sterile dressing at in-sertion site | Easily inserted; inex-pensive; low risk of side effects | Not suitable for prolonged use; must rotate sites q 2-3 days; cannot administer incompat-ible drugs simultaneously; often lasts only 1 day with irritating drugs |
| Landmark | | Sterile dressing change 3 × weekly; heparin flush 1-2 × daily | Lasts 2-10 weeks in one site; soft, pliable Silastic | Difficult to insert unless veins are excellent; catheter life may be decreased if used for blood draws; dressing changes cannot be done in-dependently |
| **PERIPHERALLY IN-SERTED CENTRAL VENOUS CATHETER (PICC LINES)** Arm vein insertion with tip at (but not in) right atrium | Need IVs frequently; need drugs likely to cause phlebitis | Sterile dressing changes 1-3 × weekly Heparin flushes 1-2 × daily Accessed via external injection cap | Can be inserted or re-moved by a trained nurse in outpatient setting; can be used for blood draws; can stay in place up to 1 yr; easier to insert and less expensive than central venous catheters; painless access | Dressing changes cannot be done independently; some activity restrictions second-ary to exterior placement; potential complications in-clude vessel perforation, migration into wrong vessel; tend to slip partially out (if do so, do not reinsert; rather, secure with tape in new position); care costs of-ten high because of frequent dressing changes and flushes |

*The frequency of heparin flushes, dressing changes, and site changes varies greatly between agencies and institutions. Practice patterns should be based on an established agency policy that has been approved by the medical advisory board.

*Continued.*

**Table 4-6** Intravenous access options—cont'd

| Type of access line | Indications | Access and care* | Advantages | Disadvantages |
|---|---|---|---|---|
| **EXTERNALLY TUNNELLED CENTRAL VENOUS CATHETERS** | Need for frequent IV access; need for potentially sclerosing or incompatible drugs | | | |
| Hickman (inserts on anterior chest, tunneling to subclavian vein, with tip at or near right atrium; anchored in place by a cuff that becomes imbedded into the tissue after about 4 weeks) | | Painless access via external injection cap; heparin flushes daily to qod; frequent (i.e., qod) dressing changes; clean technique (or no dressing at all) may be adequate once healed | Can use for blood draw; some have 2-3 separate lines so can administer incompatible drugs simultaneously; can remain in place months to years; low risk of accidental removal or ascending infection once cuff adhesions form | Technically difficult to insert; must be inserted by physician in surgery; some activity restrictions secondary to exterior placement; some discomfort with removal secondary to adhesions; care costs high |
| Groshong | | Saline flush once weekly; dressing changes 3 × weekly | As above, but easier care; no need for heparin | As above |

| | | | | |
|---|---|---|---|---|
| **IMPLANTABLE VENOUS ACCESS DEVICES** | Frequent IV therapy; poor veins | | | |
| Portacath (subcutaneous placement on anterior chest, tunneling to subclavian vein with tip in superior vena cava; pediatric sizes may be preferable for very thin adults) | | Accessed using right-angled Huber needle through skin and portal septum; antibiotic levels may be inaccurate if drawn from port. Permits approximately 2000 accesses; heparin flushes approximately q 4 weeks when not in use | Fully implanted, therefore lower infection rate, minimal care needs, no interference with physical activities. Esthetically more pleasing than external lines; some have dual lines permitting simultaneous administration of incompatible drugs; can use for blood draws; require dressings only when port is accessed with needle | Requires needle stick for each access; permanent lump more apparent in wasted patients and is esthetically upsetting for some; must be inserted and removed in surgery |
| PAS-Port (subcutaneous port site on forearm, threaded up basilic or cephalic vein with tip in superior vena cava; smaller lumen than Portacath) | | Permits approximately 1000 accesses; heparin flushes approximately q 2 weeks when not in use; while in use must change needle and dressing weekly and flush q 3-7 days with heparin | Smaller than Portacath and often easier to conceal | Dressing changes and accessing cannot be done independently; obstructed more easily due to smaller lumen |

Potential complications of venous access lines include the following:

- Venous thrombosis at catheter tip
    Edema secondary to impaired venous return
    Increased risk of embolus
- Infection
    At site of entry
    Septicemia
- Venous phlebitis
- Embolization secondary to catheter break-off
- Catheter migration into wrong vessel
- Perforation of vessel
- Portal pocket cellulitis
- Pneumothorax

Nursing care strategies for the home care patient with an acute respiratory tract infection are presented in Table 4-7.

## Prevention of Respiratory Tract Infection

Prevention of respiratory tract infection is an important aspect of nursing care of the patient with chronic lung disease. Strategies to prevent respiratory infections in the patient with chronic lung disease include maintenance of airway clearance, general supportive measures, thorough cleaning of respiratory equipment, immunization, and rarely chemoprophylaxis. Patients with four or more exacerbations each year may benefit from prophylactic antibiotic therapy (Murphy, 1992). Preventive measures are summarized in Table 4-8. Influenza, pneumococcal, and *Haemophilus influenzae* vaccines are available and should be administered to home care patients (MMWR, 1991). Protocols for administration follow.

### Influenza Vaccine

It is recommended that home care agencies develop and implement a policy for the routine administration of influenza vaccine to patients and staff each year in the fall, preferably in November.

■ *Indications.* Persons at increased risk for serious consequences from a lower respiratory tract infection include the following:

- The chronically ill (especially those with pulmonary, heart, renal, or liver disease or diabetes)
- The elderly (over 65 years of age)
- Those with compromised immune systems
- Caregivers and family members of persons at risk
- Medical personnel working with persons at risk

■ *Contraindications.* Contraindications to the use of the influenza vaccine include the following:

- History of allergy to eggs, chickens, chicken feathers, or chicken dander (vaccine made from highly purified egg-grown viruses)
- Prior toxic reaction to flu vaccine
- History of allergy to thimerosol (preservative in vaccine)
- Acute or febrile illness
- Active neurologic disease (consult physician about patient stability)

■ *Adverse Effects.* The adverse effects of the influenza vaccine include the following:

- Commonly, soreness at injection site for 1 to 2 days
- Infrequently, fever, malaise, or myalgia starting 6 to 12 hours after vaccine and persisting for 1 to 2 days
- Rare immediate allergic response such as local wheal and flare or airway hyperreactivity

In addition, the following should be noted:

- Vaccines cannot cause influenza as made from inactivated viruses.
- An increased incidence of Guillain-Barré syndrome has not been seen with any strain since the 1976 swine flu.

■ *Precautions.* The following precautions are needed:

- Vaccine must be refrigerated.
- Screen patient for contraindications and discuss possible side effects in advance.
- Have epinephrine 1:1000 available in case of anaphylaxis.

■ *Administration.* The recommendations for administration are as follows:

- Adult dose, 0.5 ml IM deltoid or midlateral thigh (increased side effects with subcutaneous administration)

**Table 4-7**   Nursing interventions for the patient with acute respiratory tract infection

| Problem or need | Intervention |
| --- | --- |
| Effective use of medications | Teach patient and caregiver proper administration of prescribed medications. |
| | Observe for effectiveness of therapy by decreased signs and symptoms of acute infection. |
| | Increase frequency of inhaled bronchodilators for increased bronchospasm or wheezing. |
| | Check with physician about adjunctive corticosteroid therapy if patient is already using maximal doses of bronchodilators or is experiencing side effects and is unable to increase the dosage sufficiently to reduce symptoms. Overuse of bronchodilators without antiinflammatory agents increases risk of death. Patients who are receiving maintenance corticosteroid therapy may need to increase the dose temporarily. |
| | Antipyretic drugs such as Tylenol every 4 to 6 hr may be necessary to reduce discomfort from high fevers. |
| | Consider possibility of drug interactions. Antibiotics such as erythromycin decrease hepatic clearance and can cause an increase in serum levels of other drugs, such as theophylline, that are cleared by the liver. It may be necessary to obtain blood for a serum theophylline level and adjust the dose accordingly if antibiotic therapy is instituted. |
| Adequate intake of food and fluids | Encourage adult patients to drink approximately eight large glasses (2 qt) of liquids each day unless fluid restrictions are necessary because of heart or renal failure. |
| | *Offer juice and water to young children and infants hourly.* |
| | Adequate fluids are particularly important to prevent dehydration if the patient is febrile. |
| | Frequent small meals may be indicated if a respiratory tract infection causes patients to feel more short of breath while eating. |
| | High-calorie food supplements may be appropriate after meals or at bedtime if patients are unable to maintain adequate dietary intake. |
| Adequate oxygenation | Patients may become hypoxemic during acute phase of respiratory tract infection. |
| | Monitor oxygen saturation with pulse oximeter or arterial blood gas measurement. |
| | Supplemental oxygen should be administered as necessary to maintain oxygen saturation at 90% or higher. |
| | Monitor adequacy of ventilation in patients on home ventilators. It may be necessary to adjust ventilator settings temporarily during acute infection. |

*Continued.*

**Table 4-7**  Nursing interventions for the patient with acute respiratory tract infection—cont'd

| Problem or need | Intervention |
|---|---|
| Adequate secretion clearance | Increase frequency of bronchial hygiene measures, such as therapeutic coughing, postural drainage with percussion, and vibration, if patient is having difficulty clearing secretions. |
| | Review bronchial hygiene regimen with patient and caregiver to be sure that techniques are appropriate and being performed effectively. |
| | Encourage patient to take frequent deep breaths to prevent atelectasis and enhance mucociliary clearance. Incentive spirometers may motivate some patients to take deeper breaths. |
| | Oropharyngeal suctioning may be necessary for patients who are unable to clear secretions. It may be necessary to increase frequency of suctioning if patient has tracheostomy. |
| | Avoid cough suppressants that dry secretions and interfere with clearance. |
| Relief of breathlessness | Above interventions may be adequate to relieve breathlessness associated with acute infection. |
| | May be necessary to reduce or temporarily suspend exercise programs and encourage more frequent rest periods. |
| | Promote strategies such as positioning and coordination of activities with breathing to help provide relief. |
| Infection control | Maintain appropriate infection control precautions. |
| | Respiratory secretions should be discarded properly. |
| | May be necessary to increase frequency of cleaning of home respiratory therapy and ventilator equipment, suction catheters, and tracheostomy tubes, particularly if secretions are thick and copious. |
| | Home care staff, patients, and caregivers must wash their hands carefully before and after administering treatments and providing care. Universal body substance precautions must be followed. |
| Provide necessary patient monitoring | Increase frequency of home visits during acute phase of infection for patient monitoring and support. |
| | Patients and caregivers may be less able to cope and may become excessively anxious at such times. |
| | Additional support from home care staff may mean difference between successful management at home and the need for hospitalization. |
| | Hospitalization may be necessary if patient continues to deteriorate despite optimal home care. |

**Table 4-8**    Prevention of respiratory tract infection in the patient with chronic lung disease

| Preventive measure | Nursing intervention |
| --- | --- |
| Promote airway clearance | Utilize measures presented in Chapter 7 to promote airway clearance, thereby enhancing respiratory tract defense mechanisms. |
| Decrease exposure to infection | Maintain careful hand-washing technique.<br>Avoid crowds during flu season. Avoid others who have colds or flu.<br>Maintain proper cleaning of home respiratory equipment. |
| Enhance resistance | *All children should be immunized for communicable diseases of childhood* (see Table 3-6).<br>Adults and *children* with chronic lung disease *older than 6 mo of age* should receive influenza vaccine each year in the fall. Family members and health care providers who have frequent close contact with patients should also receive annual influenza immunizations because they are less likely to transmit the virus if they have been immunized.<br>*Children over the age of 2 yr* and adults should also receive pneumococcal vaccine to prevent pneumococcal pneumonia. The pneumonia vaccine can be given the same time as the influenza vaccine. *A booster dose should be given to high-risk children 3 yr after the initial dose if they were younger than 3 yr of age when they were initially vaccinated.* A booster vaccination may also be given to adults 6 yr after the initial dose.<br>*H. influenzae* vaccine should also be given to adults with chronic lung disease and *children between the ages of 12 mo and 5 yr.* |
| Chemoprophylaxis | Chemoprophylaxis of bacterial respiratory tract infections with antibiotics has not been shown to be effective in most instances. However, some patients use antibiotic therapy to prevent bacterial bronchitis when they have a viral URI.<br>Amantadine may be effective following exposure to influenza A. The usual dosage (200 mg po, qd for 2-3 days before and 6-7 days after influenza A infection) reduces the incidence and severity of symptoms. Amantadine causes insomnia, nightmares, and ataxia. It is more toxic in patients with renal failure. Rimantadine is a less toxic alternative to amantadine.<br>*Ribavirin aerosol early in course of influenza A and B infections or RSV infections in small children may reduce the severity of the symptoms.*<br>Rifampin prophylaxis should be given to household contacts of patients with invasive *H. influenzae* disease within 1 week of exposure. The usual dose is 20 mg/kg with a maximum of 600 mg qd × 4 days.<br>Patients with HIV infection who have CD4 cell counts of less than 200 should receive prophylaxis for *P. carinii* pneumonia. Effective regimens include trimethoprim/sulfamethoxazole (Septra DS), 1 qd or 3 × week; dapsone, 50 mg qd; and aerosol pentamadine, 300 mg/mo. |
| General supportive measures | Turn patients who are confined to bed every 2 hr; elevate head of bed while eating and drinking; encourage coughing and deep breathing.<br>Elevate head of bed of patients with gastroesophageal reflux to prevent nocturnal aspiration. Avoid food and fluids 2-4 hr before retiring. |

• *Dosage schedule for children*

| Age | Dose |
|-----|------|
| 6-35 mo | 0.25 ml in 1-2 doses |
| 3-8 yr | 0.5 ml in 1-2 doses |
| 9-12 yr | 0.5 ml in 1 dose |
| >12 yr | 0.5 ml in 1 dose |

• *Children under 12 years of age should receive split-virus vaccine.*

*Two doses are recommended if the child is receiving the vaccine for the first time. Doses should be 1 month apart. Influenza vaccine should not be given within 3 days of DTP immunizations.*

### Pneumococcal Vaccine

The pneumococcal vaccine confers protection for 23 types of pneumococci, which are responsible for 80% of all bacteremic pneumococcal diseases in the United States. It is recommended for the same patients as those who should receive the influenza vaccine, especially those with chronic lung disease.

■ *Adverse Effects.* The adverse effects include redness and soreness at the injection site for 1 to 2 days in approximately 50% of patients.

■ *Administration.* The recommendations for administration are as follows:
• Administer at any time of year
• Can be given concurrently with flu vaccine at different site
• Usual dose, 0.5 ml IM deltoid or lateral thigh

### *Haemophilus influenzae* Type b Vaccine

*Children less than 5 years of age develop over 85% of cases of invasive H. influenzae disease* (MMWR, 1991). Adults at greatest risk for invasive *H. influenzae* disease are those with chronic pulmonary disease and other conditions that predispose them to infections with encapsulated bacteria.

■ *Adverse Effects.* The adverse effects include the following:
• Local reactions
• Fever, weakness, nausea, vertigo, and myalgias

■ *Administration.* The recommendations for administration are as follows:
• *Recommended for children between 2 months and 5 years of age*
• Can be administered at same time as influenza and pneumococcal vaccines, but at a different site

### REFERENCES

Anthonisen NR et al: Antibiotic therapy in exacerbations of chronic obstructive pulmonary disease, *Ann Intern Med* 106:196, 1987.

Douglas RG: Pathogenic mechanisms in viral respiratory tract infections. In Sande MA, Hudson LD, Root RK, editors: *Respiratory infections,* New York, 1986, Churchill Livingstone.

Geppert EF: Recurrent pneumonia, *Chest* 98:739, 1990.

Hodson ME: Antibiotic treatment aerosol therapy, *Chest* 94(2 suppl):156S, 1988.

Hoiby N: *Haemophilus influenzae, Staphylococcus aureus, Pseudomonas cepacia,* and *Pseudomonas aeruginosa* in patients with cystic fibrosis, *Chest* 94(2 suppl):97S, 1988.

Kuzemko JA: Home treatment of pulmonary infections in cystic fibrosis, *Chest* 94(2 suppl):162S, 1988.

Levy J: Antibiotic therapy in cystic fibrosis: evaluation of efficacy, *Chest* 94(2 suppl):150S, 1988.

Montgomery AB et al: Aerosolized pentamidine as sole therapy for PCP in patients with AIDS, *Lancet* 2:480, 1987.

Murphy TF, Sanjay S: Bacterial infection in chronic obstructive pulmonary disease, *Am Rev Respir Dis* 146:1067, 1992.

Update on adult immunization, recommendations of the immunization practices advisory committee, Centers for Disease Control, *MMWR* 40:40, 1991.

### SUGGESTED READINGS

Camp-Sorrell D: Advanced central venous access selection, catheters, devices and nursing management, *J Intravenous Nurs* 13:361, 1990.

Morton JW, Kerrebijn KF: Antibacterial therapy in cystic fibrosis, *Med Clin North Am* 74:837, 1990.

Niederman MS, editor: Respiratory infections, *Clin Chest Med,* vol 8, 1987.

# CHAPTER 5

# SPECIAL CONSIDERATIONS IN ASTHMA MANAGEMENT

AMY L. PADAVICH • SUSAN G. MARSHALL

Asthma is a disorder of the tracheobronchial tree characterized by reversible, variable, and intermittent airway inflammation and obstruction. Bronchial hyperreactivity ("twitchy airways") is a key feature of the disease. The National Center for Health Statistics (1989) estimates that asthma affects 11.6 million Americans of all age groups, or 3% to 4% of the population of the United States. *Asthma is very common in childhood, with a prevalence in children in the United States estimated to be between 3% and 8.5%* (Woolcock, 1988). *Although it may improve during adolescence,* it commonly reappears during the adult years (Cropp, 1985). For many individuals, the problem persists undiminished throughout adulthood. It may also appear for the first time in adulthood, sometimes following a viral respiratory illness and often in association with chronic bronchitis, in which case it is referred to as asthmatic bronchitis. An alarming increase in deaths from asthma over the past decade mandates greater understanding and more scrupulous management of this pervasive disease.

Patients with asthma present special challenges for the home care nurse. Because asthma is an illness characterized by periods without respiratory symptoms, patients are often tempted to stop taking the routine medication they need to prevent exacerbations. In addition, reduction of environmental irritants and allergens is a major component of asthma control, and home care nurses are in an ideal position to evaluate the patient's home for the presence of these triggers. Patients and their families often need considerable education and support to achieve the changes in behavior that will best control the disease.

## ETIOLOGY

The underlying mechanisms of asthma are believed to include the release of chemical mediators leading to inflammation and edema of the bronchial mucosa, contraction of bronchial smooth muscle (bronchospasm) and increased production of mucous secretions. Each of these factors contributes to narrowing of airways (Fig. 5-1).

### Immunoglobulin System

The immunoglobulin system functions as a mediator between the environment and the body's defense mechanisms. It is a complex system designed to detect and eliminate foreign substances from the body. When exposed to an antigen or allergen (substances in the environment capable of evoking immunologic responses), the immunoglobulin system releases specific antibodies (molecules that react

**87**

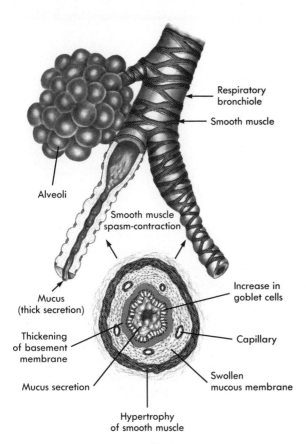

Respiratory bronchiole

Smooth muscle

Alveoli

Smooth muscle spasm-contraction

Mucus (thick secretion)

Increase in goblet cells

Thickening of basement membrane

Capillary

Mucus secretion

Swollen mucous membrane

Hypertrophy of smooth muscle

**Fig. 5-1** With bronchial asthma, bronchiole is obstructed on expiration, particularly by muscle spasm, inflammation, edema of mucosa, and thick secretions. (From Wilson SF, Thompson JM: *Respiratory disorders,* St Louis, 1990, Mosby.)

with a specific antigen) designed to defend the host, some of which have the potential to cause severe allergic reactions.

There are five classes of immunoglobulins (IgM, IgA, IgG, IgE, and IgD), each with its own function and each present in various body tissues. The class associated with allergic reactions is immunoglobulin E (IgE). In most people, serum IgE levels are very low, reaching a concentration of 10 to 100 ng/ml in healthy adults. People with atopic (allergic) diseases may have high IgE levels.

## Agents Capable of Provoking an Asthma Episode
### Allergens

An asthma episode can be triggered by both allergens and irritants. Many allergens present in the everyday environment have the potential to cause an allergic reaction, given early, repeated, and intense exposures. The sensitivity is dose related, so that the greater the exposure the greater the allergic response. Examples of common allergens are summarized in the following:

*Animal allergens*
- Cats are especially allergenic, but dogs, mice, horses, guinea pigs, and rabbits may also cause reactions.
- Antigens are found in animal saliva, urine, hair, and dander (epithelial fragments).

*Feathers*
- Sensitivity to feathers themselves or to contamination of the feathers with mites can cause an allergic reaction.
- The allergic response is increased when feather-filled products are older or have been stored for long periods.

*Kapok*
- Seed hair from kapok trees is often used to stuff throw pillows and sleeping bags.
- Kapok is more allergenic when older, suggesting contamination with mites.

*Housedust*
- Housedust is composed of a number of potential allergens including animal dander, indoor molds, vegetable fibers, food particles, algae, dirt, insect parts, and feces of a microscopic creature called the housedust mite.
- Human epithelial scales are the preferred growth substrate for dust mites, which therefore are found in the greatest concentration in bedding, mattresses, and furniture stuffing.
- Mite concentration is highest in bedrooms of homes in warm, humid environments, and is lower at high altitudes.
- Dust mite feces are a potent allergen and are small enough to be inhaled into the lower respiratory tract.
- Parts or feces of cockroaches, termites, ear-

wigs, bedbugs, beetles, moths, flies, ants, wasps, ticks, and sowbugs may be allergens.

*Pollens*

- Pollens are produced just before and after the flowering of plants.
- Pollens are the predominant cause of seasonal allergies.
- The concentration of pollen in the air varies with the time of day.
- The concentration can be almost as high in urban as in rural areas because of the efficiency of wind currents.
- Deciduous trees, grasses, and weeds are the most important allergen-producing plants.
- Ragweed is most troublesome in late August and September and is one of the most important causes of allergic rhinitis and bronchial asthma in the United States.

*Molds*

- Molds and the fungal spores they produce are ubiquitous and survive under most conditions.
- The spore content of indoor air is similar to outdoor air and can be reduced, but not eliminated, by air conditioners.
- The indoor mold concentration may increase in garbage containers, food storage areas, upholstery, wallpaper, damp basements, cool-mist vaporizers, and greenhouses.
- Molds are often the precipitating allergen in occupational asthma in farmers, grain workers, mushroom harvesters, paper mill workers, and tobacco strippers.

*Food*

- A food allergy must be distinguished from an intolerance: a food allergy is an IgE-mediated response to a specific food; a food intolerance is a nonimmunologic response to food involving local gastrointestinal factors.
- True food allergies are more common in infants and children and often become less symptomatic over time.
- The allergic response may include rhinitis, asthma, skin reactions, gastrointestinal problems, or anaphylaxis.
- Common food allergens in children are cow's milk, soy, eggs, wheat, fish, and peanuts.

- Common food allergens in adults are shellfish and nuts.

**Irritants**

Whereas an allergen causes asthma through the mechanism of an IgE-mediated immune response, an irritant does so on a nonimmunologic basis. Sometimes it is difficult to distinguish an allergic response from an irritant response. In someone with bronchial hyperreactivity all kinds of inhaled substances can be irritating enough to trigger asthma. Examples of common irritants include the following:

*Cigarette smoke*

- Cigarette smoke is a major irritant, capable of activating airway disease.
- Increased bronchial reactivity can last for hours after exposure to even passive (i.e., side stream) smoke.
- Cigarette smoke can potentiate additional triggers that may not have been sufficient to cause bronchospasm alone.
- The elevated IgE levels in smokers and in children of smokers suggest that smoking may facilitate sensitization.

*Air pollution*

- Asthmatics are highly sensitive to air pollution, specifically to increased levels of nitrogen dioxide, sulfur oxides, and ozone.
- Sensitivity is enhanced by exercise, changes in temperature (especially cold), and dry air.
- Wood stove smoke and high concentrations of dust can also trigger asthmatic symptoms.

*Strong odors and fumes* (Shim, 1986)

- Perfume, cologne, cooking smells, automobile exhaust, gas stove fumes, fresh paint, hairsprays, household cleaners, fabric softeners, insecticides, and volatile chemicals may induce asthma in sensitive individuals (if you can smell it, it can be an irritant).

*Nonisotonic aerosols*

- Most asthmatics experience a significant decrease in forced expiratory volume in 1 second ($FEV_1$) after inhalation of water (a hypotonic solution) or 3% to 5% saline (a hypertonic solution).

*Miscellaneous*
- Other potential irritants include cold, dry air; gastroesophageal reflux; inhalation of acid aerosols; and cola drinks, cold drinks, and ice.

## Other Factors

Other factors that have been shown to induce or aggravate asthma are presented below. Exposure to a combination of factors, either allergic or irritant, may initiate or complicate an asthma reaction. For example, some persons with asthma may be sensitive to certain allergens or irritants only when they are suffering from a respiratory infection.

*Infection*
- Viral respiratory tract infections, especially with agents such as influenza A, respiratory syncytial, parainfluenza, and corona viruses, frequently aggravate asthma and may trigger the onset of asthma in someone with no prior history.
- Fungal, parasitic, and bacterial infection may also precipitate asthma.
- *Otitis media, allergic rhinitis, and sinusitis are triggers in children* and adults.

*Weather*
- Changes in the weather can induce asthma. A proposed mechanism is that humidity and rainfall increase the concentration of antigens in the atmosphere (Lancet, 1985).
- A drop in temperature may trigger asthma, most likely caused by rapid heat loss from the respiratory mucosa (Kamakura, 1985).

*Emotions*
- Nervous tension, denial, hostility, fear, anger, and stressful events may aggravate or initiate an attack in some people; however, emotions do not cause asthma.

*Exercise*
- Of people with asthma, 70% to 80% will experience bronchoconstriction approximately 6 to 8 minutes after strenuous exercise (Anderson, 1985).
- Some types of exercise (e.g., running) are

more asthmagenic than others (e.g., gymnastics, swimming).

*Endocrine factors*
- Some women, usually those with more severe asthma, have increased symptoms just before and during menses (Eliasson, 1986).
- Symptoms often decrease during adolescence and pregnancy.

*Nonallergic hypersensitivity to drugs and chemicals*
- Aspirin, aspirin-containing products, and nonsteroidal antiinflammatory drugs are known to cause or exacerbate asthma.
- Aspirin sensitivity is often associated with a syndrome of nasal polyps, rhinitis, and sinusitis.
- Aspirin sensitivity is sometimes associated with sensitivity to tartrazine (FD&C yellow dye No. 5) and benzoates (common food additives).
- Monosodium glutamate (MSG), sulfites, and sulfur dioxide used as preservatives may trigger asthma.

## Role of the Sympathetic and Parasympathetic Nervous Systems

Both the sympathetic and parasympathetic nervous systems play a role in the pathogenesis of asthma and may partially explain the bronchial hyperreactivity seen in persons whose asthma is not allergic in nature. In other words, either an increase in sensitivity to parasympathetic nervous system stimulation or an insensitivity to β-adrenergic stimulation could result in asthma.

## Classification of Asthma
### Allergic Asthma

Allergic, or "extrinsic," asthma occurs in allergic (atopic) patients and implies an IgE-mediated phenomenon. *It accounts for the majority of cases of asthma, especially in children* and younger adults, who can frequently identify substances (triggers) such as inhalants or foods that are likely to initiate an episode. People with allergic asthma may have positive responses to skin tests, whereas people with nonallergic asthma will not.

Patients may be allergic to a wide variety of provoking stimuli or to only very specific allergens. For example, "seasonal" or "pollen" asthma occurs only at times of the year when specific pollens are present. People with occupational asthma experience symptoms in response to specific triggers in the workplace that may or may not be allergic in nature.

### Nonallergic Asthma

A patient with symptoms of asthma but no evidence of allergy or atopy is said to have nonallergic, or "intrinsic," asthma. Adult onset asthma is more likely to be nonallergic in nature.

## Early, Late, and Dual Asthmatic Reactions

Early or immediate reactions generally occur within 5 to 10 minutes of exposure and last from 1½ to 2 hours. They are typically caused by histamine, methacholine, exercise, cold air, irritants (cigarette smoke), and possibly emotional stress. Late reactions generally start 3 to 8 hours following an exposure and last a variable amount of time. Late asthmatic reactions are usually caused by pollens, molds, animal dander, housedust mites, dusts, and industrial chemicals (Lemanske, 1988).

Dual asthmatic reactions include both early- and late-phase responses. Both phases are characterized by symptoms including cough, wheeze, and dyspnea. However, the late phase of the reaction is generally more prolonged and severe than the early phase.

## ASSESSMENT
## Presenting Complaints

The diagnosis of asthma is generally based on the following presenting complaints:
- Cough
- Wheeze
- Chest tightness
- Shortness of breath
- Exercise intolerance

- Chronic chest "rattle" or recurrent chest "congestion"
- Persistent cough and/or tight chest with colds
- Recurrent croup, bronchiolitis, bronchitis, or pneumonia

Symptoms may be worse at night. Cough is often the primary and sometimes the only symptom in children and adults. Symptoms of status asthmaticus (severe wheezing and dyspnea that is not responsive to usual acute therapy with bronchodilators) are increased dyspnea; paroxysmal coughing; anxiety or agitation; use of sternocleidomastoid muscles for breathing (shoulders appear raised); refusal of food and drink; and occasionally, posttussive emesis. This is a medical emergency.

## Physical Examination

If asthma is mild to moderate, there may be cough, mild tachycardia, and tachypnea with or without expiratory wheezing on auscultation. If asthma is more severe, there are increased cough and dyspnea, marked use of accessory muscles of respiration, intercostal retractions, flaring of the nostrils, inspiratory and expiratory wheezing, and hyperresonance on percussion. In very severe asthma (status asthmaticus), cough and dyspnea are more profound, color may be poor, breath sounds may be inaudible, and wheezing may be diminished or absent. Pulsus paradoxus greater than 20 mm Hg is an ominous sign.

## Spirometry and Peak Flow

Select measures of pulmonary function can be obtained readily at home using a portable spirometer or peak flow meter. Expiratory flow rates are decreased in patients with asthma. Those with unstable asthma may benefit from once or twice daily monitoring of peak expiratory flow rates. A slow insidious or a sudden decline of 20% from baseline can guide early interventions, which may abort an incipient asthma episode. Use of these devices in the home can enhance self-management of asthma symptoms (Janson-Bjerklie, 1988) (see Chapter 2). If asthma is severe, the patient may be unable to perform a forced expiratory maneuver.

**Table 5-1**   Arterial blood gas measurements in asthma

| Severity of asthma | pH | Paco$_2$ | Pao$_2$ |
|---|---|---|---|
| Mild | Normal | Normal | Normal |
| Moderate | Increased | Decreased | Decreased |
| Severe | Normal | Normal | Significantly decreased |
| Very severe | Decreased | Increased | Significantly decreased |

From Schroeder FA: *Current medical diagnosis and treatment*, San Mateo, Calif, 1990, Appleton & Lange.

## Arterial Blood Gases

Arterial blood gas findings in mild to very severe asthma are summarized in Table 5-1.

## Methacholine Challenge Testing

Both the diagnosis of asthma and the severity of bronchial hyperresponsiveness can be determined in the pulmonary function laboratory by methacholine challenge testing. Inhaled bronchodilators must be withheld for 6 hours before the test. After baseline pulmonary function testing, a known concentration of methacholine (a cholinergic agent that causes bronchospasm in people with asthma and usually no response in a normal person) is inhaled. Lung function is measured at timed intervals after the inhalation of methacholine to identify changes. People with highly reactive airways experience a significant (greater than 20%) reduction in spirometry with even a low challenge dose of methacholine.

## Skin Testing

Skin testing, done in the clinic setting by a physician or nurse with specialized training, can be used to determine whether an individual is atopic and to identify specific allergens. It is important to note, however, that not all atopic individuals have asthma and not all individuals with asthma are atopic. If skin testing has been done, the nurse is encouraged to request results from the referring physician. Results of skin tests are used to plan environmental control measures and treatment.

## NURSING INTERVENTIONS

Treatment of chronic asthma includes medications for the control of symptoms, identification and removal of allergic and irritant factors, and identification and alleviation of any associated conditions that may lead to exacerbations, work or school absenteeism, or interference with performance in work and school. Education regarding the disease and its usual course and treatment is of paramount importance. Acute exacerbations must be identified and treated promptly.

### Medications

The pharmacologic management of asthma is aimed at both prevention of symptoms and treatment of exacerbations and is summarized in the following:

| Chronic Therapy | Acute Exacerbations |
|---|---|
| Inhaled cromolyn sodium | Inhaled β-adrenergic agents |
| Inhaled or oral β-adrenergic agents | Oral or IV steroids |
| Oral theophylline | Oral or IV theophylline |
| Inhaled or oral steroids | Inhaled atropine |
| Inhaled ipratropium bromide or (occasionally) atropine | Subcutaneous or IV β-adrenergic agents |

Regular use of medication in chronic asthma therapy helps to control symptoms and prevents acute exacerbations. Antiinflammatory agents such as cromolyn and steroids are particularly helpful in the control of chronic asthma. Because asthma symptoms are often worse at night, adjustments in the timing of medication may be required (Li, 1985). Some patients state that they obtain benefit from the use of antihistamines. Although these medications are thought to be of little use in asthma, they may assist in controlling symptoms of rhinitis and postnasal drip, which can trigger asthma. A full discussion of medications used in the treatment of asthma is found in Chapter 6.

The home care nurse's role is to teach patients the appropriate use of each medication, stressing the importance of continuing the regimen even when symptom free. It is especially important to observe the patient's technique when using inhaled medications (e.g., metered dose inhalers), since ineffective use is extremely common. A spacing device is often needed. The use of spacers is discussed in Chapter 14.

## Treatment of an Asthma Exacerbation

Patients with asthma need to be under the regular care of a physician so that they may learn to recognize the significance of their symptoms and seek treatment appropriately. Adjustments in the frequency and dosage of inhaled bronchodilators and oral or inhaled steroids will be needed if symptoms worsen. These increases should always be made in consultation with the physician and should be followed up with more frequent home care visits to evaluate the response to the adjustments in therapy.

*Asthma in a child, especially one who might not be able to retain fluids or medication, may develop into a medical emergency in hours.* Asthma also may develop quickly in adults, and early effective treatment is of great importance. If home treatment does not relieve the symptoms, the patient must be examined in the physician's office or emergency room. As a general rule, *any child needing more than six bronchodilator treatments in a 24-hour period* and any adult needing bronchodilators more frequently than every 3 hours should be evaluated by a physician. Criteria for when to call the physician are as follows:

- Significant increase in wheezing, shortness of breath, chest tightness, or discomfort
- Chest pain
- Excessive fatigue
- Persistent fever
- Presence or significant change in color, odor,

consistency, or volume of sputum; hemoptysis
- Significant (20%) drop in peak expiratory flow rate if monitored at home
- Need for inhaled bronchodilator treatments *more often than every 4 hours for children* and every 3 to 4 hours for adults
- Lack of clinical improvement following usual measures prescribed for moderate exacerbations

Death or permanent brain damage from hypoxia can occur if acute asthma is not treated properly. In most cases these complications occur because the patient, family, or physician has failed to realize the severity of the acute episode. *Adolescents are notorious for not seeking medical help early and for trying to "tough it out" on their own by using their inhalers every few minutes.* Such "abuse" of metered dose inhalers may keep a patient from seeking medical attention until an exacerbation is severe and more difficult to control.

## Prevention of Asthma Exacerbations
### Reducing Allergens and Irritants in the Home

The first line of therapy is to eliminate or reduce the asthma triggers in the patient's environment, if they are known. Generally, allergen control efforts are begun in the bedroom because individuals typically spend more time there than in any other room. The box on p. 94 describes measures for a dust-free bedroom that are appropriate for anyone believed to be sensitive to housedust or housedust mites. Some of these measures are relatively easily achieved, usually reduce asthma symptoms, and disrupt the patient's life very little. Starting with the least disruptive and least expensive measures is prudent. *For example, washing stuffed animals that can be machine washed will decrease dust mite exposure; however, removal of stuffed animals from the child's room may be necessary and the family and child may need support through this process.* If simple measures are unsuccessful, more extensive measures such as removal of a woodstove, replacing a furnace, or finding a new home for a pet may be needed. General suggestions for

---

### Allergen Control Measures for the Bedroom

Keep all clothes in closets, never lying about the room. Keep closet and all other doors closed. In humid areas, keep a light burning in the closet to reduce mold growth. Do not put moth balls or camphor in closets. Avoid storing blankets, woolens, or other dust catchers in closets; if woolen clothes are kept in room, enclose in plastic zipper bags.

Avoid ornately carved furniture, books, or bookshelves; they are great dust catchers.

Avoid upholstered or stuffed furniture. Wood, metal, or plastic is best.

Wood or linoleum flooring is preferred. If rugs are used, they should be short pile and washed monthly. Damp dust floors twice weekly with disinfectant solution to prevent growth of mold spores. Air the room well after vacuuming.

If using a humidifier, avoid high humidity. Mites grow best at 75% to 80% relative humidity and cannot live at less than 50% humidity. Use a humidity gauge to maintain relative humidity at 40% to 50%.

Have few toys and no stuffed animals in the room. Permit no perfumes, talc, cosmetics, or flowers in the room.

Have few pennants, pictures, or other dust catchers on the wall. Walls should be painted or papered with washable wallpaper. Inspect for swelling that may indicate collection of mold.

Use fully sealed allergen-proof encasings for pillows, mattress, and box springs. These can be obtained commercially from such companies as Allergen Proof Encasing, Inc., Eastlake, Ohio. Vacuum mattress and pillow covers frequently. Never store anything under the bed.

Use washable cotton or synthetic blankets instead of fuzzy-surfaced or wool ones. Wash blankets in hot water every 2 weeks.

Use easily laundered cotton bedspread instead of chenille.

Do not use kapok, feather, or foam rubber pillows. Use Dacron or other synthetics and wash monthly. Foam rubber grows mold, especially in damp areas.

Air conditioning may be helpful, but intake filters must be cleaned and disinfected regularly. HEPA-type air cleaners can remove airborne dust particles. Inexpensive tabletop models are not effective. If sensitive to pollens, keep windows closed, especially in the summer. Check that windows close tightly.

Do not use venetian blinds.

Clean window coverings every 3 to 4 weeks. Curtains should be washable.

Furnace vents should be closed off or covered with a filter or several layers of cheesecloth to reduce dust circulation. Move the bed as far away from the vent as possible. Use electric heater or baseboard heat in lieu of forced air, if possible.

---

Modified from *How to desensitize a room,* AH Robins Company, Richmond, Va, 1971, The Company; and *Dust control in the bedroom,* Allergy Control Products, Inc, Ridgefield, Conn, 1987.

reducing allergens and irritants throughout the household include the following:

*Measures to decrease irritants*

- Prohibit smoking in the home.
- Avoid room deodorizers, insect or aerosol sprays, and tarpaper.
- Avoid strong perfumes and scented fabric softeners.
- Avoid wood-burning stoves.
- Avoid oven cleaners and other strong chemicals.
- Listen to air pollution reports; on air alert days, stay indoors, keep windows closed, and decrease activity.

*Measures to decrease dusts and dander*

- Avoid sitting on overstuffed furniture.

- If possible have another person dust and vacuum; if not, wear a well-fitting face mask while cleaning. Damp dusting is best.
- If possible, avoid being in the house during cleaning and for 3 to 4 hours afterward.
- Keep animals and birds out of the house if possible. At minimum, keep them out of the bedroom and off furniture.
- Clean furnace regularly and change filters at least once a month.
- If using forced air heat, consider purchasing a central electrostatic filter.

*Measures to reduce molds*
- If possible, keep relative humidity low.
- Consult physician about need for air purifier, air conditioner, or electrostatic filter. *Consumer Reports* is a good source of information regarding reliable brands.
- Keep such equipment clean; wash or replace filters regularly.
- Avoid the use of a cool-mist vaporizer because mold grows readily in these devices.
- Clean refrigerator drainage tray (located under the refrigerator) regularly.
- Minimize number of houseplants.
- Use ventilation fans; repair leaks and eliminate areas of seepage; dehumidify excessively damp areas and treat with fungicides (e.g., Lysol, Clorox, zephiran chloride aqueous solution) to retard growth.

### Reducing Allergens and Irritants in Other Environments

Attention must also be paid to other environments the patient frequents. Suggestions to make traveling by automobile more comfortable include the following:

- Prohibit smoking in the car.
- Whenever possible, keep car window closed or travel in an air-conditioned vehicle.
- Try to plan trip routes to bypass sources of excessive pollution, such as refineries or large industrial plants.
- Avoid excessive motor vehicle exhaust (e.g., rush hour traffic, heavily traveled highways,

frequent stoplight intersections). Keep at least four car lengths behind vehicles, especially when they leave blue exhaust. Do not drive closely behind diesel buses or trucks.
- Avoid freshly tarred highways.
- Avoid farms and roadside areas being sprayed with insecticides or weed abatement chemicals. If you cannot avoid them, close the windows.
- When refueling, have passengers with asthma stay inside the car with the windows rolled up.
- If pollen sensitive, avoid riding in automobiles, especially in the countryside, before 11 AM and after 6 PM because these are periods of highest pollen concentration.

### Physical Conditioning

Although exercise neither prevents nor reduces the severity of asthma, a regular exercise program may be beneficial in several ways. It tones muscles, helps maintain the patient in a better overall state of health, and reinforces a sense of "normalcy," thereby improving self-esteem and quality of life. Home exercise programs are discussed in Chapter 9 and are a useful approach for the homebound older asthmatic patient. *However, when children and young adults with asthma are referred for home care, it is usually because their disease is poorly controlled. These patients are rarely homebound and will benefit from encouragement to exercise outside the home.* Swimming, especially in a heated pool, is an excellent sport for patients with asthma. In addition, the inhalation of moist, warm air may reduce the airway hyperresponsiveness that so often occurs with other forms of exercise. However, excessively high levels of chlorine in the pool may be an irritant and aggravate bronchospasm. Other beneficial forms of exercise include running, jogging, or cycling. It is important for the asthmatic with exercise-induced bronchospasm to use inhaled bronchodilators approximately 20 minutes before exercise.

### Immunotherapy

Immunotherapy or desensitization injections may be appropriate for major environmental allergens that cannot be avoided, such as pollens and dust. The efficacy of immunotherapy is well established for allergic rhinitis and has shown increasing benefit in patients with asthma (Fink, 1985). Immunotherapy should be considered when skin testing demonstrates positive reactions to specific antigens; when specific environmental control measures have been attempted and have failed to adequately control the symptoms; and when the patient is willing to commit to frequent visits to the physician over a long course of desensitization.

## Education

Medical noncompliance is a common problem, especially in the adolescent with asthma, and has potentially serious consequences (see Chapter 21). Factors contributing to noncompliance include denial or minimalization of the seriousness of the disease (which can be easy, given the intermittent nature of the symptoms), teenage rebelliousness, and a strong need not to be different from one's peers. Thus education is the single most important intervention in dealing with asthma and one of the most important functions of the home care nurse. The patient's, family's, and caregiver's perceptions, beliefs, and anxieties may be modified by education, thereby improving communication, judgment, and compliance. Through education, misconceptions and concerns may be brought into the open and resolved. The goal of education is to teach patients that they can control their asthma, rather than be controlled by it. Essential components of asthma education include the following:

- Simplified pathophysiology of asthma, specific to the patient
- Personal triggers (allergens and irritants) and whether to eliminate, avoid, or premedicate before exposure
- Early warning signs of an attack
- Specific actions that bring relief
- Rationale, frequency, and side effects of medications
- Decision-making skills, including when to call the doctor or go to the emergency room
- Relaxation skills
- Psychosocial and emotional aspects of living with asthma

## Asthma Camps and Support Groups

*Asthma camps offer support and education along with summer fun, and reinforce the child's ability to function as a "normal kid," enjoying the same activities as nonasthmatic peers. The camp experience may improve the fitness of children who may lead a rather sedentary life at home. Because camping offers more rewards for being well than for being ill, it may also result in better compliance (Scherr, 1985).* Adult and parent/child asthma support groups stress problem solving, help to clarify misconceptions, and reinforce learning.

It is important for the home care nurse to know about local community asthma resources and to encourage patients and their families to use them. The names and locations of excellent family asthma programs, asthma camps, and asthma support groups are often available through local offices of the American Lung Association.

## Interface with the School System

*The home care nurse can play a significant role in educating school personnel about the optimal management of the child's asthma and often have the role flexibility to do so. Outreach to schools is especially important when the child has severe disease and is often absent from school or when parental involvement in the child's care appears minimal. Home tutoring is available in most states, although childhood asthma can usually be controlled well enough to allow the child to attend school regularly.*

**REFERENCES**

Anderson SD et al: Airway cooling as the stimulus to exercise induced asthma—a reevaluation, *Eur J Respir Dis* 67:20, 1985.

Asthma and the weather (editorial), *Lancet* 1:1079, 1985.

Cropp GJ: Special features of asthma in children, *Chest* 87(1 suppl):55S, 1985.

Eliasson O et al: Morbidity in asthma in relation to the menstrual cycle, *J Allergy Clin Immunol* 77(pt 1):87, 1986.

Fink JN: Immunotherapy of asthma, *J Allergy Clin Immunol* 76:402, 1985.

Janson-Bjerklie S, Shnell S: Effect of peak flow information on patterns of self-care in adult asthma, *Heart Lung* 17:543, 1988.

Kamakura T, et al: Point process models in asthma attacks for assessing environmental risk factors, *Environ Health Perspect* 63:203, 1985.

Lemanske RF, Kaliner MA: Late phase allergic reaction. In Middleton E et al, editors: *Allergy: principles and practice,* ed 3, St Louis, 1988, Mosby.

Li JT, Reed CE: Nocturnal asthma and timing of treatment, *Am J Med* 79:10, 1985.

National Center for Health Statistics, Science and Technical Information Branch, Division of Data Services, Hyattsville, Md, 1989.

AH Robins Company: *A guide to desensitizing a room for the allergy patient,* Richmond, Va, 1971, The Company.

Allergy Control Products, Inc: *Dust control in the bedroom,* Ridgefield, Conn, 1987, The Company.

Scherr MS: Summer camps for asthmatic children. In Weiss EB, Segal MS, Stein M: *Bronchial asthma, mechanisms and therapeutics,* ed 2, Boston, 1985, Little, Brown.

Schroeder FA: *Current medical diagnosis and treatment,* San Mateo, Calif, 1990, Appleton & Lange.

Shim C, Williams MH: Effects of odors in asthma, *Am J Med* 80:18, 1986.

Woolcock AJ: Asthma. In Murray JF, Nadel JA, editors: *Textbook of respiratory medicine,* Philadelphia, 1988, WB Saunders.

## SUGGESTED READINGS

National Asthma Education Program Expert Panel Report: *Guidelines for the diagnosis and management of asthma,* NIH Pub No 91-3042, Washington, DC, 1991, US Dept of Health and Human Services.

Bierman CW, Pearlman DS, editors: *Allergic diseases from infancy to adulthood,* Philadelphia, 1988, WB Saunders.

Bierman CW, Pearlman DS: Asthma. In Chernick EL, editor: *Disorders of the respiratory tract in children,* Philadelphia, 1990, WB Saunders.

Cockcroft DW, Hargreave FE: Outpatient management of bronchial asthma, *Med Clin North Am* 74:797, 1990.

Janson-Bjerklie S et al: Clinical markers of asthma severity and risk: importance of subjective as well as objective factors, *Heart Lung* 21:265, 1992.

Larter NL, Kieckhefer G: Asthma. In Jackson P, Vessey J, editors: *Primary care of children with chronic conditions,* St Louis, 1991, Mosby.

# CHAPTER 6

# PHARMACOTHERAPY IN CHRONIC LUNG DISEASE

GWENDOLYN J. McDONALD

Medications that reduce airway inflammation and bronchospasm, improve clearance of pulmonary secretions, and prevent further lung irritation or injury are key components of the medical management of most chronic lung diseases. One of the single most important functions of the home care nurse is to teach, supervise, and evaluate the patient's response to these medications. Inherent in this process is the ability to evaluate the adequacy of the medication regimen and suggest changes if indicated. The purpose of this chapter is to provide home care nurses with sufficient knowledge of the current pharmacologic management of chronic lung disease so that they can both educate patients regarding drug therapy and collaborate with physicians in the pharmacologic "fine tuning" that is invariably needed.

## IMPORTANCE OF MEDICATION MANAGEMENT IN HOME CARE

Management of the patient's medication regimen is of exceptional importance for several reasons:

- Most patients take several medications, increasing their risk for drug interactions.
- Patients often see several physicians, each of whom may prescribe drugs without awareness of what the others have prescribed.
- Patients tend to be older and thus at increased risk for toxicity caused by slower drug metabolism and excretion.
- Many respiratory patients have impaired memory or concentration as a result of older age,

depression, or blood gas alterations and thus are at increased risk for drug errors.
- Use of inhaled drugs involves technical skills, which usually require repeated instruction.
- Current approaches to drug therapy change constantly as new drugs are developed and more is learned about respiratory pathophysiology. Many respiratory patients are managed by physicians without specialty training in pulmonary disease, some of whom may not be fully aware of newer pharmacologic approaches.

## NURSE'S ROLE IN MEDICATION MANAGEMENT

The role of the home care nurse in the management of the drug regimen is the following:

1. *Ensure patient understanding of the drug regimen.* The nurse must review all current medications (prescribed and over the counter) with the patient or a responsible family member on the first home visit and at regular intervals thereafter. Essential knowledge for each medication includes the following:

- Name of drug and reason for its use
- Correct dose, frequency of administration, method of administration (e.g., by mouth, by inhalation), and conditions of administration (e.g., with meals, on an empty stomach)
- Important side or toxic effects and interventions to prevent or ameliorate these

- Relevant drug interactions
- How and when to reorder, if prescription is ongoing

2. *Ensure adequate technique with inhaled medications.* It is estimated that less than 40% of patients use a correct metered dose inhaler (MDI) technique (Allen, 1986). Until mastery is apparent, technique and treatment efficacy should be evaluated on each home visit. The elderly often need repeated coaching and practice sessions to achieve mastery. Teaching aids such as placebo MDIs (available from some drug representatives) can be useful. The very young and the cognitively impaired may be unable to master the technique, and a spacer or change to an updraft nebulizer will be needed. Instruction and supervision in the use of these devices are among the most important roles of the home care nurse and are discussed in Chapter 14.

3. *Evaluate efficacy and safety of the drug regimen.* The home care nurse must monitor the clinical response to each medication, observing for expected objective and subjective effects. Criteria for evaluating a drug's efficacy should be established at the onset of treatment, then used as the basis for subsequent assessments of the patient's response to the new medication. For example, whenever a new respiratory medication is prescribed, baseline symptoms such as dyspnea, wheezing, and nocturnal wakenings should be documented as specifically as possible and supported by objective measures, such as the presence of crackles, wheezes or abnormal breath sounds, daily sputum volume, peak flow rate, and oxygen saturation. Subjective and objective measures are then repeated using a time frame consistent with the predicted optimal effect for that medication. This could range from 1 hour for an inhaled β-adrenergic agent to several weeks for cromolyn and other steroid-sparing agents. The subjective response is as important as the spirometric response in most decisions regarding continuation of a respiratory medication.

The nurse must also observe for signs of toxicity and be alert to the potential for medication interactions. When several prescribing physicians are involved, the nurse must ensure that each is aware of medications prescribed by the others.

Finally, the nurse must evaluate the effectiveness of the overall medication regimen. For example, there may be medications or combinations of medications that might offer greater benefit or fewer side effects than those the patient is currently taking. Such an assessment requires a thorough understanding of current pharmacologic approaches and the needs of the patient. Any concerns regarding the regimen must then be discussed with the prescribing physician and alternatives tactfully suggested, if indicated.

It is important to remember, however, that medication regimens may differ between patients with similar diagnoses (because of both individual variations in patient response and the personal prescribing preferences of physicians) and that these differences may fall easily within the normal range of good clinical practice.

4. *Assess patient compliance with the regimen.* Lack of clinical improvement over time (as evidenced by continued cardiopulmonary instability, dyspnea, wheezing, or adventitious breath sounds) should prompt the nurse to consider poor medication compliance as a possible explanation.

Common reasons for noncompliance include lack of understanding regarding the use or importance of the drug, perceived (or actual) lack of drug efficacy, presence of unacceptable side effects, and excessive cost of drugs. Compliance issues are discussed in Chapter 21.

5. *Suggest ways to control drug costs.* These include the following:

- Using generic drug equivalents whenever possible (although not for slow-release theophylline preparations)
- Comparing prices between pharmacies
- Using mail order pharmacies when eligible, such as the American Association of Retired Persons (AARP) for persons over 55 years of age or the National Cystic Fibrosis Foundation Pharmacy for persons with cystic fibrosis (1-800-541-4959)

## BRONCHODILATORS

Over the past decade, improved understanding of underlying airway pathophysiology and the development of better drugs have changed the general pharmacologic approach to management of chronic obstructive pulmonary disease (COPD) and asthma. Methylxanthines, long a mainstay in the treatment of these diseases, are losing popularity as a result of their frequent side effects and a relatively poor benefit-to-toxicity ratio. Oral $\beta_2$-bronchodilators have also lost favor because of frequent side effects. Longer-acting, aerosolized $\beta_2$-selective agents and inhaled steroids are prescribed instead.

### β-Adrenergic Bronchodilators
#### Pharmacologic Action and Clinical Effects

β-Adrenergic bronchodilators (β-agonists) are agents that selectively stimulate $\beta_1$- and $\beta_2$-receptors throughout the body. Their therapeutic effects result from stimulation of $\beta_2$-receptors located in bronchial smooth muscle and include bronchodilation, improved mucociliary clearance, and reduced airway hyperreactivity.

Typical side effects (predominantly tachycardia and muscle tremors) result from stimulation of $\beta_1$-receptors in the heart and $\beta_2$-receptors in skeletal muscle, peripheral blood vessels, heart, liver, and central nervous system. Therapeutic and side effects are presented in Table 6-1. Because aerosolized medication reaches its target site (the airways) directly, smaller doses can be used and side effects are less than with oral preparations.

#### Clinical Indications

β-Agonists are indicated in the treatment of chronic obstructive pulmonary diseases, especially when these are characterized by excessive secretions or bronchospasm. Examples include asthma, chronic bronchitis, asthmatic bronchitis, bronchiectasis, and (selectively) emphysema and cystic fibrosis.

#### Specific Preparations

■ *$\beta_2$-Selective Agents.* Aerosolized $\beta_2$-selective agents administered routinely or on a prn basis are now the standard of care for long-term management of reversible airway disease. They may also benefit patients with "irreversible" airway problems (i.e., emphysema). β-Agonists currently available in the United States include metaproterenol, albuterol, terbutaline, bitolterol, and pirbuterol (Table 6-2). Although manufacturers each claim superiority for their particular drug, there is little real clinical difference between them, and selection should be based on patient preference and cost (ATS standards, 1987). Adults often respond better to doses approximately double the manufacturer's usual recommended dose of 1 to 2 puffs per treatment. Four puffs every 4 to 6 hours is a fairly typical dosage pattern.

Two other agents, fenoterol and procaterol, are widely used in other countries but are not yet available in the United States. Formoterol, also unavailable in the United States, is a promising new drug with a very long duration of action (8 to 12 hours).

Oral β-agonists tend to be less expensive, are easier to use, and are effective small airway bronchodilators but have a higher incidence of side effects, especially skeletal muscle tremor. These may diminish after 2 to 4 weeks. However, in most instances the addition of an oral β-agonist adds no significant benefit to the use of an inhaled preparation alone.

■ *Non-$\beta_2$-Selective Agents.* Older sympathomimetic agents stimulate α- and $\beta_1$- and $\beta_2$-receptors. Examples include isoetharine, epinephrine, and isoproterenol (Isuprel). The clinical effect of epinephrine (adrenalin) is rapid but of short duration. Before the advent of potent inhaled agents, people with asthma were often taught self-administration of subcutaneous adrenalin for emergency use. This would be unusual today except for persons at high risk for status asthmaticus or an anaphylactic asthmatic reaction. Isoproterenol (Isuprel) is inexpensive and has a rapid onset, short duration, and potent cardiac-stimulating effects. It is no longer recommended.

Isoetharine (Bronkosol) also has a rapid onset and short duration and causes less cardiac stimulation than isoproterenol but more than metaproterenol. Tachyphylaxis (diminished responsiveness to a dose that was previously adequate) is common.

**Table 6-1**   Physiologic and clinical effects of adrenergic receptor stimulation

| Receptor | Physiologic effect | Clinical effect |
|---|---|---|
| α | Constriction of bronchial blood vessels | Decongestant effect, followed by rebound congestion with repeated doses |
| | Constriction of peripheral blood vessels | Mild increase in blood pressure and reflex slowing of heart rate |
| | Weak contraction of bronchial smooth muscle | Mild bronchoconstriction |
| | Small increase in rate and force of cardiac contraction | Slight tachycardia |
| | Reduced tone, motility of gastrointestinal tract; sphincter constriction | Urinary retention, especially with prostatic hypertrophy |
| | Inhibition of insulin secretion | |
| $\beta_1$ | Increased rate and force of cardiac contraction | Increased heart rate, cardiac output, and blood pressure; arrhythmias and palpitations (especially in presence of hypoxemia) |
| | Dilation of bronchial blood vessels | Transient drop in $Pao_2$ due to ventilation/perfusion mismatch; increase in airway congestion |
| | Reduced tone, motility of gastrointestinal tract | |
| | Stimulation of insulin secretion; lipolysis | |
| $\beta_2$ | Relaxation of bronchial smooth muscle | Bronchodilation |
| | Stimulation of ciliary motility | Enhanced secretion clearance |
| | Mast cell stabilization | Reduced bronchospasm, cough |
| | Excitation of skeletal muscles | Fine muscle tremors |
| | CNS stimulation | Nervousness, anxiety, agitation, headache, insomnia |
| | Metabolic effects | |
| |   Stimulation of glucose metabolism (glycolysis, glycogenolysis) | Slight increase in blood sugar; aggravation of diabetes mellitis; aggravation of ketoacidosis |
| |   Increased plasma concentration of lactate and ketones | |
| | Dilation of blood vessels | Mild hypotension with reflex tachycardia |
| | Uterine relaxation | Inhibition of uterine contractions |

**Table 6-2**   β-Selective sympathomimetic bronchodilators

| Drug | Available forms | Onset, peak, and duration | Comments |
|---|---|---|---|
| **METAPROTERENOL** | | | |
| Alupent (Boehringer Ingelheim)<br>Metaprel (Sandoz) | Powder suspension in a MDI*<br>200 puffs/inhaler<br>650 μg/puff<br><br>Inhalant solution<br>10 ml and 30 ml bottles of 5% solution (50 mg/ml)<br><br>Unit dose vials<br>10 mg or 15 mg/ 2.5 ml<br><br>10 and 20 mg tablets<br><br>Cherry flavored syrup<br>10 mg/5 ml | Inhaled preparations:<br>Onset: 5-30 min<br>Peak: 30-90 min<br>Duration: 3-4 hr<br><br>Oral preparations:<br>Onset: 15-30 min<br>Peak: 1-2 hr<br>Duration: 3-4 hr | An isoproterenol derivative and the first of the β-selective agents to be developed<br><br>Less β$_2$ selectivity than later agents<br><br>Side effects similar to isoetharine, (Bronkosol), but duration is longer<br><br>Solutions appropriate for use in powered nebulizers<br><br>Side effects significant with oral preparations (increased heart rate, palpitations, fine muscle tremor)<br><br>Known as orciprenaline in Canada |
| **ALBUTEROL** | | | |
| Ventolin (Allen and Hansburys)<br>Proventil (Schering) | Powder suspension in an MDI<br>200 puffs/inhaler<br>90 μg/puff<br>Ventolin Rotacaps<br>200 μg capsules<br><br>Inhalant solution<br>20 ml bottle of 0.5% solution (5 mg/ml)<br><br>Unit dose vials<br>830 μg/3 ml<br><br>Tablets<br>2 or 4 mg<br><br>Extended release tablets<br>2 or 4 mg<br><br>Orange flavored syrup<br>2 mg/5 ml | Inhaled preparations:<br>Onset: 10-15 min<br>Peak: 1-1½ hr<br>Duration: 4-6 hr<br><br>Oral preparations:<br>Onset: 15-30 min<br>Peak: 2-3 hr<br>Duration: 4-6 hr<br><br>Extended release tablets:<br>Duration up to 12 hr | Longer duration and fewer β$_1$ side effects than metaproterenol; however, side effects still prevalent with oral preparations<br><br>β-Agonist of choice for exercise-induced asthma (Berkowitz, 1986)<br><br>Rotacaps are newest method of delivery; developed in response to anticipated future restrictions on the use of freon propellants; capsules are punctured by rotohaler, releasing a powder that is then inhaled through the device<br><br>*Syrups often used in pediatrics for treatment of "one time" wheezing episodes; oral tablets are not used for children*<br><br>Oral preparations may result in hypokalemia; may inhibit uterine contractions during labor<br><br>Known as "salbutamol" outside the United States |

**Table 6-2**   β-Selective sympathomimetic bronchodilators—cont'd

| Drug | Available forms | Onset, peak, and duration | Comments |
|------|-----------------|---------------------------|----------|
| **TERBUTALINE** | | | |
| Brethaire (Geigy) | Powder suspension in an MDI 300 puffs/inhaler 200 μg/puff | Inhaled preparations: Onset: 5-30 min Peak: 2 hr Duration: 4-6 hr | Also effective for exercise-induced bronchospasm MDI* less expensive than many other preparations |
| Bricanyl (Lakeside) | 0.1% solution in normal saline (1mg/ml) for injection | Oral preparations: Onset: 15-30 min Peak: 2-3 hr Duration: 4-6 hr | No FDA-approved solutions for inhalation; parenteral solutions sometimes used for this purpose |
| Brethine Bricanyl | 2.5 mg and 5 mg tablets | | Side effects prevalent with both oral and subcutaneous use |
| | | | Subcutaneous administration gives rapid relief of bronchospasm, but is not recommended in home setting |
| **BITOLTEROL MESYLATE** | | | |
| Tornalate (Winthrop) | Aerosol solution in an MDI 300 puffs/inhaler 370 μg/puff | Onset: within 15 min Peak: ½-2 hr Duration: 5-8 hr | Longer duration than older preparations, permitting q 8 hr dosing |
| **PIRBUTEROL** | | | |
| Maxair (3M Riker) | Powder suspension in an MDI 300 puffs/inhaler 200 μg/puff | Onset: within 5 min Peak: ½-1 hr Duration: 5 hr | Less expensive than many other preparations *Not recommended for use by young children* |
| **FENOTEROL** | | | |
| Berotec (Boehringer Ingelheim) | Powder suspension in an MDI 200 puffs/inhaler 160 μg/puff | Onset: within 5 min Peak: ½-1 hr Duration: 6-8 hr | Not yet available in the United States Heavy use has been associated with increased risk of death (Spitzer, 1992) |
| **PROCATEROL** | | | |
| Pro-Air | 200 puffs/inhaler 10 μg/puff | Onset: within 5 min Peak: 1½ hr Duration: 6-8 hr | Not yet available in the United States *Not recommended for use by young children* |

*MDI* indicates metered dose inhaler. MDI doses for β₂-selective agents can be increased to 16 to 24 puffs daily for adults who are not also taking oral β-agonists (ATS Standards). FDA requires that the label on MDIs state the amount of drug reaching the patient, rather than the amount dispensed with each actuation. Thus products available in the United States may appear to have a lower dose per actuation than the same products manufactured elsewhere.

Bronkosol turns pale pink when exposed to air and can cause expectorated secretions to appear blood tinged. Patients should be warned that this is normal.

Since the advent of superior β-selective agents, nonselective inhaled preparations are rarely prescribed, although some (e.g., Primatene Mist) inexplicably are available as over-the-counter (OTC) preparations. Use of OTC inhaled bronchodilators should be discouraged.

### Storage of Aerosolized Bronchodilators

Metered dose inhalers (MDIs) are stable at room temperature. To slow deterioration, solutions for use in powered nebulizers should be kept away from heat and light and preferably refrigerated. They should be discarded if they become pink or brownish.

### Evaluating Efficacy of Inhaled Agents

Methods to evaluate the efficacy of an inhaled bronchodilator are listed in the box at right. Bronchodilator responsiveness (defined as a 15% improvement in FVC or $FEV_1$) is generally used as a criterion for efficacy. However, many patients with COPD will not experience improved spirometric values in response to a single dose, yet will benefit with long-term use (Guyatt, 1988). Thus it is generally best to reserve judgment regarding the efficacy of a new inhaled agent until the patient has used it for at least a month.

### Optimizing Therapy with Inhaled Medication

Factors such as preexisting airway patency, dose per treatment, characteristics of the aerosol delivery device, inhalation technique, and use of a spacing device affect the amount of aerosolized drug reaching the airways. Deposition from an MDI can usually be improved by adding a spacing device and increasing the number of puffs per treatment. Therefore there is no advantage in using an updraft nebulizer for most patients. An updraft nebulizer should be tried if patients are unable to use an MDI effectively even with a spacing device, or if the response remains suboptimal. longer duration of

---

> ## Criteria for Efficacy of an Inhaled β-Agonist
>
> Clinically significant improvement in FVC or $FEV_1$
> Clinically significant improvement in peak expiratory flow rate, as measured by peak flow meter
> Improvement in breath sounds
> Reduction in adventitious sounds
> Less dyspnea
> Greater ease in clearing secretions

---

each treatment (5 to 10 minutes of slow deep breaths versus two to eight puffs of an MDI), and the larger doses normally prescribed for use with nebulizers often result in more effective bronchodilation, especially in an elderly population (23 puffs Alupent MDI approximately equivalent to the usual 0.3 ml dose Alupent solution).

### Potential Risks Associated with Use

Recently an association between heavy use of inhaled β-agonists (particularly fenoterol) and an increased risk of death caused by acute asthma exacerbations was reported (Spitzer, 1992). This could represent a serious adverse medication effect. However, it is equally possible that heavy use of a β-agonist is merely a marker for more severe asthma. Heavy use of any inhaled β-agonist should alert the home care nurse to the need for increased vigilance and a thorough reevaluation of the patient's condition (Burrows, 1992; Spitzer, 1992).

## Anticholinergic Bronchodilators
### Pharmacologic Action and Clinical Effects

The autonomic nervous system is composed of both sympathetic (adrenergic) and parasympathetic (cholinergic) divisions, which act in opposition to each other. The parasympathetic fibers that innervate the lungs and airways are part of the vagus nerve, with receptors located primarily in medium and large airways. Stimulation results in the release of acetylcholine, a bronchoconstrictor. Anticholinergic drugs block the vagus nerve by binding to these cholinergic receptors, thereby inhibiting the action of acetylcholine on the parasympathetic nerve endings.

The primary beneficial effect of anticholinergic agents is airway relaxation, seen predominantly in medium and large airways. Compared with inhaled β-adrenergic agents, peak effect occurs later (½ to 1 hour) but duration is longer (4 to 8 hours, depending on dose) (Gross, 1989).

### Clinical Indications

Anticholinergic agents are most effective in select patients with stable severe COPD who have responded poorly to β-agonists (Gross, 1987; Braun, 1989). They are the agents of choice for emergency treatment of bronchospasm resulting from the use of β-adrenergic blocking agents such as propranolol and for the treatment of patients whose acute asthma has become refractory through overuse of β-agonists. They are less effective in chronic asthma therapy (Schlueter, 1986; Gross, 1987) but may enhance bronchodilator responsiveness when combined with a β-agonist. Thus they are often used as adjunctive agents.

### Specific Preparations

Ipratropium bromide (Atrovent) is a quaternary ammonium derivative of atropine, available only in a metered dose inhaler. Each canister contains 200 puffs at 18 μg/puff. The usual dose is two puffs every 6 hours (ATS standards, 1987), although some patients may need as many as four puffs per treatment for optimal effect (LeDoux, 1989). A similar preparation, oxitropium bromide, is available in Europe.

Subcutaneous solutions of atropine diluted with 2 to 3 ml of saline solution are occasionally prescribed when children or adults are unable to use an MDI. The atropine solution is administered by nebulizer, often in combination with a β-agonist or cromolyn solution. The usual dose is 1 to 2.5 mg every 6 to 8 hours. A solution of Atrovent (500 μg/2.5 ml) should be available soon and will be preferable to atropine.

### Side Effects

Side effects with ipratropium and oxitropium are negligible, in part because they do not cross the blood-brain barrier. Aerosol eye contact can cause pupillary dilation, blurred vision, and (for people with narrow-angle glaucoma) potentially harmful increases in intraocular pressure. Thus patients are advised to close their lips around the inhaler and close their eyes during inhalation.

Side effects of atropine solution are more prevalent and may include dry mouth, a bitter metallic aftertaste, tachycardia, palpitations, light-headedness, and blurred vision. At higher doses patients occasionally report skin flushing, decreased bowel motility and constipation, urinary retention, and headache. Although rare, atropine psychosis has been reported.

Tachyphylaxis does not occur with anticholinergic agents, as it so often does with β-adrenergic agents (Gross, 1987). In addition, these agents do not cause pulmonary vasodilation, so $PaO_2$ does not drop, even transiently, when they are used. Paradoxic bronchoconstriction has been reported in some patients receiving ipratropium (Barnes, 1989).

## Methylxanthines

Methylxanthines are effective bronchodilators that have been used for years in the management of asthma and COPD. Currently, because of frequent side effects and the availability of better inhaled agents, they are typically used only if clinical response to other agents (long-acting β-agonists, anticholinergic agents, and inhaled steroids) is suboptimal (ATS standards, 1987).

### Pharmacologic Action and Clinical Effects

All methylxanthine preparations metabolize to the active ingredient, theophylline, which causes relaxation of smooth muscle in airways, blood vessels, and the uterus. Methylxanthines also affect cardiovascular performance, respiratory muscle function, ventilation, dyspnea, and the work of breathing. Specific physiologic and clinical effects are described in Table 6-3.

**Table 6-3**   Physiologic and clinical effects of theophylline

| Physiologic effect | Clinical effect |
| --- | --- |
| **PULMONARY** | |
| Relaxes bronchial smooth muscle | Bronchodilation |
| Increases strength and endurance of diaphragmatic contraction | Increased resistance to and recovery from diaphragmatic fatigue |
| Stabilizes mast cells, reducing histamine release | Prevents bronchospasm |
| Reduces work of breathing | Reduces dyspnea in some patients with COPD (Murciano, 1989) |
| Stimulates respiratory center and increases ventilatory response to hypoxemia | *Reduces central apneas in apnea-prone infants* |
| Stimulates ciliary motility (modest effect) | Slight enhancement of mucociliary clearance |
| **CARDIOVASCULAR** | |
| Increases heart rate | Palpitations, flushing |
| Dilates coronary vessels | Improves coronary flow |
| Increases right and left ventricular performance | Improves cardiac output |
| Stimulates vasomotor center | Mild increase in blood pressure |
| Increases renal plasma flow | Mild diuresis |
| Stimulates vagus nerve | Mild reflex drop in heart rate |
| Dilates pulmonary vessels (early in therapy) | Reduces pulmonary hypertension; may worsen ventilation/perfusion mismatching, leading to transient worsening of hypoxemia |
| **GASTROINTESTINAL** | |
| Increases gastric acid secretion, resulting in mucosal irritation | Anorexia, nausea, vomiting, epigastric pain, hematemesis, diarrhea |
| **CENTRAL NERVOUS SYSTEM** | |
| Stimulates the CNS | Tremulousness, nervousness, irritability, insomnia, *hyperactivity in children* |
| Dilates cerebral blood vessels | Headache |
| **MISCELLANEOUS** | |
| Stimulates sympathetic nervous system | Modest increase in plasma glucose and insulin production |
| Relaxes uterine smooth muscle | Slows uterine contractions during labor |

## Side and Toxic Effects

Gastrointestinal, cardiac, and central nervous system (CNS) side effects are common and often distressing, especially in children and younger adults. Gastric upset can usually be reduced by taking theophylline with food or an antacid, although this tends to slow its absorption.

The severity of side effects and risk of toxicity increase as serum levels approach the upper limits of the therapeutic range of 10 to 20 μg/ml. *Children may become hyperactive even with blood levels in the therapeutic range* (Weinberger, 1987; Furukawa, 1988).

Toxic effects are usually seen at serum levels in excess of 30 μg/ml but can also occur at lower serum levels (Aitken, 1987). Symptoms of toxicity include the following:

• Confusion and agitation
• Severe headache
• Muscle twitching; seizures
• Life-threatening arrhythmias (extrasystole, asystole, ventricular tachycardia, ventricular fibrillation)
• Cardiac arrest

With serum levels greater than 40 μg/ml, patients should be hospitalized for careful observation and treatment (Aitken, 1987).

## Clinical Indications

Oral methylxanthine preparations are most often used in the long-term management of COPD and asthma. Recently developed long-acting preparations such as Uniphyl, administered once daily in the early evening, appear to control nocturnal asthmatic symptoms (Arkinstall, 1987; Helm, 1987). *Methylxanthines are also used to treat apnea and bradycardia episodes in newborns.*

## Methylxanthine Preparations

Theophylline is available as short-acting and slow-release tablets; timed-release bead-filled capsules; ultrasustained-release tablets designed for once daily administration; and alcohol-based and alcohol-free solutions. Guaifenesin or potassium iodide are added to some preparations as expectorants (e.g., Slo-Phyllin GG syrup and Elixophyllin-KI).

Plain tablets are rapidly absorbed and can be used interchangeably. Most brands have a chewable formulation that can be divided into quarters. However, they must be swallowed rapidly to avoid a bitter aftertaste. To minimize whip-saw variations in serum level, short-acting preparations should be taken as close to every 6 hours as is practical.

Longer-acting preparations (administered two or three times daily or, for some preparations, once daily) produce a more consistent 24 hour/day serum level and therefore greater stability of symptoms throughout the day. Less frequent daily doses also result in better patient compliance. Once-daily preparations are not useful for rapid metabolizers needing 900 mg or more of theophylline daily. Sustained-release preparations must not be crushed or chewed. However, bead-filled capsules can be swallowed whole or opened up and the tiny beads sprinkled on soft food. *This is useful for children* or adults *with chewing or swallowing problems.*

*Alcohol-free syrups are especially useful for infants because small doses can be easily measured. Alcohol-based solutions increase both gastric irritation and CNS side effects and are contraindicated for children* and for adults with alcohol sensitivity or a history of alcohol abuse. Rectal solutions are not indicated for home use because of unpredictable absorption and rectal mucosal irritation.

Oxtriphylline (Choledyl) and aminophylline are theophylline derivatives and therefore have lower anhydrous theophylline contents. A 100 mg tablet of aminophylline, for example, contains only 79 mg of theophylline, and 100 mg of Choledyl contains just 64 mg.

Examples of commonly used methylxanthine preparations are presented in Table 6-4.

Caffeine, also a methylxanthine, occurs naturally in coffee, tea, cocoa, and cola. Two strong cups of coffee contain approximately 350 mg of caffeine, enough to increase measures of pulmonary function significantly (Bukowskyj, 1987). Concurrent use can add to side effects and must be

**Table 6-4** Methylxanthine preparations

| Examples of preparations | Available as | Comments |
|---|---|---|
| **RAPIDLY ABSORBED PREPARATIONS** | | |
| Theophylline (Slo-Phyllin; Rorer) | 100, 200 mg scored tabs | |
| Theophylline (Theolair; 3M Riker) | 125, 250 mg scored tabs | Theolair is more expensive because of its individual foil packaging |
| Aminophylline (Aminophyllin; Searle) | 100, 200 mg tabs | 100 mg aminophylline = 79 mg anhydrous theophylline |
| **ALCOHOL-FREE ORAL LIQUIDS** | | |
| Theophylline (Slo-Phyllin GG syrup; Rorer) | 150 mg theophylline and 90 mg guaifenesin/15 ml | All are sugar free |
| Theophylline (Theolair liquid; 3M Riker) | 80 mg/15 ml | |
| Theophylline (Aerolate; Fleming) | 50 mg/15 ml | |
| **ALCOHOL-BASED ORAL LIQUIDS** | | |
| Theophylline (Elixophyllin Elixir; Forest) | 80 mg/15 ml in 20% alcohol base | |
| Theophylline (Elixophyllin KI; Forest) | 80 mg theophylline and 130 mg potassium iodide/15 ml in 10% alcohol base | |
| Oxtriphylline (Choledyl Elixir; Parke-Davis) | 100 mg oxtriphylline/5 ml in 20% alcohol base | 100 mg oxtriphylline = 64 mg anhydrous theophylline |
| **BEAD-FILLED TIMED RELEASE CAPSULES** | | |
| Theophylline (Slo-Bid Gyrocaps; Rorer) | 50, 100, 200, 300 mg caps | Slo-Bid Gyrocaps may have a longer duration than other bid preparations |
| Theophylline (Theo-Dur sprinkles; Key) | 50, 75, 125, 200 mg | Absorption of Theo-Dur sprinkles affected greatly by food; always take about 5 min prior to eating; take whole with a glass of cold water or sprinkle on a teaspoon of soft food; *not recommended for children because highly variable erratic absorption* |
| Theophylline (Aerolate; Fleming) | 65, 130, 260 mg | |
| **INTERMEDIATE-ACTING SLOW-RELEASE TABLETS** | | |
| Theophylline (Theo-Dur; Key) | 100, 200, 300, 450 mg tabs, scored | |
| Theophylline (Quibron-T/SR; Bristol) | 300 mg, scored | Quibron-T/SR is scored so it can be divided into halves or thirds |

**Table 6-4** Methylxanthine preparations—cont'd

| Examples of preparations | Available as | Comments |
|---|---|---|
| Theophylline (Theolair SR; 3M Riker) | 200, 250, 300, 500 mg scored | Dose dumping can occur if Theolair SR is taken with water only; *in children, food slows absorption* |
| Oxtriphylline (Choledyl SA; Parke-Davis) | 400, 600 mg tablets in wax base | 400 mg of Choledyl SA = 254 mg of anhydrous theophylline; 600 mg tablet equivalent to 382 mg of theophylline; following release of drug, the nonabsorbable wax matrix may be visible in stool |
| **LONG-ACTING PREPARATIONS** | | |
| Theophylline (Uniphyl; Purdue Frederick) | 200, 400 mg | Absorption of Uniphyl almost doubles if taken after fatty meal; therefore patients must be consistent about when they take Uniphyl in relation to food |
| Theophylline (Theo 24; Searle) | 100, 200, 300 mg | Absorption of Theo 24 highly erratic; dose dumping can occur if taken with food |

considered when evaluating patient response to therapy. Although not advocated for routine management of patients with asthma, multiple strong cups of coffee may provide emergency interim relief for bronchospasm until more appropriate medication can be obtained.

### Dosage Guidelines

A typical daily dose for a nonsmoking adult is 10 to 12 mg of theophylline per kilogram of body weight (roughly 600 to 800 mg). It is usually administered in divided doses twice daily. The dose is generally increased by about 50% for smokers. It is reduced by 25% to 50% for hypoxemic patients or those with liver dysfunction, and by 30% to 50% for patients undergoing concurrent cimetidine therapy (ATS standards). *Starting doses for children are titrated according to weight and age.*

The doses described in the preceding are only estimates. Because of wide variations in absorption, metabolism, and excretion, both within and between individuals, an optimal maintenance dose can be determined *only* by serum theophylline

levels. An optimal dose is that which results in a serum level between 10 to 20 μg/ml, although if symptoms are controlled at lower levels, there is no reason to push the dose higher, *especially in children*. A serum level at the high end of the normal range is associated with greater clinical efficacy but also with more side effects and greater risk for toxicity.

### Protocol for Serum Theophylline Level

A serum theophylline level is usually determined *after five to six doses for children* and 3 to 4 days after initiating theophylline therapy for adults, using the protocol described in Table 6-5. Thereafter serum levels are reevaluated as follows:

- If symptoms suggest either toxicity or an inadequate dose
- With a significant change in clinical status (e.g., increased right ventricular failure)
- When starting or stopping a drug known to affect blood levels (e.g., cimetidine, erythromycin)
- If the patient stops or restarts smoking

**Table 6-5**    Measurement of serum theophylline level

| Protocol | Implications of subtherapeutic serum level |
| --- | --- |
| **PEAK LEVEL** | |
| For short-acting preparations, draw 1 hr after dose | Suggests inadequate dose or noncompliance; if respiratory symptoms are not relieved, increase dose or frequency of administration |
| For slow-release preparations, draw 4 hr after dose | |
| **TROUGH LEVEL** | |
| Draw 1 hr prior to next scheduled dose | Suggests too wide a fluctuation in serum level; if respiratory symptoms are not relieved, may need a longer acting preparation or a higher dose; must know peak level to increase dose safely |
| **DOCUMENTATION ON LABORATORY SLIP** | |
| Name and dose of medication | |
| Time of last dose | |
| Time specimen was drawn | |

**Table 6-6**    Factors affecting theophylline absorption

| Factor | Clinical effect |
| --- | --- |
| Concomitant administration with food, especially high-fat, high-carbohydrate diet | Usually slower, more complete absorption, but marked variability between individual preparations; dose dumping (rapid absorption with sudden, potentially dangerous increases in serum level) with some products |
| Alcohol base to preparation | More rapid absorption |
| Slow-release preparations | More gradual absorption with more consistent serum levels throughout the day |

- When changing to another brand of a long-acting preparation
- Routinely, approximately once a year for adults, *every 6 months for children in a rapid growth spurt*

### Factors Affecting Serum Theophylline Level

The serum theophylline level is determined by the rate and adequacy of drug absorption, metabolism, and excretion. Factors affecting theophylline absorption are described in Table 6-6. Factors such as age, smoking, concurrent medications, liver dysfunction, a concurrent viral respiratory tract infection, and diet can dramatically alter the rate at which theophylline is metabolized and excreted (Table 6-7). When metabolism is increased, serum levels drop more quickly and the dose may need to be increased. Conversely, when theophylline metabolism is slowed, serum levels readily build and toxic effects can occur at doses that were formerly well tolerated.

Patients with pulmonary heart disease are especially vulnerable to fluctuations in serum level associated with hepatic dysfunction. In this population, any further respiratory insult such as an infection may lower PaO$_2$ enough to precipitate overt right ventricular failure. This in turn may worsen hepatic congestion, impair hepatic function, and precipitate theophylline toxicity.

*Children over 1 year of age typically need more frequent doses with a higher dose per body weight than do adults. However, risk of toxicity is increased with a febrile viral illness. Seizures and permanent brain damage have occurred when children with flu syndromes were treated with usual pediatric doses of theophylline.*

Women in the third trimester of pregnancy may require a smaller dose because of theophylline binding associated with the physiologic hypoalbuminemia of pregnancy (Connelly, 1990).

The clinician must be particularly alert to symptoms of toxicity whenever a patient begins cimetidine therapy because clearance can be reduced by 40% after a single dose. Ranitidine is a preferable choice of drug for treatment of gastric hyperacidity. Theophylline is best avoided by patients with a seizure disorder because of its inherent seizure potential and its interactive effects with phenytoin.

## Precautions Regarding Drug Substitutions

More than with other classes of drugs, sustained-release theophylline preparations cannot be interchanged nor can less expensive generic preparations be substituted with any certainty of equivalency (Hendeles, 1989). This is because the anhydrous theophylline content, rate of absorption, and half-life vary greatly between products. When changing from one long-acting preparation to another, drug efficacy and side effects must be reevaluated even if the stated dose is the same.

## Management of Increased Nocturnal Symptoms

Airways are subject to normal circadian changes that include increased reactivity and decreased caliber during the early morning hours, roughly 3 to 4 AM (Clark, 1987). These changes are undetectable in most individuals, but can precipitate a clinically significant drop in FEV$_1$ and peak flow rate,

**Table 6-7**   Factors altering theophylline clearance

| Slower clearance (reduce theophylline dose) | More rapid clearance (increase theophylline dose) |
|---|---|
| Liver dysfunction | |
| Neonates and the elderly | Children over 1 year of age |
| Cessation of smoking (tobacco or marijuana) | Smoking—40% to 100% increase in rate of metabolism |
| Febrile respiratory illness | |
| Low-protein, high-fat, or high-carbohydrate diet | High-protein, low-carbohydrate diet |
| | High-intake of charcoal-broiled beef |
| Hypoalbuminemia of pregnancy (third trimester) | |
| Flu vaccine (modest effect only) | |
| Medications (Hendeles, 1985) | Medications |
| Cimetidine—40% slower after a single dose | Rifampin—50% to 75% faster |
| Allopurinol—25% slower at doses >600 mg daily | Phenytoin (Dilantin)—50% to 75% faster after 10 days |
| Troleandomycin (TAO)—50% slower | Carbamazepine (Tegretol)—100% faster |
| Erythromycin—25% slower after 5 days | Phenobarbital—in high doses, 25% faster after 3 to 4 weeks |
| Oral contraceptives containing estrogen—30% slower | |
| Clindamycin | |

early morning wheezing, and dyspnea in an asthmatic. Nocturnal symptom control may be further compromised by nighttime alterations in the absorption of sustained-release theophylline preparations. Theophylline absorption is slower in the supine position (Warren, 1985), and *some individuals, notably children between 6 and 16 years, achieve lower serum levels after bedtime doses of bid slow-release preparations than they do after comparable morning doses* (Szefler, 1986). Thus serum concentrations of prescribed theophylline preparations may be lowest at the precise time that optimal levels are most needed. If theophylline is used, better symptom control can often be achieved by timing the evening dose of a long-acting preparation so the peak effect will occur between 3 and 6 AM, the time of poorest airway function. For Uniphyl, this is usually about 6 PM. Other options include increasing the dose or frequency of inhaled steroids, β-agonists, or cromolyn.

In treating nocturnal dyspnea, it is also important to consider the potential role of xanthines in exacerbating the problem. Gastroesophageal reflux is a known cause of increased nocturnal wheezing and dyspnea. Because xanthines relax the lower esophageal sphincter, they often aggravate chronic reflux (Ward, 1988). Thus in some patients control of nocturnal symptoms may be best achieved by discontinuation of theophylline.

### Evaluating Efficacy of Methylxanthines

Because symptomatic improvement with theophylline may reflect benefits such as improved diaphragmatic function that cannot be measured by spirometry, lack of spirometric improvement does not necessarily mean lack of clinical efficacy. Thus a final decision regarding the continuation of therapy is reasonably based on both clinical and spirometric response following a 1-month trial.

## ANTIINFLAMMATORY AGENTS

Increased focus on the role of inflammation in asthma and COPD has led to a dramatic shift in asthma therapy—from a predominantly symptomatic approach (treatment of bronchospasm) to greater emphasis on treatment of the underlying inflammatory process. Early use of steroids, especially aerosolized preparations, is the hallmark of current asthma therapy. However, steroid side effects remain a problem. Thus interest in the use of other drugs with antiinflammatory or steroid-sparing effects (such as cromolyn, ketotifen, methotrexate, and parenteral gold) has also increased.

### Corticosteroids
#### Pharmacologic Action and Beneficial Effects

Corticosteroids relax bronchial smooth muscle by reducing inflammation and the release of vasoactive amines and other mediators and by potentiating the effect of β-adrenergic sympathomimetics. They are highly effective in blocking both early- and late-stage asthmatic responses, and they reduce bronchial hyperreactivity to allergen challenge. They reduce inflammation and airway edema by reducing exudation and the migration of inflammatory cells to the area and by decreasing leakage of fluid from blood vessels. They also reduce mucous volume and improve mucociliary clearance.

By means that are not clearly understood, steroids tend to produce a mild euphoria and an improved sense of well-being. Coexisting extrapulmonary problems such as arthralgias or rhinorrhea also improve with systemic administration. The early and effective use of steroids is believed to reduce morbidity and mortality of acute exacerbations of asthma (Hargreave, 1988).

#### Clinical Indications

The following are clinical indications for the use of corticosteroids:
- Acute and chronic asthma — "first-line" therapy, aerosolized agents preferred
- COPD, characterized by some degree of reversibility to airway obstruction; decision to use is generally based on response to a steroid trial
- Restrictive lung diseases, such as pulmonary fibrosis or allergic bronchopulmonary aspergillosis; oral preparations only, in higher doses

## Steroid Trial

A steroid trial is usually needed to identify adult patients with COPD who may benefit from chronic oral steroid therapy. The American Thoracic Society suggests the following protocol (ATS standards, 1987):

1. Optimize bronchodilator therapy using β-agonist and anticholinergic agents and theophylline as indicated. Confirm adequate theophylline levels and effective inhaler technique.
2. Obtain baseline spirometric values, then initiate prednisone, 40 mg (or its equivalent, 32 mg oral methylprednisolone), once daily for 2 to 3 weeks.
3. Repeat spirometry.
4. If measures of flow rate have improved by 15% or more, reduce dose to the lowest that will maintain this improvement. If no improvement is seen in pulmonary function values, taper and discontinue steroid dose.

Inhaled steroids are an acceptable alternative for "responders," and shorter trials (e.g., 8 days) may be sufficient to determine responsiveness.

## Side Effects

A short course of high-dose steroids (40 to 80 mg/day for adults or 1 to 2 mg/kg/day for children) poses a minimal risk of serious sequelae. However, long-term steroid use is associated with many serious side effects (Table 6-8), even at doses as low as 10 mg of prednisone daily. Suggestions for minimizing oral steroid side effects include the following:

- Initiate only after optimal use of other preparations.
- Use inhaled rather than oral preparations whenever possible.
- If oral steroids are required:
  Use lowest dose that controls symptoms.
  Give full daily dosage in one dose in the morning.
  Implement an alternate day dosing schedule.
  Add inhaled steroids (e.g., four puffs every 6 hours) in an attempt to reduce oral dose.

## Minimizing Adrenal Suppression

As little as 10 mg of prednisone or 500 to 600 μg of aerosolized beclomethasone administered daily for 2 weeks is sufficient to suppress adrenal function (Toogood, 1982). Approximately 10 to 25 mg of endogenous cortisone is produced by the adrenal gland each day, following a diurnal pattern of increased secretion during the late hours of sleep. For most people this peak occurs between 4 and 8 AM. Exogenous steroids taken near the end of or following the peak period cause less interruption of the normal diurnal pattern and therefore less suppression of the pituitary-adrenal axis. Thus steroids are usually administered once daily in the morning. People who sleep during the daytime hours (e.g., night shift workers) quickly readjust adrenal function to match their new sleep-wake cycle and must be counseled that, once they are back to work again, they should be taking their full daily dose on awakening in the late afternoon.

Alternate-day dosage, in which the entire 2-day dose is administered on alternate mornings, also markedly reduces adrenal suppression by presenting an interval day when no exogenous steroid is introduced. Conversely, divided doses (bid or tid) tend to increase adrenal suppression. Although divided doses may improve a patient's response in the acute situation, they should be avoided for maintenance therapy.

## Steroid Taper

A short course of high-dose oral steroids is often used to reverse an asthma or COPD exacerbation. However, the dose should be tapered back to baseline levels as soon as possible. An example of a typical "steroid taper" follows:

Prednisone, 40 mg daily for 2 days
Reduce to 20 mg daily for 2 days
Reduce by 5 mg every 3 days until patient is back to usual daily dose

More frequent home care visits are needed during steroid tapers to assess the patient's response. If symptoms worsen, the physician must be notified and the dose may need to be temporarily increased, then tapered again more gradually.

**Table 6-8**  Side effects of steroid use

| Side effect | Impact on patient | Measures to reduce impact on patient |
|---|---|---|
| Skeletal muscle weakness and wasting | Leg weakness<br>Decreased exercise capacity | |
| Short term: leg muscle weakness | | Encourage regular conditioning exercises to improve muscle tone. |
| Long term: myopathies, especially of shoulder muscles and hip girdle | | Encourage regular conditioning exercises to improve muscle tone. |
| Impaired inflammatory response | Impaired wound healing | Provide scrupulous care of wounds to prevent infection and maximize healing. |
| | Increased susceptibility to infection, especially TB and fungal infections | |
| | May reactivate old TB by breaking down inflammatory wall | Consider prophylactic TB therapy (INH) if history of old TB or if PPD positive. |
| | Masking of usual signs of infection (e.g., redness, swelling, fever) | Increase alertness to subtle indicators of infection. |
| Endocrine effects | | |
| Increased liver glycolysis leading to hyperglycemia and glycosuria | Can precipitate diabetes or worsen preexisting diabetes:<br>Diet-controlled patient may need an oral glycosuriside<br>An oral medication-controlled patient may need insulin | If taking high-dose steroids or if symptomatic:<br>Monitor blood sugar or urine sugar and acetones.<br>Limit carbohydrate intake if indicated.<br>Treat with oral glycosurisides or insulin if necessary. |
| Effects on reproductive hormones | Menstrual irregularities and virilism in women, impotence in men | |
| Increased appetite, possibly caused by increased glycolysis | Weight gain<br>A beneficial effect if malnourished<br>A problem if obese | Capitalize on improved appetite to encourage increased intake, if malnourished.<br><br>Encourage decreased caloric intake if obese. |
| Altered serum electrolytes and acid base status caused by minerocorticoid effects:<br>Sodium retention | Increases fluid retention, especially in patients with preexisting right ventricular failure<br>Can worsen preexisting hypertension | No added salt diet; monitor blood pressure; observe for evidence of increased fluid retention. |

**Table 6-8**  Side effects of steroid use—cont'd

| Side effect | Impact on patient | Measures to reduce impact on patient |
|---|---|---|
| $K^+$ loss with metabolic alkalosis | Hypokalemia: Contributes to skeletal muscle weakness May precipitate digoxin toxicity, especially in patients taking $K^+$-wasting diuretics | Monitor serum $K^+$ and replace if necessary. Increase dietary $K^+$ intake. |
| Changes in mood and mental functioning Short term: | | |
| Euphoria | Initial and often beneficial euphoria common | Capitalize on feelings of euphoria to encourage patient to increase activities and involvement in self-care. |
| Psychosis | Overt steroid psychosis develops in some patients even with short-term therapy, although usually at higher doses | |
| Long term: behavior changes, including paranoia, suicide attempts | | |
| Irritation of gastric and esophageal mucosa | Nausea, vomiting, epigastric pain, discomfort, gastritis, esophagitis Exacerbation of preexisting ulcer disease may cause major gastrointestinal bleeding, even with short-term use | Initiate prophylactic use of a (low prophylactic use of a (low $Na^+$) antacid, if history of ulcer disease. Take oral preparations with food. |
| Restlessness, insomnia (short term) | Increased anxiety, mild sleep deprivation | Encourage sleep-enhancing behaviors (see Chapter 12). |
| Suppression of pituitary-adrenal axis with long-term use in doses greater than 5-10 mg daily | Impaired ability to respond physiologically to increased stress | Increase endogenous steroid dose at times of increased stress (e.g., surgery, infection, trauma) both during and for up to 1 year after discontinuation of steroid therapy. Instruct patient to wear Medic Alert bracelet or obtain wallet card to identify patient as steroid dependent. Slow steroid taper for those who have been maintained on greater than 10 mg per day. |
| | Adrenal insufficiency, Addison's crisis, if steroids are tapered too quickly | |

*Continued.*

**Table 6-8**   Side effects of steroid use—cont'd

| Side effect | Impact on patient | Measures to reduce impact on patient |
|---|---|---|
| Osteoporosis, especially in postmenopausal women (Lukert, 1990) | Spontaneous fractures, especially of:<br>Ribs, from coughing<br>Vertebrae, resulting in severe, often unmanageable back pain | $Ca^{++}$ and vitamin D supplements may help.<br><br>Teach controlled cough techniques.<br>Perform chest percussion with care. |
| Causes or exacerbates ophthalmologic problems<br>Short term: increased intraocular pressure leading to worsening of glaucoma<br>Long term: cataracts, exophthalmos | Impaired vision | Maintain close monitoring of ophthalmic pressures, if patient has history of glaucoma; ophthalmologic consultation needed for management of any ophthalmologic problems. |
| Cushingoid changes in body appearance<br>Acne<br>Increased facial hair<br>Central obesity with "buffalo hump"<br>"Moon" face<br>Stretch marks on limbs, trunk | Impaired self-image | Provide supportive interventions to improve patient's self-esteem and body image. |
| Increased capillary fragility and thin, fragile skin | Petechiae and easy bruising | Teach measures to prevent skin abrasions and soft tissue bruising. |
| Growth suppression in children (although children tend to "catch up" once steroid therapy is discontinued) | Short stature; impaired self-image | Keep dose as low as possible, especially during growth-spurt years. Use aerosolized agents in lieu of oral medication, and use steroid-sparing agents (e.g., cromolyn) in lieu of steroids when possible. |

Once a successful tapering schedule has been identified, it will often be effective with subsequent exacerbations. Thus "reliable" patients may be taught to implement their usual steroid burst-taper schedule with future exacerbations. Routine steroid tapering orders can also be integrated into the home care plan, permitting nursing staff to implement needed treatment without delay.

Patients who have been on high doses for long periods will need to be tapered very slowly and watched closely for evidence of glucocorticoid withdrawal symptoms (see box on p. 117). Adrenal recovery may take as long as 9 months following 2 to 4 months of steroid use.

---

### Symptoms of adrenal insufficiency caused by steroid withdrawal (addisonian-like syndrome)

Weakness, fatigue, headache, malaise
Anorexia, nausea, weight loss
Depression
Orthostatic hypotension, dizziness, fainting
Hypoglycemia
Increased susceptibility to stress
Rhinitis, conjunctivitis, myalgias, arthralgias (i.e., exacerbations of primary or secondary diseases)
Skin desquamation

---

### Drug and Disease Interactions

Phenytoin (Dilantin), barbiturates, and some tranquilizers (diazepam, hydroxyzine, nitrazepam) increase steroid metabolism and excretion; concurrent use may require an increase in the steroid dosage. Macrolide antibiotics (e.g., troleandomycin [TAO], erythromycin) and high doses of salicylates tend to potentiate the activity of steroids. Concurrent use of steroid-sparing agents such as cromolyn, methotrexate, and ketotifen often permit the reduction of the steroid dose.

Hepatic insufficiency impairs conversion of prednisone to prednisolone, thereby increasing the steroid half-life and the risk of side effects. Patients with hypoalbuminemia may develop side effects more readily because they have less serum albumin available to bind with the hydrocortisone.

### Steroid Preparations

■ *Oral Preparations.* Prednisone is inexpensive and the most frequently prescribed of oral steroids. It is converted by the liver to prednisolone, the form in which it is biologically active. Prednisolone use may be preferable in patients with liver dysfunction because it does not require liver conversion. Two other intermediate-acting preparations, methylprednisolone (Medrol) and triamcinolone

(Aristocort), are occasionally prescribed. Dexamethasone (Decadron) is a long-acting steroid with much greater antiinflammatory potency than other agents and is therefore given in smaller doses. Its chief disadvantage is increased risk for adrenal suppression resulting from its very long (36 to 54 hours) half-life.

■ *Inhaled Preparations.* Aerosolized steroids are most effective in patients with chronic asthma. Those with chronic bronchitis tend to respond poorly, especially in the presence of thicker, more purulent secretions. Pretreatment with oral steroids may enhance the efficacy of aerosolized steroids in this group. The chief advantage of aerosolized steroids is reduced systemic absorption, resulting in fewer side effects and less adrenal suppression.

Available preparations are presented in Table 6-9. High-potency preparations such as budesonide (Pulmicort) and beclomethasone (Beclo-Forte) are widely used in other countries and appear to provide better asthma control for those who cannot reduce the oral steroid dose with standard inhalers.

### Strategies for Use of Inhaled Steroids

When an oral steroid dose reaches 15 mg a day or more, an inhaled steroid is often added in an effort to reduce or discontinue the oral dose. Deposition is enhanced if aerosolized steroids are administered 15 to 20 minutes after use of an inhaled bronchodilator. Patients should be warned not to expect immediate relief of dyspnea with an inhaled steroid because it is not a "bronchodilator" like other inhalers they may be using.

Side effects of inhaled steroids are minimal and easily prevented, especially if a spacer is used (Table 6-10). If oral steroids are discontinued at the time inhaled steroids are started, systemic antiinflammatory benefits will be lost, and symptoms (such as nasal stuffiness and arthralgias) that existed before steroid therapy often recur.

Inhaled steroids are significantly more expensive than prednisone and require skill in the use of a metered dose inhaler. *The increased cost and teaching efforts are well justified, especially for children* and postmenopausal women, if the oral

**Table 6-9** Inhaled steroid preparations

| Preparation | Inhaler characteristics | Usual dose | Comments |
|---|---|---|---|
| **BECLOMETHASONE** | | | |
| Oral metered dose inhalers (MDIs)<br>Vanceril (Schering)<br>Beclovent (Allen & Hanburys) | 200 puffs per MDI<br>50 μg per puff | 1-4 puffs tid to qid, to maximum of 2000 μg per day | A micronized powder; therefore increases cough and wheezing in about 20% of asthmatics causing reduced compliance with therapy<br>6 to 8 puffs daily = 7 to 8 mg of prednisone<br>Adrenal suppression at doses of >1600 μg daily (Li, 1989) |
| Beclo-forte (Glaxo)* | 200 puffs per MDI<br>250 μg per puff | 1-2 puffs bid, or 1 puff qid, not to exceed 1 g daily | Potency 5 times U.S. preparations<br>Weak systemic activity; no significant adrenal suppression at 1 g daily |
| Intranasal inhalers<br>Vancenase AQ (Schering)<br>Beconase AQ (Allen & Hanburys) | 200 puffs per MDI<br>42 μg per puff | 1 puff each nostril, 2-4 times daily | Nasal pump spray units must be "primed" with 3-4 actuations before medication delivered to patient<br>Nasal MDI also available<br>Shake before use |
| **TRIAMCINOLONE** | | | |
| Azmacort (Rorer) | 200 puffs per MDI<br>100 μg per puff | Adults: 2-4 puffs tid to qid, to maximum of 1600 μg per day<br>Children: 1-2 puffs tid to qid to maximum of 1200 μg per day | Prednisone derivative<br>Incorporates a spacer<br>Less cough and wheezing than with beclomethasone (Shim, 1987)<br>Discard after 240 activations because of inconsistent dosing after this many puffs |
| **FLUNISOLIDE** | | | |
| Oral metered dose inhaler<br>AeroBid (Forest) | 100 puffs per MDI<br>250 μg per puff | 2-4 puffs bid to maximum of 2000 μg per day | Longer acting, therefore can administer bid |
| Intranasal inhaler<br>Nasalide (Syntex) | 200 puffs per inhaler<br>25 μg per puff | 2 puffs each nostril bid to tid, to maximum of 300 μg daily | For symptoms of allergic rhinitis (note that dose per puff is one tenth that of AeroBid) |

**Table 6-9**   Inhaled steroid preparations—cont'd

| Preparation | Inhaler characteristics | Usual dose | Comments |
|---|---|---|---|
| **BUDESONIDE** | | | |
| Pulmicort (Astra)* | 200 puffs per MDI 100 or 200 μg per puff | 200 to 400 μg bid, to maximum of 1600 μg daily | High potency preparations Available as a MDI or a turbuhaler |
| Pulmicort Pediatric* | 50 μg per puff | | Turbuhalers deliver dry powder only (i.e., no propellants); are breath actuated and therefore require no coordination |
| | | | 200 μg preparation equivalent to Beclo-forte in potency |
| | | | Fewer systemic side effects at high doses than other preparations (Toogood, 1990) |

*Not yet available in the United States.

**Table 6-10**   Side effects of inhaled steroids

| Side effect | Management |
|---|---|
| Increased cough, especially with beclomethasone (Shim, 1987) | Use inhaled bronchodilator first |
| Reflex bronchospasm (Toogood, 1990) | Use with spacer Inhaled bronchodilator prn |
| Sore throat, hoarseness, "weak" voice | Rinse mouth after inhalation |
| Oral candidiasis | Prevention: Rinse mouth after inhalation Use a spacer Treatment: Mycostatin oral swish |

dose can be significantly reduced as a result. When cost is an important factor and the patient's condition can be managed with 5 mg of prednisone daily or less, the use of inhaled steroids is probably not justified.

## Cromolyn Sodium

Cromolyn is used to prevent rather than treat bronchospasm. Its mechanism of action is not fully understood but may include mast cell stabilization with inhibition of the release of histamine and other inflammatory mediators. It also has a beneficial effect on nonspecific bronchial hyperresponsiveness (Petty, 1989; Mellon, 1989). Unlike sympathomimetic bronchodilators that reverse the early asthmatic response, cromolyn blocks both early and late responses (McFadden, 1987; Mellon, 1989). Its long duration of action adds to its preventive efficacy.

### Clinical Indications and Benefits

Clinical indications for cromolyn are listed in Table 6-11. *Cromolyn has gained wide acceptance*

**Table 6-11**   Clinical indications for cromolyn

| Clinical indications | Comments |
| --- | --- |
| Allergic asthma | Drug of choice |
| | Has potential steroid-sparing effects |
| | *May reduce cost of care for children* (Ross, 1988) |
| Exercise-induced bronchospasm | Drug of choice |
| Adult onset, nonallergic asthma (Petty, 1989) | May help some patients |
| Delayed allergic response associated with allergic alveolitis (e.g., aspergillosis, bird fancier's lung) | |
| Seasonal allergic rhinitis (hay fever) | Nasal and ocular administration |
| | Must begin before pollen season (Schwartz, 1986) |

**Table 6-12**   Cromolyn preparations (Intal [Fisons])

| Preparation | Comments |
| --- | --- |
| Metered dose inhaler Two sizes: 112 puffs/inhaler 200 puffs/inhaler 800 μg/puff | Micronized powder, but associated with minimal side effects; therefore the preferred method of administration (ATS standards) |
| Powder capsules 20 mg, for use with spinhaler turboinhaler | A micronized powder |
| | Increased prevalence of side effects, including cough and bronchospasm; therefore may require preadministration of bronchodilator |
| | Spinhaler must be replaced approximately every 6 mo |
| Nebulizer solution Unit dose ampules containing 20 mg in 2 ml of purified water for use in updraft nebulizer | A solution rather than a powder therefore less irritating |
| | Can be mixed with inhaled bronchodilator solution for simultaneous administration, but use within 60 min of mixing |
| | Unit dose preparations more expensive |

*in the United States for the treatment of asthma in children*, but it has only recently gained popularity for adults with asthma (McFadden, 1987). A cromolyn trial may also be indicated for allergic rhinitis. *Telltale signs of allergic rhinitis in young children include frequent rubbing or twitching of their noses.*

### Side Effects

Side effects of cromolyn are minimal, and toxicity is virtually absent. Increased cough, dyspnea, and bronchospasm are sometimes associated with the use of the micronized powders, but these can usually be controlled with prior inhalation of a bronchodilator. Other reported side effects include a dry, irritated throat and mouth.

### Preparations and Dose

Cromolyn preparations are presented in Table 6-12. The usual dose is two puffs from a metered dose inhaler, or 20 mg of the powder capsules or nebulizer solution, four times daily and before exercise (if patient has exercise-induced bronchospasm) or before exposure to a known allergen.

Nedocromil sodium (Tylade) is undergoing clinical trials and is likely to be available soon. Preliminary findings do not suggest any advantage over its parent agent, cromolyn.

### Key Points for Effective Use

The key points for effective cromolyn use include the following:

• Proper use of spinhaler: The spinhaler contains

tiny prongs that puncture the cromolyn capsule. The patient's inhalational force then activates a tiny propeller within the device, which disperses the powder. Patients are instructed to use a high inspiratory flow rate followed by a 10-second breath hold. Peak effect should occur in 5 to 30 minutes with a duration of 4 to 6 hours.

- Measures that enhance compliance
  Advise patients that symptomatic improvement may not be seen for up to 6 weeks of regular use, and offer frequent encouragement to continue with treatment.
  Can be mixed with a $\beta_2$-solution to simplify administration via nebulizer.
  Frequency of dosing can often be reduced to two or three times daily, once initial control has been achieved.
- If the patient is taking inhaled medications of other classes, use the following sequence: bronchodilator → cromolyn → steroid.
- Begin treatment at least a week before seasonal allergen exposure; use 30 minutes before exposure to a specific known allergen and 15 minutes before exercise.
- With an acute respiratory infection, the patient may need to add or enhance bronchodilator and steroid therapy but should not discontinue cromolyn.

## Methotrexate

Low-dose methotrexate may be indicated for a very few, highly steroid-dependent individuals with asthma whose steroid dose cannot be reduced by any other means. Potential benefits include a 50% reduction in the steroid dose, less coughing and wheezing, and fewer nocturnal wakenings. The usual dose is 15 to 50 mg administered intramuscularly once a week (Mullarky, 1990).

### Side Effects and Toxicity

Oral administration may cause mild transient nausea. Potential toxic effects include liver damage (suggested by transient increases in liver enzymes) and pulmonary fibrosis, and these dictate the need for careful monitoring and longer-term studies. Methotrexate is not recommended for pregnant women or patients with liver or kidney disease, pulmonary fibrosis, or a low diffusing capacity (the last being associated with increased vulnerability for fibrosis).

## ANTIHISTAMINES

People with asthma and associated rhinitis, sinusitis, or sinobronchitis are likely to do better if symptoms of upper airway inflammation and infection are controlled with nasal cromolyn, nasal steroids, antibiotics, antihistamines such as astemizole (Hismanol) or terfenadine (Seldane), or some combination of these (Friday, 1988; Holgate, 1985). Otherwise, antihistamines are not generally used in the long-term management of asthma or COPD. Oral antihistamines can impair mucociliary clearance (ATS standards).

Ketotifen (Zaditen), a potent oral antihistamine with mast cell–stabilizing properties, may have a future role in the control of allergen-induced asthma (Kasuya, 1988; Craps, 1987). It is thought to have steroid-sparing effects similar to those of cromolyn, but more studies are needed to establish its efficacy. Its main side effect, similar to other antihistamines, is sedation, especially in older patients. Ketotifen is currently unavailable in the United States.

## MUCOLYTICS

Mucokinetic agents such as guaifenesin, terpin hydrate, and saturated solution of potassium iodine (SSKI) are sometimes prescribed empirically in the hope of thinning secretions, but they have not proved effective in clinical trials. Inhaled *N*-acetylcysteine (Mucomyst) enjoyed a period of popularity over a decade ago, especially for patients with cystic fibrosis, but it has an unpleasant odor and often increases bronchospasm. It is not recommended. A recent multicenter study of the efficacy and safety of iodinated glycerol (Organidan) for chronic bronchitis did not demonstrate any objective improvement in mucus clearance following 8 weeks of treatment at 60 mg qid (Petty, 1990).

However, the subjects did report a reduced frequency and severity of cough and chest discomfort, greater ease in clearing secretions, improved well-being, and shorter duration of acute exacerbations, suggesting that, for some patients with COPD, mucolytics may offer some subjective benefit.

Clinical trials are under way for two new aerosolized drugs that may reduce sputum viscosity in patients with cystic fibrosis who have unusually thick, purulent secretions. RhDNase is a genetically engineered human enzyme that alters sputum viscosity by cutting the long strands of DNA released by the dead white blood cells that constitute purulent sputum. Preliminary data from a multicenter study of patients with cystic fibrosis suggest there is significant symptomatic and spirometric improvement with minimal side effects following twice daily inhalation treatments (Aitken, 1992 and personal communication). Amiloride, a sodium channel–blocking agent, acts by altering sodium transport across the membranes of epithelial cells, thereby presumably "rehydrating" viscous secretions. In a pilot study of 14 adults with cystic fibrosis, deterioration of pulmonary function was slowed and mucus viscosity improved following 25 weeks of qid therapy (Knowles, 1990).

## DRUGS USED FOR PULMONARY FIBROSIS

Patients with severe pulmonary fibrosis are often treated with high doses of prednisone—for example, 1 to 1.5 mg/kg/day for 2 to 3 weeks, tapering to 40 mg daily (Raghu, 1987). If this does not halt the progression of the disease, an oral immunosuppressive agent such as azathioprine (Imuran), 3 mg/kg/day (not exceeding 200 mg daily), or cyclophosphamide (Cytoxan), 1 to 2 mg/kg/day, may be added. Like steroids, they act by inhibiting inflammation. However, the response to therapy is typically slower—that is, 3 to 6 months as compared with 2 to 4 weeks for steroids. Although the side effects of azathioprine are fewer, both drugs increase the risk for cancer and opportunistic lung infections associated with neutropenia. Liver toxicity and penicillin-like allergic

reactions may occur with azathioprine; bladder irritation, bone marrow toxicity, and further pulmonary damage can occur with cyclophosphamide. Patients receiving these drugs require careful monitoring and common sense precautions to prevent infection.

**REFERENCES**

Aitken ML, Martin TR: Life-threatening theophylline toxicity is not predictable by serum levels, *Chest* 91:10, 1987.

Aitken ML et al: Recombinant human DNase inhalation in normal subjects and patients with cystic fibrosis, *JAMA* 267:1947, 1992.

Allen SC, Prior A: What determines whether an elderly patient can use a metered dose inhaler correctly? *Br J Dis Chest* 80:45, 1986.

American Thoracic Society: Standards for the diagnosis and care of patients with chronic obstructive pulmonary disease (COPD) and asthma, *Am Rev Respir Dis* 136:225, 1987.

Arkinstall WW et al: Once-daily sustained release theophylline reduces diurnal variation in spirometry and symptomatology in adult asthmatics, *Am Rev Respir Dis* 135:316, 1987.

Barnes PJ: Muscarinic autoreceptors in airways: their possible role in airway disease (editorial), *Chest* 90:1220, 1989.

Berkowitz R et al: Albuterol protects against exercise-induced asthma longer than metaproterenol sulfate, *Pediatrics* 77:173, 1986.

Braun S et al: A comparison of the effect of ipratropium and albuterol in the treatment of chronic obstructive airway disease, *Arch Intern Med* 149:544, 1989.

Bukowskyj M, Nakatsu K: The bronchodilator effect of caffeine in adult asthmatics, *Am Rev Respir Dis* 135:173, 1987.

Burrows B, Lebowitz MD: The beta-agonist dilemma, *N Engl J Med* 326:558, 1992.

Clark TJH: Diurnal rhythm of asthma, *Chest* (suppl) 91:137S, 1987.

Connelly TJ et al: Characterization of theophylline binding to serum proteins in pregnant and nonpregnant women, *Clin Pharmacol Ther* 47:68, 1990.

Craps LP: Ketotifen: its role in preventing allergic inflammation and bronchial hyperresponsiveness, *Immunol Allergy Pract* 9:11, 1987.

Friday GA, Fireman P: Sinusitis and asthma: clinical and pathogenetic relationships, *Clin Chest Med* 9:57, 1988.

Furukawa C et al: Cognitive and behavioral findings in children taking theophylline, *J Allergy Clin Immunol* 81:83, 1988.

Gross NJ: Anticholinergic agents in COPD, *Chest* (suppl) 91:52S, 1987.

Gross NJ et al: Dose response in ipratropium as a nebulized solution in patients with COPD, *Am Rev Respir Dis* 139:1188, 1989.

Guyatt GH et al: Acute response to bronchodilators: an imperfect guide for bronchodilator therapy in chronic airflow limitation, *Arch Intern Med* 148:1949, 1988.

Hargreave FE: The drug treatment of asthma: how can it be better applied? *Postgrad Med J* 64(suppl):74, 1988.

Helm SG: Diurnal stabilization of asthma with once-daily evening administration of controlled-release theophylline: a multiinvestigator study, *Immun Allergy Pract* 9:414, 1987.

Hendeles L: Slow release theophylline: do not substitute, *Am Pharm* NS29:2, 1989.

Hendeles L, Massanari M, Weinberger M: Update on the pharmacodynamics and pharmacokinetics of theophylline, *Chest* (suppl) 88:103S, 1985.

Holgate ST, Emmanuel MB: Astemizole and other H-1 antihistaminic drug therapy of asthma, *J Allergy Clin Immunol* 76:375, 1985.

Kasuya S, Izumi S: Steroid-sparing effect of ketotifen in steroid dependent asthmatics: a long period evaluation of 12 patients, *Pharmacotherapeutics* 5:177, 1988.

Knowles MR et al: A pilot study of aerosolized amiloride for the treatment of lung disease in cystic fibrosis, *N Engl J Med* 322:1189, 1990.

LeDoux EJ et al: Standard and double dose ipratropium bromide and combined ipratropium bromide and inhaled metaproterenol in COPD, *Chest* 95:1013, 1989.

Li JTC, Reed CE: Proper use of aerosol corticosteroids to control asthma, *Mayo Clin Proc* 64:205, 1989.

Lukert BP, Raisz LG: Glucocorticoid-induced osteoporosis: pathogenesis and management, *Ann Intern Med* 112:352, 1990.

McFadden ER: Cromolyn: first-line therapy for chronic asthma? *J Respir Dis* 8:39, 1987.

Mellon MH: *Childhood asthma: effective pharmacotherapy to reduce morbidity and prevent mortality (symposium highlights),* Princeton, 1989, Excerpta Medica.

Mullarky MF, Lammert JK, Blumenstein BA: Long-term methotrexate treatment in corticosteroid-dependent asthma, *Ann Intern Med* 112:577, 1990.

Murciano D et al: A randomized controlled trial of theophylline in patients with severe COPD, *N Engl J Med* 320:1521, 1989.

Petty TL: The National Mucolytic Study: results of a randomized, double-blind placebo-controlled study of iodinated glycerol in chronic obstructive bronchitis, *Chest* 97:75, 1990.

Petty TL et al: Cromolyn sodium is effective in adult chronic asthmatics, *Am Rev Respir Dis* 139:694, 1989.

Raghu G: Idiopathic pulmonary fibrosis, *Chest* 92:149, 1987.

Ross RN et al: Cost-effectiveness of including cromolyn sodium in the treatment program for asthma: a retrospective record-based study, *Clin Ther* 10:188, 1988.

Schlueter DP: Ipratropium bromide in asthma: a review of the literature, *Am J Med* 81(suppl 5A):55, 1986.

Schwartz HJ: The effect of cromolyn on nasal disease, *Ear Nose Throat J* 65:449, 1986.

Shim CS, Williams MH: Cough and wheezing from beclomethasone dipropionate aerosol are absent after triamcinolone acetonide, *Ann Intern Med* 106:700, 1987.

Spitzer WO et al: The use of beta agonists and the risk of death and near death from asthma, *N Engl J Med* 326:501, 1992.

Szefler SJ: Erratic absorption of theophylline from slow-release products in children, *J Allergy Clin Immunol* 78:710, 1986.

Toogood JH: Steroids and cromolyn for treatment of chronic asthma, *Chest* 82(suppl 1):43S, 1982.

Toogood JH: Complications of topical steroid therapy for asthma, *Am Rev Respir Dis* 141(suppl):S89, 1990.

Ward PH et al: Complications of gastroesophageal reflux (specialty conference), *West J Med* 149:58, 1988.

Warren JB, Cuss F, Barnes PJ: Posture and theophylline kinetics, *Br J Clin Pharmacol* 19:707, 1985.

Weinberger M: Effects of theophylline on learning and behavior: reason for concern or concern without reason? *J Pediatr* 111:471, 1987.

## SUGGESTED READINGS

American Thoracic Society: Standards for the diagnosis and care of patients with chronic obstructive pulmonary disease (COPD) and asthma, *Am Rev Respir Dis* 136:225, 1987.

Cockcroft DW, Hargreave FE: Outpatient management of bronchial asthma, *Med Clin North Am* 74:797, 1990.

Hudson LD, Monti CM: Rationale and use of corticosteroids in chronic obstructive pulmonary disease, *Med Clin North Am* 74:661, 1990.

Lemanske RF, Joad JP: Uses of beta-agonists in asthma: a comparison, *J Respir Dis* (suppl), June 1989, p S28.

Levinson H, Reilly PA, Worsley GH: Spacing devices and metered dose inhalers in childhood asthma, *J Pediatr* 107:662, 1985.

National Asthma Education Program: *Guidelines for the diagnosis and management of asthma,* DHHS Pub No 91-3042, Bethesda, Md, 1991, Department of Health and Human Services.

Schlueter DP: Ipratropium bromide in asthma: a review of the literature, *Am J Med* 81(suppl 5A):55, 1986.

Simon PM, Statz EM: Drug treatment of COPD, *Postgrad Med* 91:473, 1992.

Ziment I: Pharmacologic therapy of obstructive airway disease, *Clin Chest Med* 11:461, 1990.

# CHAPTER 7

# AIRWAY CLEARANCE

JOAN TURNER

Retained secretions may cause serious problems for the patient with chronic lung disease. The respiratory muscle effort necessary to maintain ventilation when secretions obstruct airways increases the work of breathing and the sensation of dyspnea. Alveolar hypoventilation (from partial or complete obstruction of airways caused by retained secretions) and worsening ventilation-perfusion inequalities cause hypoxemia and hypercapnia. Retained secretions also increase the likelihood of pneumonia, lung abscesses, bronchiectasis, and atelectasis.

Promotion of airway clearance is a primary goal of respiratory home care. The significance of ineffective airway clearance, assessment of airway clearance problems, and appropriate nursing interventions are discussed in this chapter.

## ETIOLOGY

The effects of chronic lung disease on normal airway clearance mechanisms are summarized in Table 7-1. In general, airway clearance is impaired if the diameter of the airways is reduced, if the volume and viscosity of respiratory tract secretions are increased, if ciliary motility is decreased, and if effective cough mechanisms are inhibited. These problems increase the likelihood of acute exacerbations that further inhibit airway clearance and lead to respiratory failure. Other factors that inhibit effective clearance of airway secretions are summarized in Table 7-2. Respiratory tract infection is discussed in detail in Chapter 4.

## ASSESSMENT

The evaluation of ineffective secretion clearance in the patient with chronic lung disease is based on the knowledge of what is normal for that patient. *The signs and symptoms of increased work of breathing in children are presented in Chapter 3.* It is important for the nurse to evaluate the following:

- Change in symptoms
    Increased chest congestion
    Increased cough
    Increased dyspnea
    Increased wheezing
    Increased or decreased sputum production
- Changes in signs
    Thickening or discoloration of secretions
    Decreased breath sounds on auscultation
    Adventitious breath sounds, e.g., crackles, audible wheezes, and rhonchi
    Increased respiratory rate
    Reduced expiratory flow rates with spirometry or peak flow meter
    Reduction in oxygen saturation on oximetry or worsening arterial blood gas levels
    Increased frequency of respiratory tract infections and fever

The effectiveness of interventions to enhance airway clearance may be determined by improvement in the signs and symptoms noted above. Initially the sputum volume increases as retained secretions are cleared and stabilizes as effective bronchial hygiene is maintained.

**Table 7-1**    Etiology of ineffective airway clearance in chronic lung disease

| Disease | Mechanisms of ineffective clearance |
| --- | --- |
| Emphysema | Reduced cough effectiveness because of decreased expiratory flow rates from airway collapse and air trapping; loss of cilia |
| Chronic bronchitis | Increased amounts of thick, purulent mucus; reduced airway diameter because of inflammation of bronchial mucous membranes and accumulation of secretions; loss of cilia |
| Asthma | Bronchoconstriction resulting in decreased airway diameter; thick tenacious mucus; inflammation of bronchial mucous membranes |
| Cystic fibrosis | Thick purulent secretions; inflammation of bronchial mucous membranes; reduced ciliary motion; bronchiectatic cysts |
| Bronchiectasis | Dilation and destruction of bronchial walls from recurrent inflammation and infection |
| Primary ciliary dyskinesia | Structural abnormalities of cilia causing less effective motion |

**Table 7-2**    Other factors that impair the clearance of secretions

| Factor | Mechanisms of ineffective airway clearance |
| --- | --- |
| Respiratory tract infection | Increased thick purulent secretions; reduced airway diameter from inflammation of bronchial mucosa; reduced ciliary activity |
| Allergens and irritants | Hypersecretion of mucus; inflammation of bronchial mucosa; bronchoconstriction; depression of ciliary activity; anaphylaxis in extreme cases |
| Poor nutrition | Reduced cough effectiveness because of respiratory muscle fatigue and weakness |
| Dehydration | Thick, viscous mucous secretions; mucus that may remain attached to secretory duct, inhibiting clearance |
| Tracheostomy | Mucosal crusting causing bleeding, infection, and airway obstruction because normal humidification mechanisms of upper airways bypassed |
| More than 4 L/min oxygen without humidification | Mucosal drying that may lead to crusting, bleeding, infection, and airway obstruction |
| Mechanical obstruction of airway (e.g., from tumor, foreign body, enlarged lymph node) | Obstruction of large airway that is usually an emergency requiring surgery or removal of foreign body by bronchoscopy; partial obstruction that may cause decreased clearance of secretions |
| Neuromuscular disease | Reduced cough effectiveness because of respiratory muscle weakness and decreased ability to keep glottis closed long enough to generate sufficient airway pressure for explosive discharge of air; blunted gag reflex predisposing patient to aspiration |
| Young age | Small airway diameter |
| Old age | Reduced expiratory flow rates because of decreased elastic recoil of lungs and chest wall |

## NURSING INTERVENTIONS

Several strategies may be used in the home to promote airway clearance and are referred to as bronchial hygiene measures. The maintenance of adequate nutrition and hydration, the avoidance of allergens and irritants, the treatment of bronchospasm, and the prevention and treatment of infection are of the utmost importance and are fully discussed in other chapters.

In the past, aerosolized mucolytic agents such as acetylcysteine were prescribed to reduce the viscosity of pulmonary secretions, but they were not particularly effective. A new medication, aerosolized DNase, has been shown to reduce the viscosity of pulmonary mucus and to enhance secretion clearance in early studies in patients with cystic fibrosis (Aitken, 1992). If further studies support the effectiveness of this therapy, it will be used more extensively in the future.

Patients who produce excessive secretions (30 ml/day or more) and those with acute respiratory infections may benefit from special techniques, including therapeutic coughing, forced exhalation techniques, autogenic drainage, positive expiratory pressure, and postural drainage with chest percussion and vibration. One or a combination of these strategies may be most appropriate for a given patient. The home care nurse should work with the patient, the caregivers, and the physician to determine what interventions are most effective.

### Therapeutic Coughing

Coughing is a symptom of disease and the most effective way to clear abnormal secretions from the lungs. Coughing may cause side effects, including breathlessness, vomiting, bradycardia, heart block, headache, syncope, chest and abdominal muscle strain, rib fractures, and urinary incontinence (Sackner, 1988). A technique of coughing that may enhance secretion clearance in weak or debilitated patients and in those who experience side effects from coughing is summarized in the box at right.

#### Abdominal Push Maneuver

Patients with spinal cord injuries, extreme weakness, or paralysis of the chest and abdominal mus-

---

| **Therapeutic Coughing Technique** |
| :-- |
| 1. Sit upright with both feet firmly supported. |
| 2. Take a few deep, relaxed breaths while sitting upright. |
| 3. Exhale through pursed lips. |
| 4. Inhale slowly and deeply. |
| 5. Lean forward while producing two to three short, consecutive coughs from deep in the chest. The short cough maneuvers should be made on the same exhalation. A pillow can be held tightly against the abdomen to provide support with contraction of the muscles of the abdomen and permit a stronger cough. |
| 6. Take a few more relaxed breaths. |
| 7. Repeat the cough maneuver two or three times until secretions are raised. |

---

cles can be assisted to cough by another person who performs an abdominal push maneuver (Braun, 1984). The assistant places his or her hands on the abdomen of the patient and instructs the patient to breathe in as deeply as possible and to exhale forcefully. While the patient is exhaling, the assistant quickly and firmly pushes the abdomen up against the diaphragm to facilitate airway clearance. This maneuver should not be performed within 2 hours after meals because it may cause patients to vomit and aspirate. Care should be taken not to apply excessive pressure that could cause bruising and damage to abdominal organs.

### Forced Exhalation Techniques

Forced exhalation or huffing has been shown to enhance secretion clearance in patients who produce at least 30 ml of sputum each day (Sutton, 1983). Some patients may be able to clear secretions effectively with forced exhalation techniques alone or in conjunction with postural drainage, instead of percussion and vibration. The technique consists of a series of short, quick exhalations, or "huffs," with the glottis open, starting at midlung volume and continuing to residual volume. Huffs should follow a slow, deep inhalation with a breath hold of 1 to 3 seconds, alternating with a few relaxed breaths. As secretions move to the upper airways, they can be cleared by coughing or huffing at high lung volumes. It is thought that the dynamic compression of the airways created by the maneuver facilitates the movement of secretions toward the mouth.

## Positive Expiratory Pressure

Positive expiratory pressure (PEP) is a technique that uses a resistive device to apply positive pressure to the airways during exhalation. The degree of resistance that is applied can be measured in centimeters of water. PEP may be used as an alternative to postural drainage with percussion and vibration. *It can be performed by children older than 4 years of age*. The equipment and treatment techniques are presented in Chapter 14.

## Postural Drainage

Postural drainage consists of positioning the patient so that gravity enhances the drainage of lung segments. It is advocated for patients who produce at least 30 ml of secretions daily and are unable to clear their secretions effectively with coughing alone (Kirilloff, 1985). It is performed with percussion and vibration or forced exhalation techniques. Postural drainage positions are shown in Fig. 7-1. *Adaptations for infants and young children are shown in Fig. 7-2*. Patients with bronchiectasis and lung abscesses can be instructed to drain only the affected lung segments. However, most patients with chronic lung disease (especially cystic fibrosis) have generalized lung involvement and should use as many positions as necessary at least once a day to clear secretions. Drainage should begin with the superior segments and progress toward the lung bases. Patients should be positioned with the knees flexed and the legs supported in good alignment with pillows. A flat pillow should be placed under the small of the back when the patient is in the supine position for support. The knee-chest position (Fig. 7-3) is surprisingly well tolerated by patients with COPD because there is no pressure on the chest or abdomen. It may be easier for patients to assume the knee-

chest position than to climb on top of a pile of pillows. A modified postural drainage position where the patient lies flat or on one side with the head level with the body may be appropriate for the patient who is weak or frail or becomes breathless in a head-dependent position.

Special tilt tables or hospital beds are best for the most head-dependent positions. However, many patients can assume the proper position with pillows, newspapers, or folded blankets when appropriately arranged. A 12-inch stack of newspapers can be tied together and padded with a pillow for comfort. A well-stuffed backrest cushion turned upside down can also be effective. It is generally not safe for patients to hang over the side of the bed to perform postural drainage. Also, ironing boards should not be used as tilt tables because they are too narrow and are not stable. Instructions for performing postural drainage are presented in the box on p. 131.

## Percussion and Vibration

Percussion and vibration consist of clapping, shaking, and compression maneuvers applied to the chest wall during postural drainage to enhance secretion clearance. The techniques require training, practice, and reasonable physical stamina; however, most caregivers can learn them. Thus far studies have not demonstrated any advantage of postural drainage with percussion and vibration as compared to postural drainage with forced exhalation techniques (Kirilloff, 1985). However, percussion and vibration may enhance secretion clearance in weak or debilitated patients who cannot perform forced exhalations.

Chest wall percussion or clapping can be performed manually by cupping both hands (Fig. 7-4) to create a tight seal between the cupped hands and the surface of the patient's skin and then by rapidly clapping the chest wall. If performed correctly, this produces a rhythmic hollow sound. The resultant percussion waves that are transmitted through the chest wall are thought to help dislodge the secretions. Clapping is performed over each lung segment for approximately 2 minutes as that segment is drained (i.e., the hands should not move

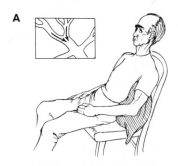

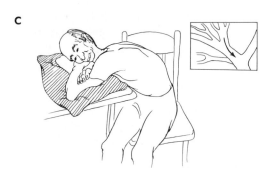

Apical segments upper lobes. Patient leans back at 30° angle; percuss between clavicle and top of scapula on each side.

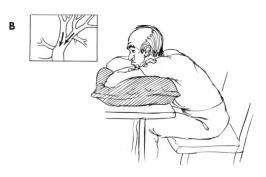

Posterior segments upper lobes. Patient leans forward at 30°-45° angle; percuss over upper back above scapula.

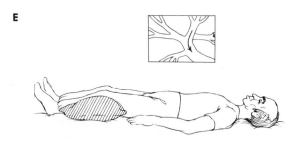

Alternate position left upper lobe apical posterior segment. Patient rotates over pillow with head elevated 45°; percuss upper back on left.

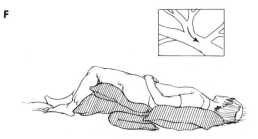

Alternate position right upper lobe posterior segment. With bed flat, patient rotates 45° from prone position; percuss upper back on right.

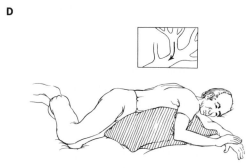

Anterior segments upper lobes. Percuss between clavicle and fourth rib on each side of chest.

Lingula left upper lobe. Hips elevated 12-14 inches and patient rotated 45° to right; percuss anterior chest just below fourth rib or nipple area.

**Fig. 7-1**    Postural drainage positions for adults. Positions for upper lobes include **A** through **E**. Positions for lower lobes include **H** through **L**. Lingula (**F**) is part of left upper lobe. Drainage of right middle lobe is depicted in **G**.

G

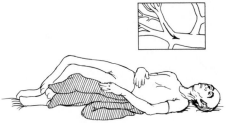

Right middle lobe. Hips elevated to 12-14 inches and patient rotated 45° to left; percuss anterior chest just below fourth rib or nipple.

H

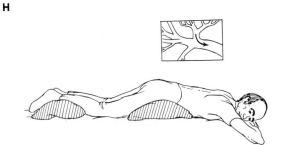

Superior segments lower lobes. Patient lies prone with one or two pillows under hips; percuss area below tip of scapula on each side of spine.

I

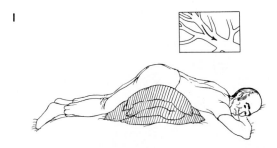

Posterior basal segments lower lobes. Elevate hips 14-18 inches; percuss over lower ribs on each side of spine.

J

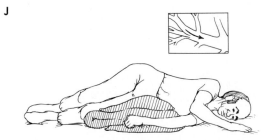

Lateral basal segment right lower lobe. Elevate hips 14-18 inches and rotate slightly forward; percuss over upper portion of lower ribs along posterior axillary line.

K

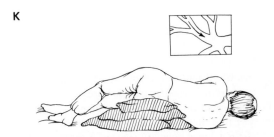

Lateral basal segment left lower lobe. Elevate hips 14-18 inches and rotate slightly forward; percuss over upper portion of lower ribs along posterior axillary line.

L

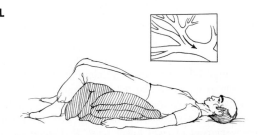

Anterior and medial segments lower lobes. Supine position with hips elevated about 14 inches; percuss over lower ribs in anterior axillary line. (Alternate position is to rotate slightly back from positions J and K.)

**Fig. 7-1, cont'd.**

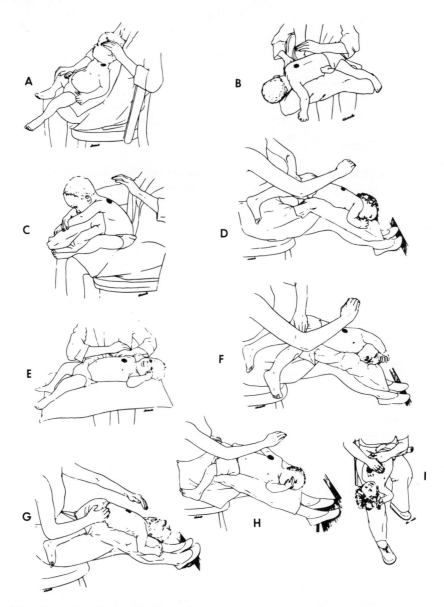

**Fig. 7-2**  Bronchial drainage positions for major segments of all lobes in infant. Procedure is most easily carried out on caregiver's lap. Dark circle on chest indicates area to be cupped or vibrated. **A,** Apical segment of left upper lobe. **B,** Posterior segment of right upper lobe. **C,** Posterior segment of left upper lobe. **D,** Superior segment of right lower lobe. **E,** Anterior basal segment of right lower lobe. **F,** Lateral basal segment of right lower lobe. **G,** Posterior basal segment of right lower lobe. **H,** Medial and lateral segments of right middle lobe. **I,** Lingular segments (superior and inferior) of left upper lobe. (Modified from Cystic Fibrosis Foundation: *Infant segmental bronchial drainage,* Rockville, Md, The Foundation.)

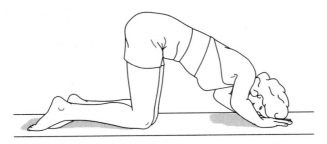

**Fig. 7-3**   Knee-chest position.

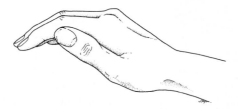

**Fig. 7-4**   Position of hand for cupping and vibrating. (From Beare PG, Myers JL: *Principles and practice of adult health nursing,* St Louis, 1990, Mosby.)

---

### Instructions for Performing Postural Drainage

1. Perform postural drainage at least 1 hour before or 2 hours after meals when the stomach is empty. If it is performed directly before meals, the patient may be too tired to eat properly. If it is performed directly after meals, it may interfere with digestion or cause the patient to vomit. *It has also been shown to increase the incidence of gastroesophageal reflux (see Chapter 13) in infants between 1 and 4 months of age* (Vandenplas, 1991).

2. Use inhaled bronchodilators (if prescribed) approximately 15 minutes before the drainage sessions. Use oxygen during postural drainage if patient becomes hypoxemic in the head-dependent position.

3. Assume each prescribed position for at least 5 to 10 minutes.

4. Have a sputum container or tissue handy for expectoration. If clear, screw-top containers are used, the secretions can readily be observed and measured.

5. Perform forced exhalation or cough maneuvers approximately every 5 minutes during the drainage and before changing to a new position.

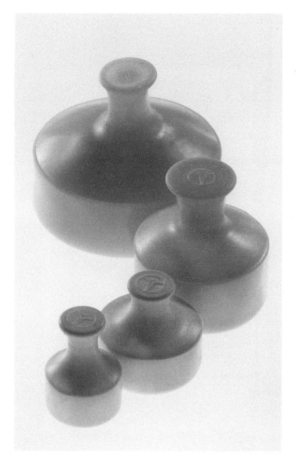

**Fig. 7-5** Manual (palm) cup for self-percussion. (Manual Percussor 240, DHD Medical Products, Canastota, NY.)

---

**Technique for Manual Vibration**

1. Place the palm of one hand on the patient's chest. Place the other hand over the back of the first hand. The fingers of both hands should be extended without touching the chest.
2. Instruct the patient to take a slow, deep breath and exhale slowly through pursed lips.
3. While the patient exhales, apply a firm, fine, vibrating pressure to the chest wall, keeping the elbows straight.
4. Repeat the maneuver four to six times.
5. Instruct the patient to cough.

---

better than clapping with the hands. Manual vibration is performed after clapping by applying pressure to the chest wall with the technique presented in the box above.

Mechanical percussors can also be used, although they are generally less effective than manual percussion and vibration. They may be useful if the caregiver is unable to perform manual vibration or for patients who resist dependence on others for help. Mechanical percussors can be purchased or rented from respiratory equipment companies.

## Autogenic Drainage

Autogenic drainage is a procedure that was developed in Europe as an alternative to postural drainage and percussion (David, 1991). The technique is beginning to generate interest in the United States, and studies to determine its efficacy are planned. It is a self-administered procedure that uses varying lung volumes, inspiratory pauses, controlled expiratory flows, and huff coughing to clear secretions. The recommended procedure requires two or three intense training sessions with an experienced therapist. *Because the technique is complicated, it is not recommended for children under 12 years of age.* Generally, a patient should continue the technique until he or she feels the airways are clear. Sessions of at least 20 to 30

all over the patient's torso). The patient should wear a single layer of light clothing to protect the skin during the clapping sessions, and the person who is performing the percussion should remove any rings. Percussion and vibration should not be performed over the heart, stomach, spine, kidneys, or women's breasts. It is probably not effective if the patient is grossly obese.

Some patients can self-percuss apical and lateral lung segments. Inexpensive percussion cups are available in neonatal, pediatric, and adult sizes (Fig. 7-5). The cups are easy to use and are often

**Table 7-3**  Potential complications of secretion clearance techniques

| Complication | Contributing factors | Comments |
|---|---|---|
| Bronchospasm | Forced exhalation | Do not exhale against closed glottis. Practice relaxed breathing after huffing. |
|  | Coughing | Practice therapeutic coughing. |
| Hypoxemia | Head-dependent position may aggravate V/Q mismatching | Measure oxygen saturation with the patient in the head-dependent position if the patient complains of severe breathlessness or develops irregular heart rate during postural drainage, or if $O_2$ saturation is known to be low. Use a modified postural drainage position if the patient experiences desaturation when the head is dependent. Check with the physician about low-flow oxygen during postural drainage if it is not prescribed. If prescribed, may need to increase the flow rate during postural drainage. |
| Breathlessness | Secondary to hypoxemia or bronchospasm (as described above) or to orthopnea | Use oxygen during postural drainage if prescribed. Use inhaled bronchodilators approximately 15 min before procedure. Try modified position. Patients with orthopnea from left ventricular failure generally cannot tolerate postural drainage. |
| Pain | Coughing | Splint the area of discomfort with a pillow or coughing belt (band of cloth approximately 4 in wide that is placed around lower chest, crossed in front and tightened during each cough maneuver). Try modified cough procedure discussed on p. 126 or substitute huff technique. |
|  | Percussion and vibration that may aggravate existing musculoskeletal problems or cause rib fractures in newborns or adults with osteoporosis | Substitute huff coughing, PEP therapy, or autogenic drainage if rib fractures, bone metastases, or chest wall muscle strain present. |
| Heartburn | Head-dependent position (may aggravate gastroesophageal reflux) | Wait at least 2 hr after meals before performing postural drainage. Try modified position. Use antacids before postural drainage. |
| Fatigue | Postural drainage | Modified, side-lying position with head supported by pillow may be tolerated. |
| Nausea and vomiting | Head-dependent position | Do not advocate head-dependent position less than 2 hr after meals or large fluid intake. |
|  | Excessive coughing | Stress controlled cough techniques. |
| Hemoptysis | Percussion and vibration | Do not perform if patient has frank hemoptysis, hemorrhage, or a recent history of either. Slightly blood-tinged sputum may be an indication of infection or strain from coughing and is not considered a contraindication for percussion and vibration. |
|  | Excessive coughing | Cough suppressant for significant frank hemoptysis. Substitute huff technique. |
| Increased intracranial pressure | Head-dependent position | Postural drainage is contraindicated in patients with head injuries, recent neurosurgery, or preexisting conditions that cause increased intracranial pressure. |

minutes twice each day are recommended. Initially the sessions may take longer; however, as patients become more skilled in the technique, the sessions take less time.

### Exercise

Exercise enhances secretion clearance in several ways. Tidal volume, alveolar ventilation, and airflow velocity are increased, propelling secretions toward the oropharynx where they can be removed by coughing or swallowing. Ventilatory muscles may also be strengthened with exercise. Vigorous exercises such as swimming, jogging, and jumping rope have been advocated for patients with cystic fibrosis as important adjuncts to postural drainage with forced exhalation or percussion and vibration (Blomquist, 1986). Adolescents and young adults are often noncompliant with time-consuming postural drainage routines. Patients who are unwilling to perform postural drainage should be encouraged to use huffing, PEP, or autogenic drainage, in addition to exercise. Such patients must be monitored frequently for adequacy of secretion clearance, increasing airflow obstruction, and signs of respiratory tract infection. Patients with respiratory muscle weakness or end-stage disease who produce excessive secretions are not able to exercise as an adjunct to other methods of secretion clearance. These patients may benefit from such devices as incentive spirometers that encourage deep breathing. These are presented in Chapter 14.

### Suctioning

Patients who have tracheostomies, significant respiratory muscle weakness, or end-stage lung disease may require suctioning to clear secretions. Appropriate techniques for suctioning in the home are presented in Chapter 16.

## COMPLICATIONS OF TECHNIQUES TO ENHANCE SECRETION CLEARANCE

There are several potential complications of techniques to enhance secretion clearance. It is important for the home care nurse to be aware of them when helping the patient establish a bronchial hygiene routine. Potential complications and strategies to prevent them are presented in Table 7-3.

### REFERENCES

Aitken ML et al: Recombinant human DNase inhalation in normal subjects and patients with cystic fibrosis, *JAMA* 267:1947, 1992.

Blomquist M et al: Physical activity and self-treatment in cystic fibrosis, *Arch Dis Child* 61:362, 1986.

Braun SR et al: Improving the cough in patients with spinal cord injury, *Am J Phys Med* 63:1, 1984.

David A: Autogenic drainage—the German approach. In Pryor JA, editor: *Respiratory care,* Edinburgh, 1991, Churchill Livingston.

Kirilloff LH et al: Does chest physical therapy work? *Chest* 88:436, 1985.

Sackner MA: Cough. In Murray JF, Nadel JA, editors: *Textbook of respiratory medicine,* Philadelphia, 1988, WB Saunders.

Sutton PP et al: Assessment of the forced expiration technique, postural drainage and directed coughing in chest physiotherapy, *Eur J Respir Dis* 64:62, 1983.

Vandenplas Y et al: Esophageal pH monitoring data during chest physiotherapy, *J Pediatr Gastroenterol Nutr* 13:23, 1991.

### SUGGESTED READINGS

Dean E, Ross J: Discordance between cardiopulmonary physiology and physical therapy, *Chest* 101:1694, 1992.

Pryor JA, editor: *Respiratory care: International perspectives in physical therapy,* vol 7, New York, 1991, Churchill Livingstone.

# CHAPTER 8

# DYSPNEA

VIRGINIA CARRIERI-KOHLMAN • SUSAN JANSON-BJERKLIE

Breathlessness in the context of disease is called dyspnea and is the most common and disabling symptom suffered by patients with chronic lung disease, cancer of the lung, and many heart diseases. This distressing symptom occurs with enormous frequency in a wide variety of clinical states.

In the past there was a tendency to focus the clinical assessment and treatment on physiologic dysfunction, rather than the symptom of breathlessness. The assessment and management of breathlessness itself are important in the care of the patient with chronic lung disease. Underlying mechanisms of dyspnea, assessment techniques, and nursing interventions are presented in this chapter.

## ETIOLOGY
### Possible Causes for Dyspnea in Chronic Lung Disease

The mechanisms producing breathlessness are multifactorial, including personal, situational, and biological factors. Once triggered, dyspnea is generated through a complex series of steps involving the activation of sensory receptors, the transmission of sensory signals to the central nervous system (CNS), and the processing of those signals by higher brain centers.

Dyspnea occurs when an individual perceives a discrepancy between the demand to breathe and the amount of ventilation actually achieved. The circumstances that may produce such a discrepancy and cause dyspnea are summarized in Table 8-1.

## Precipitants Described by Patients

Any specific trigger may precipitate dyspnea for any one individual. Factors that precipitate dyspnea can be categorized as personal, situational, and physical activities (Janson-Bjerklie, Carrieri, and Hudes, 1986). Infection, abdominal distention, increased secretions, feeling too warm or too cold, fatigue, and alcohol or cigarette use are frequently reported physical conditions that precipitate dyspnea. Dyspnea can also be triggered by talking, eating, coughing, and laughing. Actual emotional arousal, either positive or negative (e.g., being upset, excited, angry, ecstatic, anxious, or depressed), may trigger breathlessness. Certain emotions, such as panic, anger, or worry, appear to be direct correlates of acute dyspnea. Whether emotions develop as a result of dyspnea or escalate the symptom, awareness of the contribution of emotions to the intensity and frequency of distress is important.

Stressful or high-pressure situations are described by patients as a frequent trigger of dyspnea. People with allergen-sensitive or extrinsic asthma may develop shortness of breath in different seasons from exposure to grasses and molds, pollen, animal dander, dust, or air pollutants. Characteristics of weather such as extreme heat and cold or wind and fog can also initiate dyspnea.

**Table 8-1**   Etiology of dyspnea in chronic lung disease

| Cause | Mechanism | Clinical situation |
|---|---|---|
| Increased effort of respiratory muscles | Stretching of muscle spindles and tendons in inspiratory muscles, resulting in afferent signals to CNS about relationship of work of breathing and resulting volume | Weakness of respiratory muscles; hyperinflation with chronic obstructive pulmonary disease, causing shortening of inspiratory muscles and decreased efficiency of contraction; increased airflow resistance; increased dead space ventilation from airflow to poorly perfused lung segments; atelectasis from shallow breathing, accumulation of sputum, and physical inactivity; pneumonia; cancer of lung; stimulation of afferent "J" receptors in alveolar-capillary interstitium; poor conditioning of muscles from total body deconditioning, malnutrition, and hypoxemia |
| Increased respiratory drive | Causes dyspnea directly by central perception of drive to breathe or indirectly through stimulation of respiratory muscles | Increased neural activity from peripheral and central chemoreceptors when $PaO_2$ and $PaCO_2$ abnormal; hypoxemia from wasted ventilation; anxiety, anger, pain; bronchospasm caused by stimulation of irritant receptors in airway; stimulation of "J" receptors in alveolar-capillary interstitium triggers drive to breathe in interstitial fibrosis and congestive heart failure |
| Changes in central perception | Variations in pattern of breathing | Anxiety, anger, depression; mechanical behavior such as yelling or crying may trigger dyspnea by reflex mechanisms |

## ASSESSMENT

Dyspnea is a subjective perception. Only people who experience the symptom can describe or quantify the degree of dyspnea. Shortness of breath is the term most commonly used by patients to describe their breathlessness. However, a variety of other terms may more accurately describe the sensation for some (Elliott et al, 1991). Patients should be encouraged to describe the sensation in their own words, and this terminology can then be used during follow-up visits. As with other symptoms, the assessment of dyspnea at initial and follow-up home visits is important. A valid and reliable initial measure of dyspnea intensity and frequency and its impact on the patient's life will allow an accurate picture of changes in functional ability and patterns over time. The traditional seven dimensions of symptoms presented in Chapter 1 can be used to obtain an accurate, thorough history of dyspnea. Important information includes the following:

- What words does the patient use to describe the sensation ("short of breath," "can't get any air," "hurts to breathe")?
- When is the symptom present (at rest, with exercise)?
- If the symptom is present only with exercise, how much exercise causes it to occur (walking up one flight of stairs; walking a half block on level ground)?
- What other factors cause dyspnea (position changes, coughing)?
- What is the severity of the symptom? Here a rating scale is useful.
- What makes the symptom better or worse?

What strategies does the patient use to decrease dyspnea?

- Are there any other sensations that accompany dyspnea (fatigue, anxiety)?

Dyspnea must be distinguished from other changes in breathing pattern such as tachypnea, hyperpnea, or hyperventilation. These changes in the pattern of ventilation may occur concurrently with dyspnea but are not synonymous with it. In addition, the relationship of dyspnea to commonly used measures of lung function, such as the $FEV_1$ or $PaO_2$, is only moderate at best. Therefore measures of pulmonary function cannot be used to measure or monitor the subjective symptom of dyspnea.

The threshold for the perception of dyspnea varies widely among patients. Similar to pain, dyspnea probably has an affective component—that is, the stimulus intensity may be the same among patients with similar lung pathology, but the distress or dyspnea felt may vary greatly.

## Behavioral Manifestations

Although dyspnea is a purely subjective sensation, the following behavioral manifestations may be observed by others:

- Increased respiratory rate
- Restlessness
- Diaphoresis
- Use of accessory muscles of respiration
- Tremulousness
- Gasping breaths
- Pallor
- Interrupted or "staccato" speech
- Large staring eyes
- Being quiet and withdrawn
- A frozen appearance
- Audible wheezing and coughing

## Physical and Emotional Sensations During Dyspnea

Physical sensations localized in the chest may be felt by patients during breathlessness; these and the emotional correlates of the sensations are important for the home care nurse to assess. These physical and emotional sensations are summarized in the box at left on p. 138. One of the most common physical sensations that dyspneic patients describe is fatigue. The degree of pervasive fatigue patients feel correlates clinically with increasing dyspnea. Indeed, some patients describe their dyspnea only in terms of fatigue. Whether fatigue provokes dyspnea or occurs as a result of dyspnea is unknown.

*Specific statements that children have made describing dyspnea and the physical symptoms and emotional sensations they feel are presented in the box at right on p. 138. Necessary changes in activity as the result of breathlessness are upsetting to children, as is evident in quotations such as "it ruins my whole day" and "I can't play with anybody"* (Carrieri et al, 1991).

## Prodromal Indicators of Dyspnea

Patients may or may not have some sense that an episode of dyspnea is approaching. Prodromal sensations in the chest that have been reported by patients include the following:

- Congestion
- Cough
- Chest tightness
- Parched sensation
- Fever, chills
- Clammy sensation
- Flushed sensation
- Euphoria
- Depression
- Anxiety
- Change in behavior, such as in taking a higher dose of medication

## Dyspnea Severity or Intensity

To measure the patient's perception of the intensity of dyspnea several instruments may be useful.

### Visual Analogue Scale

The Visual Analogue Scale (VAS) (Wewers, 1990) is a vertical or horizontal line of a measured distance (10 cm or 100 mm). The scale is anchored at either end of the line by descriptive words, such

## Physical and Emotional Sensations During Dyspnea

**PHYSICAL SENSATIONS**

Suffocation
Chest tightness
Pain
Congestion
Associated generalized sensations: fatigue, gastrointestinal distress, palpitations, flushing, concentration and memory problems, vertigo

**EMOTIONAL SENSATIONS**

Anxiety
Anger
Claustrophobic reactions
Worry
Panic

## Indicators of Dyspnea in Children

**DESCRIPTIONS**

"Can hardly breathe"
"Fighting to get my breath in and out"
"Wheezy"
"Struggling to breathe"

**PHYSICAL SYMPTOMS**

Vomiting
Hurting
Vibrating chest
Stomach bubbles
Tired

**EMOTIONAL SENSATIONS**

Mad
Scared
Upset
Uncomfortable
Feeling rotten

From Carrieri VK et al: *Nurs Res* 40:81, 1991.

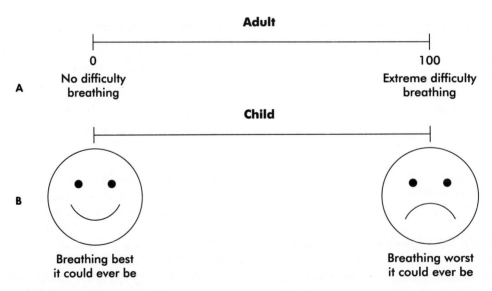

**Fig. 8-1** The 100 mm Visual Analogue Scales (VAS) for measuring intensity of dyspnea. **A,** Adult. **B,** Child.

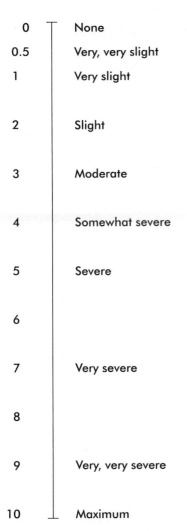

| 0 | None |
| 0.5 | Very, very slight |
| 1 | Very slight |
| 2 | Slight |
| 3 | Moderate |
| 4 | Somewhat severe |
| 5 | Severe |
| 6 | |
| 7 | Very severe |
| 8 | |
| 9 | Very, very severe |
| 10 | Maximum |

**Fig. 8-2** Modified Borg Scale for measuring perceived breathlessness. (From Borg G: *Med Sci Sports Exerc* 14:377-381, 1982.)

as "not at all breathless" and "extremely breathless" (or whatever specific words the patient uses to describe the sensation). The patient marks a slash on the line at the point representing the degree of breathlessness felt. The VAS is both reliable and valid, and it is sensitive enough to detect small changes in the intensity of dyspnea. *Children can rate their shortness of breath on a modified VAS,*

*with a happy and sad face as anchors (Fig. 8-1).* Two VAS scales can be used, one to measure dyspnea intensity and another to measure the distress the symptom causes the patient, a model that has been used to measure pain.

### Modified Borg Scale

The Modified Borg Scale (Fig. 8-2) is a 10-point categoric scale that ranks breathlessness from "none at all" to "maximal." This scale can be used to report the usual daily dyspnea or the intensity of the symptom during specific activities in or outside the home.

### Exercise Walking Test

The 6- and 12-minute distance (6 MD and 12 MD) walking tests can be used to evaluate the degree of breathlessness associated with exercise performance and are simple, reproducible methods for assessing exercise tolerance when sophisticated equipment is unavailable. It should be remembered that these tests measure exercise or functional ability, not dyspnea itself; however, dyspnea can be measured at the end of the test. The use of exercise walking tests in the home is presented in Chapter 9.

## NURSING INTERVENTIONS

Therapies are directed at decreasing dyspnea by altering one or more of the proposed etiologic factors.

### Decreasing the Sense of Increased Respiratory Muscle Effort
#### Energy Conservation

Teach and encourage patients to use strategies to conserve energy, simplify work, and pace themselves. The nurse should always consider referring the patient to an occupational therapist if dyspnea interferes significantly with the patient's activities of daily living. Strategies for pacing and energy conservation are presented in the box on pp. 140 and 141. Strategies for reducing dyspnea while eating are discussed in Chapter 11 and during sexual activity in Chapter 19.

# Strategies for Work Simplification and Energy Conservation

## GENERAL WORK SIMPLIFICATION

Always use breathing control while walking.

Sit during as many activities as possible.

Use slow, smooth, flowing movements. Rushing only increases discomfort.

Organize activities and try to do them in the same manner at all times. Repetition of the same methods will increase proficiency and save time and energy.

Organize work space. Plan ahead and position tools. Throw away things that are not used.

Preplan activities. Try a daily or weekly schedule.
Is there too much to do on any day?
Are heavy tasks alternated with light ones?
Are heavy tasks distributed throughout the week?
Are there plans for other members of the family?
Each person should know what he or she has to do for the household and when.

Evaluate activities. It is not necessary always to do things the same way.
Can the task be broken into steps?
Can any steps be eliminated?

Do not carry equipment if it can be pushed. Slide, do not lift; push, do not pull. Maintain good posture. Bend at the knees, not at the waist. Eliminate unnecessary motions.

Consider the best time for each activity. If morning is the most difficult time, do as much as possible the evening before. For example, bathe in the evening instead of the morning.

Always exhale with the strenuous part of the activity or with the part of activity requiring motion toward the body. Use the pursed lip technique when exhaling.

A slow, steady rate of work with short rest periods will get the job done with less fatigue. Remember that fast walking takes one and a half times as much energy as slow walking; walking up stairs takes seven times as much energy as walking on level ground.

## REST

Frequent short rest periods are of more benefit than fewer long rests. They prevent undue fatigue and allow more energy for other activities. Stop working and rest before exhaustion.

## DISTRIBUTION OF WORKLOAD

Heavy work for short periods may require too much energy at one time. Avoid straining and do not try to do a two-man job alone.

## PHYSICAL CONDITIONING

It pays to keep in good physical condition through regular, moderate activity.

## COOKING AND MEAL PREPARATION

Sit as much as possible. Avoid overreaching. Avoid unnecessary steps and processes.

Gather all necessary food and utensils from cupboards and refrigerator. Use recommended breathing pattern for reaching up into cupboard, inhaling when raising arms and exhaling when bringing arms down. Also exhale when stooping to lower cupboards. Break this activity into steps if necessary.

After all necessary items have been placed on counter or cart, transfer them to work area where it is possible to sit at a table or at a counter with a high kitchen stool.

Try to work with arms close to body.

Allow plenty of time to prepare meals to avoid rushing. Extra time will allow for rest periods if needed.

Set the table in the same manner used for gathering items for meal preparation. If table is small, stay in one position to set the table. If reaching across the table causes difficulty, inhale when extending arms across the table and exhale when returning arms to body. If the table is large, set one side at a time.

Use an electric mixer, if one is available, rather than mixing by hand.

Use paper napkins instead of linen ones and placemats instead of a tablecloth.

Prepare extra portions of food and freeze the excess for future use. Use prepared, frozen, or prepackaged foods and one-dish casseroles.

Serve food in baking dishes to avoid an excess of dirty dishes.

Use aluminum foil and oven bags when possible to eliminate unnecessary scrubbing.

Soak pots in hot water and detergent to eliminate need for vigorous scouring.

Wash dishes while sitting on a high kitchen stool, opening the cupboard beneath to allow for leg room. Scalding the dishes and allowing them to air dry will eliminate the need for towel drying. Rest before returning dishes to cupboard.

If possible, use the counter to slide heavy pots and other articles to avoid unnecessary carrying. If objects must be carried, use both hands and keep objects close to body.

# Strategies for Work Simplification and Energy Conservation—cont'd

## CLEANING

Allow the entire day for large cleaning projects.

Clean one room at a time and do not be distracted by another room that also needs cleaning.

Use a long-handled dustpan and sponge mop to clean floors. Use tongs to pick up objects from the floor. Inhale while pushing the mop away and exhale while pulling it toward body. Use the same breathing pattern while vacuuming.

Dusting may cause difficulty because the dust itself may be an irritant or contain allergens. Do not use spray wax because this may also be an irritant. Instead, use a cream or paste wax for polishing furniture. Some dusting may be done while sitting. Work in a pattern around the room.

Windows can be washed using the recommended breathing pattern when reaching is necessary. Do not use spray cleaner; water and vinegar work as well. A long-handled squeegee with a rubber blade will minimize reaching.

When objects must be moved from the room being cleaned, put them in a basket or on a rolling tea cart for later distribution. Do not run from one room to another when cleaning.

If furniture must be moved, have someone else move it.

Cleaning out cupboards can also be done using a systemized technique. Use a pattern of inhaling to reach and exhaling as objects are brought down, and vice versa. Again, avoid spray cleaners.

Remember to organize activities throughout the week, thus saving energy and reducing fatigue. Always work in a slow, methodical pattern. Take note of the motions used and see if any can be eliminated or revised to make work easier.

Organize your home, keeping items in the most convenient places and always returning them there.

## BEDMAKING

Start to make bed before getting up by pulling covers up snugly, then folding them back on one side, just enough to get up, *or*

Make one side of the bed at a time. When changing bed linen, put the bottom sheet, top sheet, blanket, and spread on before tucking in overhang.

When shaking out or smoothing bed linen, inhale while extending arms and exhale while pulling toward body.

Stoop instead of bending at the waist, and sit whenever possible.

Install casters or rollers on legs of bed if possible, but be sure to lock them when not moving bed.

The bed will be easier to make if only the head is against the wall.

Lightweight and electric blankets are easier to move than heavy bedclothes. Down comforters are warm and lightweight, and they eliminate the need for extra blankets.

## WASHING AND IRONING

If possible, use a rolling laundry cart. Sort clothes on a table, not on the floor.

If laundry facilities are in the basement, keep a chair for waiting in the area to avoid frequent trips up and down the stairs.

Put front-loading washer on blocks to raise the opening and thus eliminate unnecessary bending.

Always sit to iron with the board at lap level.

Slide the iron, do not lift it or set it on end. Place it on an asbestos pad while adjusting clothes on the board.

Do not iron clothes unnecessarily. Sheets, towels, and underwear can be folded instead of being ironed. Select wrinkle-free or synthetic fabrics for wardrobe.

Organize the distribution of ironed or dried clothing so that only one trip is necessary.

## BATHING AND DRESSING

Showers take less energy than baths. Sit on a stool in the shower.

Bathe with lukewarm water instead of hot water, which generates steam and makes some people feel short of breath.

Use oxygen, if prescribed, while bathing.

Use a terry robe instead of drying with towel.

Use hair dryer to dry between toes.

Gather all clothes and accessories together and sit while dressing.

Tools for putting on socks or shoes, electric tooth brushes, and grab rails in the bathroom can be used to decrease the work of breathing.

Velcro fasteners, loose-fitting clothes, front-opening clothes, and slip-on shoes require less energy to don.

Dress the lower part of the body first because this takes more energy. Try not to bend over, but bring feet up instead.

Modified from Wilson B: *Pacing and energy conservation in pulmonary rehabilitation,* Occupational Therapy Department Rehabilitation Center, General Hospital of Port Arthur, Thunder Bay, Ontario, Canada.

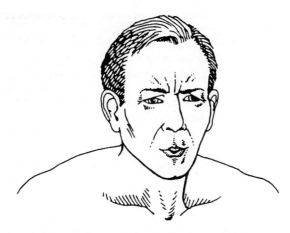

**Fig. 8-3**   Pursed-lip breathing. (From Phipps WJ et al: *Medical-surgical nursing: concepts and clinical practice,* ed 4, St Louis, 1991, Mosby.)

### Pursed Lip Breathing

Pursed lip breathing (Fig. 8-3) decreases dyspnea in some patients, probably because it makes them breathe in more slowly and exhale more completely, thereby decreasing the respiratory rate and increasing the tidal volume (Lareau and Larson, 1987). This type of breathing adds slight positive pressure to the airways during exhalation, which may decrease air trapping by preventing the collapse of some of the small airways that typically occurs during exhalation. Patients should be instructed to perform the following:

1. Inhale normally through the nose.
2. Purse lips as if about to whistle.
3. Exhale slowly and gently through pursed lips.

If patients are unable to purse their lips, they can be instructed to exhale through a fist held up to their mouths. Patients are often instructed to count to two while inhaling and to four while exhaling. Although exhalation should take at least twice as long as inhalation, instructions that require a patient to artificially alter the natural inspiratory time or to concentrate on counting may inhibit the respiratory pattern instead. It is usually more effective to simply reinforce a long, slow, gentle exhalation and let inspiration "take care of itself." Patients should be warned not to breathe too deeply, which can cause dizziness. They should also be taught not to exhale too vigorously because forced exhalations increase airway collapse and may trigger bronchospasm.

Most patients with chronic lung disease adopt a pursed lip breathing pattern naturally, indicating that it is a physiologically adaptive response. However, many need some instruction in the correct technique, and most need coaching to use pursed lip breathing with increased dyspnea and to coordinate it with specific activities.

### Paced Breathing

Paced breathing is the coordination of inspiration and pursed lip breathing on expiration with activities such as walking, stair climbing, bending, and lifting. Activities are paced to match the ventilatory capacity, and the patient is instructed to (1) breathe in while at rest before performing a strenuous activity such as lifting an object and (2) exhale slowly and gently through pursed lips while doing the work. The patient should be encouraged to focus on the prolonged exhalation and should be explicitly warned against breath holding while exerting. Holding the breath while exerting constitutes a Valsalva-like maneuver that increases intrathoracic pressure and impairs cardiac return, contributing to a subsequent drop in cardiac output that can increase dyspnea and perceived effort.

Instruction in the use of pursed lip breathing with stair climbing is an excellent way to reinforce the value of pacing and coordinated breathing. Patients should be instructed to inhale while standing at rest before climbing stairs and exhale as they slowly climb one, two, or three steps. They should stop to inhale, then exhale as they slowly climb again. When they become stronger or exertional dyspnea decreases over time, they may progress to climbing the full flight of stairs without rest stops. However, they should always use pursed lip breathing on exhalation as they climb. Patients need to practice these strategies with the nurse or therapist, and the pursed lip breathing technique should be reinforced during home health care visits.

## Diaphragmatic Breathing

Diaphragmatic breathing has long been a component of rehabilitation training for the patient with chronic obstructive lung disease, although scientific evidence of its physiologic efficacy is lacking. In diaphragmatic breathing, breathing is performed in such a way as to maximize diaphragmatic excursion in preference to increasing the use of accessory muscles of respiration. Theoretically, this is helpful only for patients who can demonstrate at least minimal diaphragmatic excursion on physical examination. It is unlikely to be useful for the patient with a low fixed diaphragm, although some still find this type of breathing relaxing, calming, and useful during either relaxation exercises or panic control. The reduced abdominal volume that results from an inward movement of the abdominal wall (with or without active tightening of abdominal muscles) presumably forces the abdominal contents upward against the diaphragm, passively assisting upward diaphragmatic excursion.

Diaphragmatic breathing instruction may focus on either front expansion or lower side rib breathing. Specific instructions for the patient for front expansion are the following (Golemb, 1983):

1. Assume a comfortable position, either lying down or reclining on a comfortable chair.
2. Place the right hand on the center of the stomach and the left hand on the upper chest to help detect movement of the diaphragm and the accessory muscles of breathing.
3. Inhale through the nose and feel the abdomen rise gently as the diaphragm moves downward.
4. Purse the lips and exhale slowly while feeling the stomach muscles draw the abdomen inward.
5. Rest.

There are two alternate methods of diaphragmatic breathing: (1) lace the fingers of both hands across the abdomen, pressing in with the hands during exhalation to maximize abdominal excursion, *or* (2) place a book on the upper abdomen so that the desired abdominal movement is made more obvious to the patient who can readily see the book rise and fall with each breath.

The patient should be given specific instructions for lower side rib breathing (Moser et al, 1983):

1. Assume a comfortable sitting position and put the hands on the sides at the base of the ribs.
2. Breathe out slowly through pursed lips while the ribs move inward.
3. Breathe in slowly through the nose and allow the ribs to expand outwardly against the hands.
4. Rest.

Lower side rib breathing presumably assists diaphragmatic excursion by enhancing the movement of the ribs to which the diaphragm is attached.

The potential yet unconfirmed benefits of diaphragmatic breathing include increased tidal volume, decreased oxygen cost of breathing, and less dyspnea (Hodgkin, 1984). However, it may be that the perceived benefits of diaphragmatic breathing have more to do with pursed lip breathing or general relaxation than with any specific effect on the diaphragm. It is also possible that the use of abdominal muscle contraction to "assist" the upward excursion of the diaphragm actually adds to the overall work of breathing.

As with any intervention of unknown merit, a pragmatic approach is probably best. If instruction in diaphragmatic breathing appears to offer the patient some relief of dyspnea, it should be encouraged; if not, it should be abandoned.

## Inspiratory Muscle Training

Training to strengthen inspiratory muscles may decrease the sensation of dyspnea in patients with weakened respiratory muscles who do not have severe hyperinflation (Harver, Mahler, and Daubenspeck, 1989). Techniques for ventilatory muscle training are discussed in Chapter 9.

## Position Changes

Patients with COPD often position themselves in the forward leaning position when they feel dyspneic. This position may be achieved while sitting by leaning forward with the arms supported on a table or the arms of a chair (tripod position). These positions stabilize the upper chest, while still allowing freedom of movement of the lower chest.

The leaning forward position permits the abdominal organs to drop away from the diaphragm and may decrease assessory muscle use, thus producing subjective relief of dyspnea by permitting better diaphragmatic excursion and improving the diaphragm's length-tension ratio. Patients should be advised to choose the most comfortable position for each activity and to sit down whenever possible and avoid bending or stooping. Many patients discover for themselves their "best" position and should be encouraged to assume this position whenever dyspnea increases. It is important to recognize that patients usually assume the position of most comfort and physiologic benefit to their breathing (Lareau and Larson, 1987).

### Exercises

Physical reconditioning or total body exercise training improves exercise tolerance and decreases dyspnea. Exercises may help reduce the sensation of dyspnea by building up the strength of particular muscles and reducing the oxygen consumption of muscles. Exercises for the home care patient are presented in Chapter 9.

### Medications

Bronchodilators and corticosteroids may be administered to reduce the effort of breathing and to relieve the sensation of dyspnea when reversible bronchoconstriction is present. When airflow obstruction is irreversible, medications such as narcotics are sometimes used to depress the perception of dyspnea. The use and benefits of medications for airflow obstruction are discussed in Chapters 5 and 6.

## Decreasing Respiratory Drive

Treatments that decrease respiratory drive such as supplemental oxygen and oral narcotics have been used for the treatment of other disease processes in the past and currently are being studied to determine their use for the relief of dyspnea.

### Oxygen Therapy

Oxygen as a treatment for dyspnea per se is in the experimental phases of study. Clinically, hypoxemic patients may experience a significant reduction in dyspnea and an increase in their quality of life when on a regimen of low-flow oxygen. However, not all hypoxemic patients experience reduced dyspnea with oxygen. Although the value of oxygen therapy is accepted in chronically hypoxemic patients, the value of oxygen for the relief of dyspnea when the $PaO_2$ is above 55 to 60 mm Hg is less apparent. In a British study, however, supplemental oxygen was shown to increase walking distance and improve exercise-induced dyspnea in patients with near normal resting $PaO_2$ values (Woodcock, Gross, and Geddes, 1981). More controlled studies are needed to identify those patients whose dyspnea decreases with oxygen. It may be helpful to increase the oxygen flow rate during exertion in patients who desaturate with exercise.

### Oral Narcotics

Opiates decrease the perception of breathlessness and increase exercise tolerance (Light et al, 1989). This type of therapy is still considered experimental. Potential benefits such as decreased respiratory drive, improved efficiency of exercise, and decreased dyspnea may be offset clinically by the risk of respiratory depression and side effects, although the actual incidence of respiratory depression has been low in most studies. If opiates are prescribed for severe dyspnea, the patient should start with a low dose (5 mg of hydrocodone or 30 mg of codeine) three times a day and, if necessary, increase the dose slowly with constant supervision until there is a measured decrease in dyspnea (Stulberg, 1986). Morphine sulfate has long been a standard treatment for pain in end-stage lung cancer patients. The efficacy of this medication in relieving severe dyspnea in lung cancer or end-stage pulmonary disease is being studied and is often used to relieve intractable dyspnea as death nears.

## Altering the Central Perception of Breathlessness

Management strategies that help to decrease the perception of dyspnea may be successful clinically. Similar to pain, strategies that help the patient to feel in control of the symptom or to distract them from the symptom seem to decrease the sensation.

### Desensitization

One approach to "desensitizing" the patient to exertional dyspnea is to encourage ambulation to the point that severe dyspnea occurs, coaching the patient, breath by breath, in pursed lip breathing techniques until comfort is regained (Levine, Weiser, and Gillen, 1986). If this technique is done in a supportive environment with someone the patient trusts, the fear of dyspnea decreases and patients gain confidence in their ability to control the symptom through their own actions. It is also important to teach spouses or significant others to coach the patient so they can reinforce the pursed lip breathing techniques while the patient's skill and confidence are increasing. Few controlled research studies have tested this intervention independently. Such strategies have been studied primarily within large pulmonary rehabilitation programs.

### Panic Control Measures

The panic that may accompany the sensation of dyspnea often exacerbates the sensation. It may be possible to help the patient control panic by permitting initial rapid, panting respirations, then by gradually coaching the patient, breath by breath, to slow the respiratory rate by extending the expiratory time. The coaching should continue until the patient relaxes.

### Distraction

Although as yet unstudied in patients with chronic lung disease, the use of distraction as a means of decreased awareness of dyspnea holds some promise. Examples of distractors include performing mental arithmetic, simple physical tasks such as moving objects into different positions, listening to music, or watching television.

### Relaxation Techniques

When anxiety and apprehension augment dyspnea, patients with COPD may benefit from relaxation techniques that can reduce emotional stress. In the laboratory, biofeedback and relaxation have reduced respiratory rates and increased tidal volumes in some patients (Sitzman, 1983). Relaxation techniques can be used on a daily basis or in panic control situations alone. Most types of relaxation include the following components:

- A quiet environment, with or without soft, slow music
- A comfortable position in bed or in a comfortable chair
- Loose, nonrestrictive clothing
- Breathing with slow, abdominal breathing, using relaxed pursed lip breathing

Relaxation techniques often incorporate some type of word or imagery that is repeated or thought in a systematic fashion over and over again. Another approach is the Jacobsen method in which the patient tightens specific muscles in sequence (e.g., moving from feet, legs, pelvis, chest, arms, and finally to the face), holds and concentrates on the tension, and then slowly relaxes while feeling the tension leave the muscles (Sexton, 1987). The patient can also be encouraged to routinely relax a certain part of his body, such as the shoulders and neck muscles, using exercises such as shoulder shrugging, elbow circling, and head circling. A variety of specific relaxation training strategies are available and published in detail (Sexton, 1987). It is important to practice these techniques in a step-by-step manner with the patient and to reinforce them with each visit. Twenty-minute sessions twice a day are suggested. Relaxation tapes are an effective tool to reinforce training. These are available commercially, but they may be even more effective if the nurse records an actual home care training session for the patient to use on his or her own.

Other psychophysiologic techniques used clinically for dyspnea control include visual imagery, biofeedback, and transcendental meditation. These strategies must be individualized for the patient; some patients are helped by meditation, others have their own methods of relaxation and can be encouraged to practice their technique every day so that they are prepared to use it in situations of severe dyspnea. The use of guided imagery is discussed in Chapter 22.

## Adult Self-Care Strategies for Managing Dyspnea

**IMMEDIATE STRATEGIES**

Position and motion
  Move slower
  Lie down or sit
  Keep still: stay quiet
  Positioning
Breathing strategies
  Diaphragmatic breathing
  Relaxation techniques
  Pursed lip breathing
Physical distancing from aggravating factor
  Self-selected medications
  Acute self-isolation
  Tension-reduction strategies
  Seeking social support
  Distraction-diversion

**LONG-TERM ADAPTIVE CHANGES**

Changes in activities of daily living (ADLs)
  Changes in methods of dressing, bathing, and
    eating
  Use of devices
  Transfer of ADLs to others
  Change in living arrangement

Activity modification
  Advanced planning
  Change in time of activity
  Planned decrease in activity
  Establishing "breathing stations"
Health-directed behaviors
  Exercise
  Weight control if obese
  Change job to one less taxing
  Self-selected treatments
  Relaxant drugs
  Adjusting medications
Home remedies
  Fans for better ventilation
Protective behaviors
  Leaving smoke-filled room
  Asking others not to smoke
  Not going to high altitudes
  Emphasizing the positive
  Distancing self from emotional situations or feel-
    ings
Tension-reduction
Social self-isolation
Seeking social support

### Patient-Reported Strategies

■ *Adults.* Strategies that adults have reported as helping them control their dyspnea are summarized in the box above (Janson-Bjerklie, Carrieri, and Hudes, 1986). Many of these strategies have already been discussed.

■ *School-Age Children. When questioned about strategies they use when their "breathing feels bad," children with asthma have been able to identify the following techniques (Carrieri et al, 1991):*

• *Self-adjusting medications*
• *Taking fluids*
• *Seeking out another person or place for assistance*
• *Altering physical activity, posture, or environment*

• *Resting or sleeping*
• *Changing position*
• *Going inside or outside*
• *Doing breathing exercises and chest percussion*
• *Coughing and breathing deeply*
• *Relaxing or reducing emotional activity*
• *Doing activities that are distracting*
• *Trying not to think about breathing*

### Education

Although the effect of education on dyspnea is unknown, knowledge has been shown to decrease anxiety, fear, and other symptoms. Clinical observations confirm that, when patients are given information about their illness or dyspnea management, their anxiety and related symptoms decrease. Clinically, it has been observed that the perception of personal self-efficacy or control does help buffer pain, and presumably this is also true of dyspnea. Knowledge may decrease dyspnea by increasing the patients' belief that they can control the symptom with the techniques they have learned.

An organized problem-solving approach should be used with patients to help them develop strategies to cope with dyspnea. The nurse and patient should build on what the patient does for himself or herself to decrease shortness of breath, extending and expanding these skills with strategies known by the clinician and used by other patients. Describing the sensations related to dyspnea helps patients believe they have control by clarifying what they should expect, by showing them how important their role is in decreasing the symptom, by finding meaning in the symptom for them, and by acknowledging the importance of techniques they have learned on their own.

Patients should be taught about the nature of the symptom itself and the pathophysiologic processes that may be the reason for the onset of their dyspnea. As with all coping strategies, knowledge about medications and the role of each drug in decreasing dyspnea is important because patients often manipulate multiple medications on a daily basis. Education during subsequent visits should include all strategies previously described, such as pursed lip breathing, breathing exercises, energy conservation, graduated exercise regimens, relaxation, and panic control. Most important is listening to the patient and family to give them information about their concerns, to answer questions they may have about what they can do and how short of breath they can be, and to support any strategies they have developed on their own.

## REFERENCES

Borg G: Psychophysical basis of perceived exertion, *Med Sci Sports Exerc* 14:377, 1982.

Carrieri VK et al: The sensation of pulmonary dyspnea in school-age children, *Nurs Res* 40:81, 1991.

Elliott MW et al: The language of breathlessness, *Am Rev Respir Dis* 144:826, 1991.

Golemb K: *Better breathers club panic control workbook,* ed 3, San Diego, 1983, California College of Respiratory Therapy.

Harver A, Mahler DA, Daubenspeck JA: Targeted inspiratory muscle training improves respiratory muscle function and reduces dyspnea in patients with chronic obstructive pulmonary disease, *Ann Intern Med* 111:117, 1989.

Hodgkin JE, Zorn EG, Connors GL: *Pulmonary rehabilitation: guidelines to success,* Boston, 1984, Butterworth.

Janson-Bjerklie S, Carrieri VK, Hudes M: The sensations of pulmonary dyspnea, *Nurs Res* 35:154, 1986.

Lareau S, Larson JL: Ineffective breathing pattern related to airflow limitation, *Nurs Clin North Am* 22:179, 1987.

Levine S, Weiser P, Gillen J: Evaluation of a ventilatory muscle endurance training program in the rehabilitation of patients with chronic obstructive pulmonary disease, *Am Rev Respir Dis* 133:400, 1986.

Light RW et al: Effects of oral morphine on breathlessness and exercise tolerance in patients with chronic obstructive pulmonary disease, *Am Rev Respir Dis* 139:126, 1989.

Moser K et al: *Shortness of breath: a guide to better living and breathing,* St Louis, 1983, Mosby.

Sexton DL: Relaxation techniques and biofeedback. In Hodgkin JE, Petty TE, editors: *Chronic obstructive pulmonary disease: current concepts,* Philadelphia, 1987, WB Saunders.

Sitzman J et al: Biofeedback training for reduced respiratory rate in chronic obstructive pulmonary disease: a preliminary study, *Nurs Res* 32:218, 1983.

Stulbarg MSL: Treatment of dyspnea: a physiological approach. In Sbarbaro JA: *Clinical challenge in cardiopulmonary medicine: a continuing education series from the American College of Chest Physicians,* 1986, American College of Chest Physicians.

Wewers ME, Lowe NK: A critical review of visual analogue scales in the measurement of clinical phenomena, *Res Nurs Health* 13:227, 1990.

Woodcock AA et al: Oxygen relieves breathlessness in "pink puffers," *Lancet* 1:907, 1981.

## SUGGESTED READINGS

Carrieri VK, Janson-Bjerklie S: Strategies patients use to manage the sensation of dyspnea, *West J Nurs Res* 8:284, 1986.

Gift AG: Dyspnea, *Nurs Clin North Am* 25:955, 1990.

Mahler DA, editor: *Dyspnea,* Mt Kisco, NY, 1990, Futura.

Sweer L, Zwillich CW: Dyspnea in the patient with chronic obstructive pulmonary disease: etiology and management, *Clin Chest Med* 11:417, 1990.

# CHAPTER 9

# ACTIVITY TOLERANCE

JANET JONES • THEDA RICKERSON-WONG

Adults and children with chronic lung disease should remain physically active despite their lung disease, yet the cycle of dyspnea and progressive deconditioning often physically limits patients beyond what their disease state warrants. The purpose of this chapter is to identify the causes of reduced activity tolerance in patients with chronic lung disease, to emphasize the importance of exercise, and to present exercise programs that can be readily implemented in the home. Simple exercise techniques and encouragement from home care staff can help patients become more active with less dyspnea, feel more in control of their disease, and enjoy life more fully.

Many individuals with chronic lung disease gradually limit their activity to avoid the frightening dyspnea that often occurs with physical exertion. This avoidance of activity leads to a downward spiral of deconditioning with worsening dyspnea at ever decreasing levels of activity (Fig. 9-1). Unless intervention reverses this trend, deconditioning can and often does progress until the individual becomes a "respiratory cripple."

## ETIOLOGY
## Exercise Response in Chronic Obstructive Pulmonary Disease

Because of altered lung mechanics, individuals with chronic lung disease differ from normal individuals in their work of breathing, response to exercise, and training adaptations to an exercise program. Work of breathing for patients with chronic obstructive pulmonary disease (COPD) may be 10 to 20 times greater than for a normal person, even at rest. During exercise the cost of breathing is further magnified, with the respiratory muscles alone consuming up to 40% of the oxygen available for the entire body. The etiologic factors of this increase in work of breathing in COPD are summarized in Table 9-1.

Unlike in normal individuals, ventilation is the limiting factor to exercise for patients with advanced COPD. During exercise, COPD patients often reach their maximum voluntary ventilation long before they achieve their maximum cardiac output; thus breathlessness often becomes intolerable before a normal target heart rate is reached. In this situation the intensity of exercise required to achieve cardiac and skeletal muscle conditioning is not possible and the training effects noted in normal individuals are often not seen.

## Exercise Response in Asthma

Individuals with asthma often have a completely reversible disease; that is, pulmonary function values are normal in the absence of an acute exacerbation. However, exercise itself can trigger bronchospasm in patients with asthma. Indeed, a specific protocol of quick, intensive exercise with an immediate stop is often used to diagnose asthma. The characteristic pattern in exercise-induced bronchospasm (EIB) in the patient not receiving med-

**Table 9-1** Etiologic factors of increased work of breathing in obstructive lung disease

| Pathophysiology | Alteration in mechanics |
| --- | --- |
| Destruction of lung parenchyma | Small airway collapse on exhalation; hyperinflation |
| Flattened diaphragm | Mechanical disadvantage causes less effective contraction; inspiratory muscles of rib cage and expiratory muscles assume more active role in respiration (Martinez, 1990) |
| Hyperinflation | Reduced elastic recoil of lungs and chest wall; requires active contraction of abdominal muscles for exhalation |

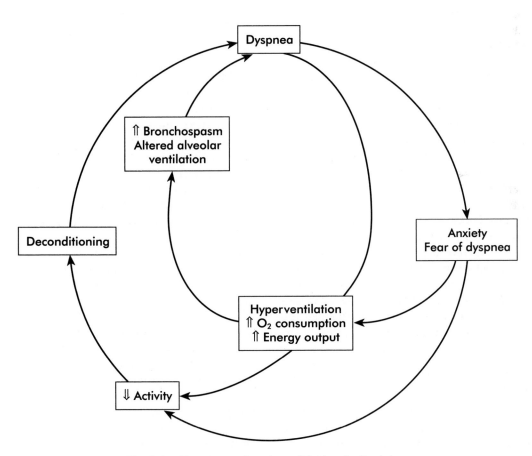

**Fig. 9-1**   Dyspnea-anxiety deconditioning feedback loops.

**Table 9-2**    Exercise tests

| Type of test | Rationale | Advantages |
| --- | --- | --- |
| Informal (6- or 12-min walking test) | Establish exercise prescription; basis to compare tests and monitor progress | Permits observation of patient during exercise in his usual setting; inexpensive; takes minimal time and equipment; nonthreatening to patient |
| Formal (bicycle, treadmill with continuous cardiopulmonary monitoring) | Establish diagnosis; identify and quantitate exercise limitation; establish disability status; monitor electrocardiograph for abnormality; monitor oxygen saturation; establish exercise prescription | Provides more information on physiologic response to exercise; emergency equipment available if adverse response to exercise; may provide objective evidence of need for less strenuous work; facilitates vocational counseling and retraining |

ication is bronchodilation during early exercise, followed by bronchoconstriction several minutes after exercise is stopped. Individuals with EIB often try to avoid breathlessness by avoiding exercise and fall into the same "dyspnea-deconditioning" cycle as those with COPD.

### Exercise Response in Restrictive Lung Disease

Whereas obstructive disease limits exercise by reducing airflow, restrictive disease limits exercise by preventing full lung or chest wall excursion. When patients with restrictive lung disease exercise, tidal volume cannot increase beyond a given level and the individual compensates by increasing the respiratory rate. However, the increased respiratory rate only partially compensates for the reduced tidal volume, and exercise becomes limited by ventilation. During exercise the patient with restrictive lung disease may breathe at rates of 50 breaths per minute or more with tidal volumes that may equal total inspiratory capacity. This degree of tachypnea is not seen in normal individuals and, when observed, suggests the presence of restrictive disease.

### ASSESSMENT

It is important to evaluate the patient's exercise ability before an exercise-training program is prescribed. This initial evaluation often can be made informally in the patient's home using pulse oximetry to monitor oxyhemoglobin desaturation during exercise and to help differentiate fatigue caused by deconditioning from that due to desaturation. Many patients with COPD can improve ventilation-perfusion matching and oxygen saturation during exercise; however, a significant number experience desaturation. Patients who experience desaturation with exercise are limited in the amount and intensity of exercise they can perform unless supplemental oxygen is prescribed. Pulse oximetry can also be used to determine the amount of supplemental oxygen needed to restore oxygen saturation to an acceptable level.

A referral for formal laboratory exercise testing can provide helpful information for the home care provider. Formal testing establishes safe heart rate limits and may identify exercise-induced dysrhythmias or ischemic electrocardiographic changes that could place the patient at increased risk. Formal and informal exercise tests appear in Table 9-2.

## Timed Walking Tests

The timed walking test is a simple and inexpensive measure of exercise capacity and can readily be carried out in the home (McGavin, 1978). A section of the patient's house (ideally, a long hallway or room) is measured, and increments of 10 feet are marked with masking tape. Patients then are asked to walk as far as possible in either 12 minutes (12-minute walking test) or 6 minutes (6-minute walking test). They are instructed to stop and rest if severe dyspnea occurs but to resume walking as soon as dyspnea has subsided; they should walk at the fastest comfortable pace, continuing to the end of the time period. Heart rate is recorded at baseline and during and at the completion of the test. If the patient's heart rate becomes irregular or if other symptoms such as dizziness or chest pain develop, testing should be discontinued. The distance covered during the allotted time is calculated and the average pace is recorded in feet per minute. This initial walking rate establishes the pace at which the patient feels comfortable, and the distance walked can serve as the basis for the initial home exercise "prescription." The goal is to increase the pace and duration of walking as the patient's exercise tolerance improves. Serial walking tests allow patients to see the progress they have made during their exercise programs. The addition of pulse oximetry provides valuable information concerning oxygen desaturation with exercise and should be done routinely if an oximeter can be obtained for home use.

## NURSING INTERVENTIONS

The role of the home care nurse in improving the exercise capacity of the deconditioned respiratory patient can be summarized as follows:

- Determine the baseline exercise capacity.
- Develop an exercise plan in consultation with the patient's physician, especially when exercise is associated with oxygen desaturation.
- Set realistic exercise goals with the patient.
- Instruct, supervise, and motivate the patient in the implementation of the exercise program. It is important to demonstrate the exercises;

observe the patient during exercise; coach the patient in proper breathing techniques while exercising; and encourage the patient.
- Periodically evaluate the patient's exercise capacity and revise the plan or establish new goals as necessary.

## Benefits of Exercise

Exercise can result in significant benefits for patients with COPD (Holle, 1988; Petty, 1987). Patients do increase their exercise tolerance and experience less dyspnea and fatigue with exercise reconditioning. They also note an enhanced sense of well-being and reduced depression and somatic concern. Improved physical fitness allows patients to perform daily activities more independently and to better control their symptoms. Significant increases in exercise capacity have been noted even after relatively short training programs of 4 to 6 weeks, regardless of the severity of the illness.

### Postulated Mechanisms for Improved Exercise Capacity

■ *Improved Efficiency of Skeletal Muscles.* An important mechanism of improved exercise tolerance is the improved endurance of skeletal muscles as a result of the conditioning effect on the muscles themselves. Oxygen is used more efficiently by muscles that are conditioned, as compared with muscles that are not conditioned.

■ *Desensitization to Dyspnea.* Considerable controversy exists regarding the mechanism for improvement in exercise capacity in patients with COPD. Perhaps the reason exercise capacity improves without a corresponding physiologic change in lung function is that exercise in the patient with COPD is most commonly limited by the patient's *perception* of dyspnea. Desensitization to dyspnea may be a key component in improved endurance after exercise training.

■ *Improved Ventilatory Muscle Function.* Increased ventilatory muscle endurance and resistance to fatigue have been demonstrated in patients following exercise conditioning programs. Specific training of ventilatory muscles using resistive

**Table 9-3**    Reasons for patients' resistance to exercise

| Reason | Nursing interventions |
|---|---|
| **Self-image** | |
| Gradual decline in activity over years, leading to adaptation to sedentary life-style | Compare patient's functional activities to those of peers |
| May not view self as deconditioned or disabled | |
| May enjoy dependent status | Be alert to clues suggesting secondary gains of disability |
| **Exercise too demanding** | |
| Patient convinced of impossibility of success | Establish small, readily achievable goals |
| **Anxiety and fear** | |
| Fear of discomfort of dyspnea | Help patient understand that dyspnea itself is not harmful |
| Fear that dyspnea will damage lungs | |
| Fear that exercise may cause a life-threatening event such as a heart attack | Reassure patient that he or she will not be asked to exercise beyond his or her capability |
| | Start program slowly, promoting success so that patient will be motivated to continue and will progress |
| | Decondition patient's fears by encouraging exercise to point of dyspnea, then coaching, breath by breath, until comfort returns |
| **Conflicting instructions** | |
| Confusion caused by seemingly conflicting instructions that encourage patients to pace activities and efficiently ration their limited energy, while simultaneously asking them to perform strenuous exercise that is likely to cause dyspnea and fatigue | Help patient understand that increased endurance from exercise leads to increased energy and improved quality of life, but that pacing and energy conservation are also important to conserve limited energy for high-priority activities |

breathing devices has also been shown to increase inspiratory muscle strength and endurance, to reduce dyspnea (Harver, 1989), and to improve exercise tolerance (Larson, 1988; Smith, 1992).

■ *Increased Motivation.* Increased motivation is often cited as an important factor. Patients develop increased confidence in their ability to exercise when they are supervised and coached by a trusted health professional.

## Getting Started: Gaining the Patient's Confidence

The patient with chronic lung disease may resist the notion of exercise for a variety of reasons, which are summarized in Table 9-3. A high degree of trust in the nurse or physical therapist is a prerequisite for the successful initiation of an exercise program.

### Factors Contributing to Successful Exercise Programs

The following factors enhance the likelihood of success in reaching rehabilitation goals:

- Develop the exercise plan using mutual goal setting between the patient and the nurse or therapist. Determine activities the patient enjoys or used to enjoy before becoming dyspneic; integrate these into the program, either as specific exercise activities or as goals of the exercise program.

- Make the initial attempts at exercise nonthreatening. Desensitize the patient to exertional dyspnea by coaching him or her to use pursed lip breathing (see Chapter 8). Patients will be less afraid to exercise once they realize they can control the uncomfortable sensation through their own actions.
- Keep it simple.
- Measure success in small increments so the patient can see progress and feel encouraged.
- Allow the patient some control over the program: the choice of when or where to exercise and what exercise to perform. The patient must be held accountable for these choices, however. A written record helps to ensure accountability.
- Encourage the patient to exercise with a friend. This changes the focus from a medical treatment to an enjoyable social activity.

## Components of an Exercise Program

The specific components of an exercise program designed to improve activity tolerance include the following:

- Breathing retraining, with pursed lips and diaphragmatic breathing, and coordination of breathing with activity
- General muscle strengthening using upper and lower extremity and trunk muscle strengthening exercises
- Cardiopulmonary endurance conditioning with activities such as walking, stair climbing, and riding a stationary cycle
- Ventilatory muscle strength and endurance training with use of a ventilatory muscle–training device

The following elements of the exercise program should be stressed:

- Warming up and cooling down before and after vigorous exercise
- What to do about bronchospasm
- When and how to use bronchodilators before exercise
- How to use oxygen if prescribed
- How to use breathing techniques such as pursed lip breathing for panic control
- How to seek help if needed

### Breathing Retraining

Breathing retraining techniques are designed to slow the respiratory rate and increase tidal volume with exercise. They are advocated for patients with asthma and COPD but are not indicated for patients with restrictive lung disease because such patients are unable to increase their tidal volume significantly.

To overcome the air trapping that occurs with COPD and the bronchoconstriction that is associated with asthma, exhalation time must be longer than inhalation time. It is helpful to monitor the inspiratory/expiratory (I/E) ratio and coach the patient to prolong the expiratory phase so that it is at least twice as long as the inspiratory phase. As patients increase their breathing rate with exercise, they should attempt to maintain the same I/E ratio.

Because upward body movements such as stretching or raising arms over the head facilitate inspiration, patients should be encouraged to breathe in during these maneuvers. Conversely, patients are taught to exhale while lowering their arms or pulling their extremities in toward their body. Pursed lip and diaphragmatic breathing techniques and coordination of breathing with activities of daily living are discussed in Chapter 8.

### General Muscle Strengthening

Exercises to strengthen muscles are an important part of an exercise regimen, particularly in patients with muscle weakness or atrophy from bed rest or steroid use. The muscles that usually are exercised include the calf, quadriceps, hamstrings, abdominals, and upper extremity biceps and triceps. The importance of lower extremity exercise conditioning is well accepted, but only recently has evidence supporting the efficacy of upper extremity exercise become available (Celli, 1986; Lake, 1989). Activities involving the upper extremities, such as combing the hair or shaving, require increases in energy similar to those of mild exercise, even in people without lung disease (Couser, 1992). For the patient with COPD such activities can be especially fatiguing. A postulated mechanism underlying the excessive fatigue and dyspnea of upper arm activity is that several of the muscles used also act as accessory respiratory muscles. When they are being used for activities of daily living, they are less able to meet increased ventilatory demands.

Stretching should be used before resistive exercise to mobilize the rib cage and limber the muscles. Patients are encouraged to move the major muscle groups through a full range of motion, using 10 to 20 repetitions for each specific movement. Weights can be added to increase the strengthening effects. These can be easily fabricated at home using a soup can for arm raises and two soup cans, pinned securely into a tea towel or pillow case and draped over the ankle, for leg raises. Examples of stretching and strengthening exercises are presented in Fig. 9-2.

### Cardiopulmonary Endurance Conditioning

Endurance training is the major emphasis of pulmonary rehabilitation (Hodgkin, 1987). The real gains in exercise tolerance, reductions in the sensation of dyspnea, and improvements in physical functioning are made as a result of endurance training. Other components of the exercise program should be viewed as adjuncts to endurance training.

■ *Endurance Prescription.* The endurance prescription consists of four elements: frequency, intensity, time, and type. These can be easily remembered by the acronym *FITT*.

F—*F*requency: number of times per day or week

I—*I*ntensity: the pace; how hard to push

T—*T*ime: how long to exercise each session

T—*T*ype: the mode of exercise

A standard endurance training regimen is carried out five times a week for 20 to 30 minutes a session. Generally the goal is to achieve a level of exercise that maintains the heart rate at 80% to 85% of the maximum heart rate, or at 20% to 30% over the resting heart rate, without excessive fatigue or dyspnea. The maximum heart rate is the maximum rate achieved during formal exercise testing, or it may be roughly determined by the formula: $220 - age$.

Any type of activity that uses the large muscle groups can be used for endurance training. The exercise prescription for a patient with chronic lung disease may need modification to reduce the intensity in order to control the sensation of dyspnea. As the disease becomes more advanced, exercise must be of shorter duration and lower intensity to maintain dyspnea at a tolerable level. If a patient can maintain an activity for only a few minutes, increasing the frequency of the activity (e.g., up to four or five times a day) can still result in a training effect. Patients should be taught to monitor their own heart rates to ensure consistent intensity of exercise from day to day.

■ *Exercise Protocol.* An example of an exercise protocol is presented in Table 9-4. The exercise protocol should be a written plan with specific exercises and lengths of exercise time. The patient should record each day's exercise and response in an exercise log book.

■ *Choice of Activity.* The best choice of activity will vary with the individual. Walking is the most common and in most cases the most helpful activity for building endurance in patients with COPD. Improvement in walking endurance most closely correlates with improvement in activities of daily living and does not require expensive equipment. The timed walking test described previously is helpful in determining the starting point for the exercise program. The average pace and time walked during the test determine the initial intensity and duration of the exercise program. Each week the pace and duration of exercise can be increased slightly, if the patient has not become excessively dyspneic on the previous week's exercise protocol.

Alternate activities such as riding a stationary bicycle may also be good choices for exercise. In selecting an activity, it is important to consider the availability, weather dependence, patient preferences, cost and amount of equipment required, and any other patient diagnoses. It is also important to remember that training tends to be task specific. Although desensitization to dyspnea may be a general effect regardless of the type of activity, muscle strengthening is specific to the type of exercise performed. For example, individuals who train on

**Table 9-4**   Exercise protocol

| Component | Exercises |
| --- | --- |
| Warm up for 5 to 10 min | Circle head slowly to right, then to left<br>Shrug shoulders and relax<br>Roll shoulders forward and back<br>Stretch legs out |
| Exercise for specific period of time | Written plan with specific exercises incorporating all four components of FITT<br>Examples include walking, riding a stationary bicycle, stair climbing, and arm and leg exercises; for walking or stair climbing, may also want to specify the number of lengths of hallway or number of flights of stairs; for the stationary bicycle, specify amount of resistance to be used<br>Specify if weights should be added for arm and leg raises<br>Try to sustain exercise for 20 to 30 min |
| Cool-down period for 5 to 10 min | Same as warm-up exercises, with emphasis on slow stretches |
| Guidelines for stopping | Heart rate more than 20% to 30% over baseline heart rate (or in excess of 120 beats per min)<br>More than 6 premature beats per min<br>Chest pain<br>Dizziness<br>Intolerable dyspnea or fatigue |
| Guidelines for increasing exercise period | Slow, stable heart rate<br>No fatigue or dyspnea |

a bicycle use muscles that will improve their bicycling ability but will not necessarily improve walking endurance. A variety of exercises may be the best choice for many individuals because this provides a well-rounded program, trains more muscle groups, and maintains patient interest. Stair climbing coordinated with pursed lip breathing is an excellent conditioning exercise for someone with mild to moderate COPD.

■ *Incorporate Functional Activities.* As exercise tolerance improves, the exercise routine may incorporate more functional activities. For instance, once a patient has mastered several laps of walking in the house, he or she may progress to walking to the mailbox each day to get the mail. Compliance with an exercise program is usually better if the patient can see some practical benefit associated with it. It is important to remember that further increases in endurance will occur only if exercise is performed at the highest intensity possible for the entire exercise period. Thus, as the patient's exercise ability increases, the intensity of the protocol must increase proportionately.

Long-term goals of exercise conditioning are to increase exercise capacity so that home care is no longer needed. Ideal maintenance programs for the successfully reconditioned home care patient include mall walks, senior center exercise programs, and YMCA or YWCA swim programs. These provide both a social and an exercise focus, can involve the spouse as an exercise partner, and can be done despite inclement weather.

*Text continued on p. 161.*

**Trunk mobility**

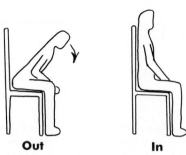

**Out**      **In**

1. Sit in chair. Lean forward from waist as you blow out. Relax and sit up as you breathe in. Repeat _____ times.

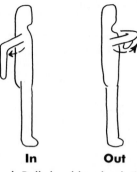

**In**      **Out**

2. Sit or stand. Pull shoulders back tightly to count of 5 as you breathe in. Relax and cross arms in front of you as you breathe out. Repeat _____ times.

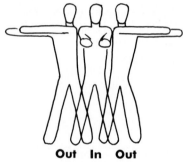

**Out   In   Out**

3. Stand up. Swing both arms to the right as you blow out. Swing both arms back to center as you breathe in. Repeat to left. Repeat _____ times.

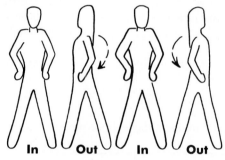

**In      Out      In      Out**

4. Stand up, with hands on hips. Turn to right as you blow out. Return to center as you breathe in. Turn to left as you blow out. Return to center. Repeat _____ times.

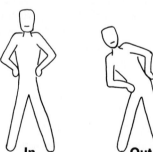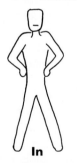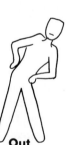

**In      Out      In      Out**

5. Stand against wall for stability. Bend at the waist to the right as you blow out. Return to upright position as you breathe in. Repeat to the left. Repeat entire set _____ times.

**Fig. 9-2**   Body conditioning exercises.

## Arm - strengthening exercises

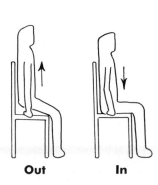

**Out**     **In**

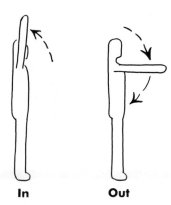

**In**     **Out**

1. Sit in chair. Lift buttocks off chair with hands and arms as you blow out.  Lower buttocks as you breathe in.  Repeat _____ times.

2. Sit or stand. Raise arms above head as you breathe in. Lower arms to sides as you blow out. Repeat. Alternately, lower arms just until they are straight in front of you. Repeat _____ times.

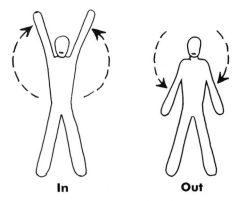

**In**     **Out**

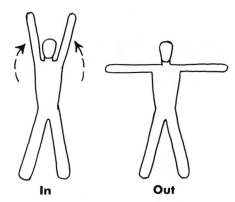

**In**     **Out**

3. Raise arms from sides above head as you breathe in. Lower arms as you blow out. Repeat _____ times.

4. Raise arms above head as you breathe in. Lower arms just to shoulder level as you breathe out. Repeat _____ times.

**Fig. 9-2, cont'd**     Body conditioning exercises.

**Arm - strengthening exercises using weights**

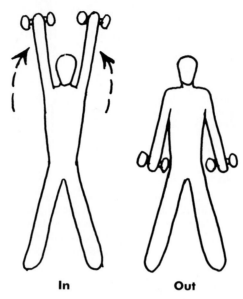

**In**          **Out**

5. Sit or stand. Keeping arms close to your body, raise 1- to 5-pound weights above your head as you breathe in. Lower weights slowly as you breathe out. Repeat _____ times.

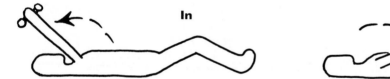

**In**          **Out**

6. Lie down, with arms at your sides and with knees bent slightly. Raise 1- to 5-pound weights above your head as you breathe in. Lower weights to sides as you breathe out. Repeat _____ times.

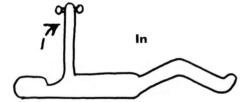
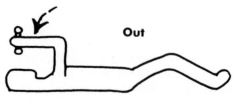

**In**          **Out**

7. Lie down with knees bent slightly. With 1- to 5-pound weights in each hand, and elbows bent, extend arms above head as you breathe in. Return to bent-elbow position as you breathe out. Repeat _____ times.

**Fig. 9-2, cont'd**    Body conditioning exercises.

**Leg - strengthening exercises**

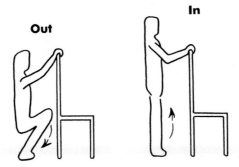

1. Hold onto back of chair. Keeping back straight, bend at knees as you blow out. Stand up as you breathe in.

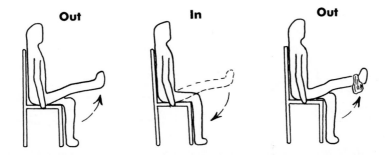

2. Sit in chair with straight back and firm seat. Raise one leg slowly as you blow out, lifting thigh off chair seat. Lower leg to floor as you breathe in. Repeat. Add weights to ankle for greater strengthening.

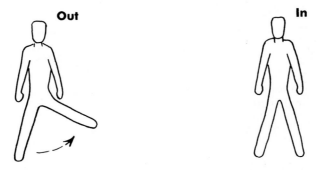

3. Stand with back straight against wall. Raise leg to one side as you blow out. Lower leg as you breathe in. Repeat.

**Fig. 9-2, cont'd**   Body conditioning exercises.

## Leg - strengthening exercises

**Out**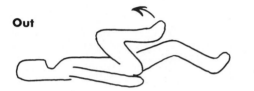

**In**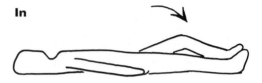

4. Lie on back with one knee slightly bent. Raise other knee to your chest as you breathe out. Lower leg as you breathe in. Repeat _____ times.

**Out**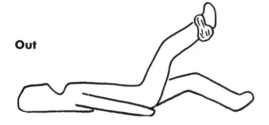

**In**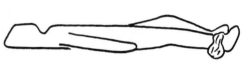

5. Lie on back with one knee slightly bent. Raise other leg slowly off bed as you blow out, keeping knee fairly straight. Lower leg as you breathe in. Repeat _____ times. Add weights to your ankle for greater strengthening.

**Out**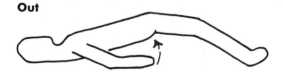

**In**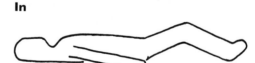

6. Lie on back with both knees slightly bent. Lift buttocks off bed as you blow out. Relax and drop buttocks as you breathe in. Repeat _____ times.

**Fig. 9-2, cont'd**    Body conditioning exercises.

## Specific Ventilatory Muscle Training

Inspiratory training devices such as the P-flex or the Pressure Threshold Breathing Device (Fig. 9-3) are used to increase the strength and endurance of inspiratory muscles. The P-flex consists of a mouthpiece attached to a one-way valve with a series of holes of progressively smaller diameters. The patient breathes in normally through the device while wearing noseclips. The inspiratory resistance is determined by the diameter of the inflow opening, while the one-way valve permits exhalation without resistance. The patient is typically started with the highest resistance that allows him or her to complete 15 minutes of breathing through the device without undue discomfort or dyspnea. Over time, smaller inflow orifice sizes are used.

If patients reduce their inspiratory flow rate while using the training device, they will reduce their inspiratory workload, thereby negating or reducing the training effect. This may help explain the conflicting results reported by those who have studied the efficacy of the devices. The Pressure Threshold Breathing Device has corrected for this problem and may prove a more effective and reliable ventilatory muscle training device (Larson, 1988).

Ventilatory muscle training may be used as an adjunct to an endurance conditioning program but alone does not provide the benefits obtained from general exercise. In addition, many patients find breathing with the devices for the required time period uncomfortable or lose interest and use them infrequently. Thus the training devices may be disappointing. However, a well-motivated patient with a good coach who uses the devices properly for a long time is likely to be rewarded with increased respiratory muscle strength and improved exercise tolerance.

## Exercise Conditioning in Children

*It may seem that children with asthma participate adequately in activities with their peers. However, many children learn to subtly avoid activity when in a group and, in fact, perform little intensive or continuous exercise. This may affect their*

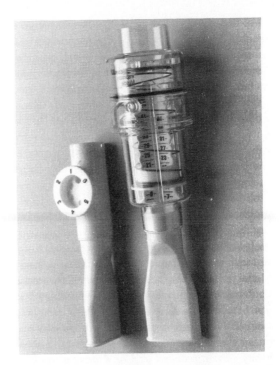

**Fig. 9-3** Inspiratory muscle training devices. *Left,* P-flex; *right,* threshold. (From Weilitz PB: *Pocket guide to respiratory care,* St Louis, 1991, Mosby.)

*body image and self-concept. The amount of regular after school active play in which a child engages can vary depending on the child's age, interests, and peers. Unless children participate regularly in an organized sport, it is difficult to know whether they are active enough. Because a patient history is of limited value in assessing exercise tolerance, direct testing and observation may be the only accurate means of assessing the child's actual exercise tolerance.*

*Children with cystic fibrosis frequently have reduced activity tolerance that may appear out of proportion to their degree of physiologic impairment. However, exercise tolerance can be normal in children with mild or moderate disease and, occasionally, in those with severe disease. Normal exercise tolerance is possible until the lung capacity is quite reduced.*

*Formal exercise testing protocols for children use a treadmill or stationary bicycle and are standardized for age, height, and sex. Testing protocols and normal values are listed in the American Hospital Association's Standards for Exercise Testing in Children (James, 1982). Formal testing is used to diagnose and quantitate the severity of disease and to monitor the effectiveness of medication programs. In most instances, however, an exercise program can be established without formal testing.*

### Exercise Prescription for Children

*It is important that children in an exercise program be involved in choosing an activity they enjoy. The goal is to maintain a maximum intensity of exercise for 15 to 20 minutes. Initially, however, children may be able to tolerate only 5 minutes of exercise with short breaks before continuing. Usually five to six exercise sessions a week are necessary to build endurance. Once the child is over the initial hurdle of endurance building, the frequency can be reduced to 3 or 4 days a week.*

■ *Components of an Exercise Program for Children. The components of the exercise program for children should include the components summarized earlier in the section on exercise in adults. The child should be taught that an increased rate and depth of breathing are normal with vigorous exercise, which will help dispel fears about exercise. Teaching aids that are entertaining and appropriate for various age groups are often available from local lung associations.*

*Walking is usually not intensive enough to provide significant exercise training unless the child is severely deconditioned or the disease is unusually severe. Swimming, bicycle riding, and distance running are all excellent forms of aerobic exercise. The long-term goal of an exercise program is to enable the deconditioned youngster to participate equally in regular athletic activity with peers. Many children with asthma or cystic fibrosis are not only deconditioned but lack the physical skills to participate successfully in athletic activities with other children. An exercise program that provides endurance conditioning and practice in*

*specific skills (such as hitting a baseball or throwing a basketball) will more effectively achieve this long-term goal. Asthma and cystic fibrosis camps provide ideal opportunities for children to participate in a wide range of normal athletic activities in an environment where they feel safe (Scherr, 1985). Success in the protected environment of camp is often all the encouragement a child needs to continue with a chosen activity following the camp experience.*

*In addition to its many other benefits, vigorous exercise greatly enhances mucus clearance in children and adults with cystic fibrosis and is advocated as a supplement to chest physical therapy. Conversely, the use of an inhaled bronchodilator or chest physical therapy before vigorous exercise may help the individual exercise better without excessive coughing and expectoration.*

*Before children with advanced cystic fibrosis are started on a rigorous exercise program, they must be evaluated for the presence of cor pulmonale and oxyhemoglobin desaturation. Oxyhemoglobin desaturation is more likely to occur with exercise if the child has a forced expiratory volume in 1 second ($FEV_1$) of less than 50% of that predicted, and it indicates the need for supplemental oxygen with exercise. The child with severe cystic fibrosis usually has less endurance and therefore will not be able to train with as much intensity as the child with asthma.*

### Interventions for Exercise-Induced Bronchospasm

Some types of exercise have been shown to elicit exercise-induced bronchospasm (EIB) more easily than others. For example, swimming is among the least provocational forms of exercise, whereas free running is among the most provocational forms. This may be because the increased humidity and warmth of the air inhaled during swimming evoke less bronchospasm than the cooler, dryer air inhaled while running.

An inhaled bronchodilator should be used before exercise. Bronchodilators and antiinflammatory medications allow most children and adults with

EIB to lead full, physically active lives with normal exercise tolerance. Medications are discussed in Chapter 6. A medication schedule that allows full exercise should be maintained, and frequent "breakthrough" bronchospasm with exercise should be viewed as a reason to modify the medication regimen.

## Modification in Exercise with Pulmonary Exacerbations

When patients experience a pulmonary exacerbation, they should temporarily cut back on their exercise program, but should begin to build back up to their previous level of exercise as soon as possible. It is especially important for patients receiving high steroid doses to maintain some degree of activity because exercise helps to counteract steroid-induced muscle weakness.

## Use of Oxygen with Exercise

The oxygen prescription for exercise is usually for the lowest flow rate that results in a saturation of 90%. Patients who experience desaturation usually increase their exercise capacity with the use of supplemental oxygen. In addition, these individuals will often, though not always, experience a decrease in exertional dyspnea. Excessively high oxygen flow rates do not enhance the patient's ability to exercise, are wasteful, and in hypercapnic patients may be harmful by decreasing the respiratory drive.

Common misconceptions and fear can surround the use of oxygen with exercise. Many patients associate the need for oxygen with worsening disease and wish to delay and avoid its use. Many avoid using it because they fear becoming dependent on oxygen or feel more vulnerable with its use. Still others incorrectly assume that they can store extra oxygen in their blood by using it for a few minutes before increasing their activity level. It is extremely important that patients be educated about the need for and appropriate use of oxygen with exercise. Patients who avoid exercise because of reluctance to use oxygen miss the potentially significant benefits of exercise conditioning.

## Benefits of Physical Therapy Referral

Because exercise conditioning is such a critical component of pulmonary rehabilitation, patients with respiratory disease should be referred to an experienced physical therapist whenever possible. The physical therapist can provide instruction, supervision, and reevaluation of the exercise regimen and reinforce its importance in the overall rehabilitation plan. Clear documentation of activity tolerance is important in the evaluation of progress.

## STRATEGIES FOR MEDICARE DOCUMENTATION

Because Medicare will not reimburse for home care unless patients are homebound, patients would theoretically have to be discharged as soon as they had increased their exercise tolerance enough to go out for walks. This situation often presents a dilemma because other care goals may not be accomplished and cardiopulmonary status may remain unstable. It is important for the nurse or physical therapist to realize that documentation of specific outside exercise (e.g., "walking two blocks on the level three times a week") will likely result in denial of payments for further visits.

If the patient is no longer homebound, cardiopulmonary status is stable, and other home care goals have been accomplished, it is appropriate to discharge the patient from home care. Patients who are stable and are no longer homebound, but who need continuing teaching and rehabilitation, should be referred to an outpatient pulmonary rehabilitation program if one is available.

*Such counterproductive reimbursement regulations do not apply to children or to many younger adults with private insurance coverage; thus exercise programs can be more freely and clearly documented for these patients.*

**REFERENCES**

Celli BR, Rassulo J, Make BJ: Dyssynchronous breathing during arm but not leg exercise in patients with chronic airflow obstruction, *N Engl J Med* 314:1485, 1986.

Couser JI, Martinez FJ, Celli BR: Respiratory response and ventilatory muscle recruitment during arm elevation in normal subjects, *Chest* 101:336, 1992.

Harver A, Mahler DA, Daubenspeck JA: Targeted inspiratory muscle training improves respiratory muscle function and reduces dyspnea in patients with chronic obstructive pulmonary disease, *Ann Intern Med* 111:117, 1989.

Hodgkin JE, Petty TL: *Chronic obstructive pulmonary disease: current concepts,* Philadelphia, 1987, WB Saunders.

Holle RH et al: Increased muscle efficiency and sustained benefits in an outpatient community hospital-based pulmonary rehabilitation program, *Chest* 94:1161, 1988.

James J et al: AHA special report: Standards for exercise testing in the pediatric age group, *Circulation* 66:1377A, 1982.

Lake FR et al: Upper and lower limb training in chronic airflow obstruction, *Am Rev Respir Dis* 139:A9, 1989.

Larson JL et al: Inspiratory muscle training with a pressure threshold breathing device in patients with chronic obstructive pulmonary disease, *Am Rev Respir Dis* 138:689, 1988.

Martinez FJ, Courser JI, Celli BR: Factors influencing muscle recruitment in patients with chronic airflow obstruction, *Am Rev Respir Dis* 142:276, 1990.

McGavin CR et al: Dyspnoea, disability and distance walked: comparison of estimates of exercise performance in respiratory disease, *Br Med J* 2:241, 1978.

Petty TL, Nett LM: *Enjoying life with emphysema,* ed 2, Philadelphia, 1987, Lea & Febiger.

Scherr MS: Summer camps for asthmatic children. In Weiss EB, Segal MS, Stein M, editors: *Bronchial asthma: mechanisms and therapeutics,* ed 2, Boston, 1985, Little, Brown.

Smith K et al: Respiratory muscle training in chronic airflow limitation: a meta-analysis, *Am Rev Respir Dis* 145:533, 1992.

## SUGGESTED READING

Gallagher CG: Exercise and chronic obstructive pulmonary disease, *Med Clin North Am* 74:619, 1990.

# CHAPTER 10

# CARDIAC DYSFUNCTION

GWENDOLYN J. McDONALD

Patients with chronic lung disease have a high incidence of cardiovascular problems, which may complicate their home care management. The two most common problems in children and adults are pulmonary heart disease (cor pulmonale) and cardiac arrhythmias. Polycythemia (an increase in the number of red blood cells) may develop in response to chronic hypoxemia and can adversely affect cardiovascular and cognitive functioning. Pulmonary embolism also may be a problem in adults with chronic lung disease and can add considerably to right ventricular workload.

Because many patients with chronic lung disease are older adults with a long history of smoking, coexisting primary cardiovascular diseases are also common. Smokers and the elderly are more likely to have systemic hypertension and coronary artery disease, which increase their risk for myocardial ischemia and infarction, left ventricular failure, and arrhythmias. These problems may be aggravated by hypoxemia, acid-base disturbances, and interventions used to treat lung disease.

Patients who have cardiovascular changes associated with chronic obstructive pulmonary disease (COPD) have a poorer prognosis. Arrhythmias may account for many COPD deaths, especially those occurring suddenly, often at night.

## PULMONARY HEART DISEASE

The terms "cor pulmonale" and "pulmonary heart disease" (PHD) are interchangeable and are used to describe the right ventricular hypertrophy and dilatation that result from disorders affecting either the structure or function of the lungs. More simply stated, it is heart disease caused by lung disease. The patient with PHD is at ongoing risk for cardiac decompensation and overt right ventricular failure.

### Etiology

The normal pulmonary vascular bed is a highly distensible low-pressure system designed to accommodate large fluctuations in blood volume with minimal changes in pulmonary artery pressure (PAP). If changes occur in the vascular bed that make it less distensible, resistance to the flow of blood from the right ventricle increases and pressure in the pulmonary arteries inevitably rises. This increase in pulmonary artery pressure is called pulmonary hypertension (PH). Patients with chronic lung disease experience many pathophysiologic changes that can alter the resistance against which the right ventricle must pump (right ventricular afterload) and the blood volume that enters the ventricle (right ventricular preload) (see the box on p. 166).

#### Factors Affecting Afterload

Of particular importance is pulmonary vascular constriction resulting from hypoxemia. Even intermittent episodes of hypoxemia, such as those that may occur with sleep or exercise, can cause

---

### Factors Contributing to Pulmonary Hypertension

**FACTORS INCREASING AFTERLOAD**

Increased pulmonary vascular resistance
   Constriction of pulmonary vascular bed as the result of hypoxemia and acidemia
   Muscularization and rigidity of pulmonary arterioles
   Destruction of pulmonary capillary bed and alveolar walls caused by emphysema
   Embolic occlusion of pulmonary capillaries
   Capillary compression caused by increased intrathoracic pressures seen with prolonged, labored expiratory efforts
Increased pulmonary venous pressure as the result of coexisting left ventricular failure
Increasing blood viscosity caused by polycythemia

**FACTORS INCREASING PRELOAD**

Increased blood volume caused by:
   Increased sodium intake or retention
   Fluid overload
Increased cardiac output caused by:
   Tachycardia
   Hypermetabolic state
   Increased blood volume

---

PHD and right ventricular failure if the episodes are severe and frequent enough. Many patients with relatively normal oxygen saturation during waking hours may desaturate precipitously during rapid eye movement (REM) sleep. These episodes of desaturation are associated with sudden sharp increases in PAP, which, if they occur often enough, can stress the right ventricle as much as if the increase in pressure were continuous. Signs and symptoms of cor pulmonale in a patient with relatively normal daytime blood gases should raise the possibility of severe nocturnal desaturation.

A significant hypoxia-induced increase in PAP may also be seen in COPD patients as a result of mild steady-state exercise and is accompanied by a reduction in right ventricular ejection fraction. The ventricular ejection fraction is the portion of blood in the ventricle that is ejected with each contraction and is normally increased with exercise. However, patients with compromised ventricular function are often unable to make the compensatory adjustments.

Afterload is further increased in the presence of left ventricular failure because any increase in end-diastolic left ventricular pressure (pulmonary venous pressure, or wedge pressure) is transferred backward through the pulmonary vascular bed.

Polycythemia (hematocrit >50% in men; >44% in women) can also contribute to development of cor pulmonale. Polycythemia occurs in response to hypoxemia, which stimulates the renal tubules to increase production of erythropoietin. Erythropoietin stimulates the bone marrow to increase the production of red blood cells. Increased red blood cell mass improves tissue oxygenation by increasing the oxygen-carrying capacity. If severe enough, however, it also increases blood viscosity and right ventricular work. Severe polycythemia (hematocrit >60%) is most often seen in patients with obesity-hypoventilation syndrome and is associated with significant myocardial depression, reduced cerebral blood flow, and increased risk for thromboemboli.

### Factors Affecting Preload

Factors that increase right ventricular preload include fluid overload and an increase in venous return resulting from exercise, fever, or other hypermetabolic states. Increased preload expands the volume of blood that the right ventricle must pump into the pulmonary artery.

### Right Ventricular Failure

The right ventricle must work harder to pump against increased resistance. If resistance increases suddenly, the right ventricle becomes distended and fails. More commonly, however, the process is slowly progressive, allowing time for the ventricular walls to hypertrophy to overcome the increase in resistance. Unless the underlying causes can be reversed, the right ventricle will eventually fatigue, cardiac output will drop, and signs and symptoms of right ventricular failure will appear.

■ *Factors Precipitating Right Ventricular Failure.* Patients with PHD tend to have no evidence of right ventricular failure as long as their cardiopulmonary status is stable. However, even a minor deterioration in cardiopulmonary stability may be enough to precipitate failure. The two most common precipitants of right ventricular failure in patients with PHD are (1) worsening hypoxemia caused by a pulmonary exacerbation such as a viral or bacterial respiratory tract infection or increased bronchospasm and (2) fluid overload caused by increased dietary sodium intake. Other potential causes include increased sodium retention resulting from high steroid dosages, diffuse pulmonary microemboli, and increased left ventricular failure.

## Assessment

### Pulmonary Heart Disease

Changes consistent with PHD are difficult to identify clinically. The medical diagnosis is usually based on radiographic and electrocardiographic (ECG) changes, cardiac examination, and newer noninvasive techniques such as echocardiography. Because early implementation of oxygen therapy can improve survival, it is important to identify early clues to PHD.

### Right Ventricular Failure

Right ventricular failure occurs when the right ventricle can no longer compensate. Cardiac output drops and blood backs up within the venous system, increasing central venous pressure and resulting in extravasation of fluid into extravascular spaces.

Most signs and symptoms of right ventricular failure result from fluid retention and are summarized in Fig. 10-1 and Table 10-1. In adults, any weight gain in excess of 1 lb a day for several days in a row or a steady weight gain over several days or weeks in the absence of any change in dietary intake suggests fluid retention. *Infants will normally grow at a rate of 10 to 30 g a day as measured over weekly gains. The growth rate for toddlers and young children is at a lower rate. Thus weight gains in excess of 30 g a day over several days for an infant, more than 20 g a day for toddlers, and more than 10 g a day for 3- to 6-year-olds are likely to indicate fluid retention.*

Edema does not appear until significant fluid retention has occurred (4 to 7 L or 10 to 15 lb weight) (Laurent-Bopp, 1991). Dependent edema is usually worse toward the end of the day or after standing for long periods and is most apparent in the feet and legs. In the bedridden patient it appears as sacral edema. Changes in mental function can result from mild cerebral edema. With rest and by elevating the extremities, extravascular fluid is reabsorbed into the vascular bed and diuresis occurs. Nocturia is a frequent complaint in right ventricular failure as a result of reabsorption diuresis and hormonal effects, which result in increased glomerular filtration of electrolytes at night.

Hepatomegaly, ascites, and abdominal complaints are due to mesenteric and hepatic engorgement with transudation of fluid into the abdomen. Ascites is a late finding and should be monitored by regular measurement of abdominal girth. Liver engorgement can be identified by palpation and percussion of the liver borders. The liver is usually tender to palpation and feels firm, smooth, and enlarged. Impaired liver function may be evident by increased serum glutamic-oxaloacetic transaminase (SGOT), lactate dehydrogenase (LDH), and bilirubin values.

The cardiac findings of right ventricular failure are best appreciated by palpation or auscultation of the left sternal border or (in patients with marked hyperinflation) of the epigastrium. A deep inspiration presents the failing right ventricle with an increased volume of blood and often makes an $S_3$ gallop more apparent.

## Nursing Interventions

Goals of nursing care of the patient with PHD and right ventricular failure are to improve oxygenation and reduce fluid retention. Interventions are listed at the top of p. 170.

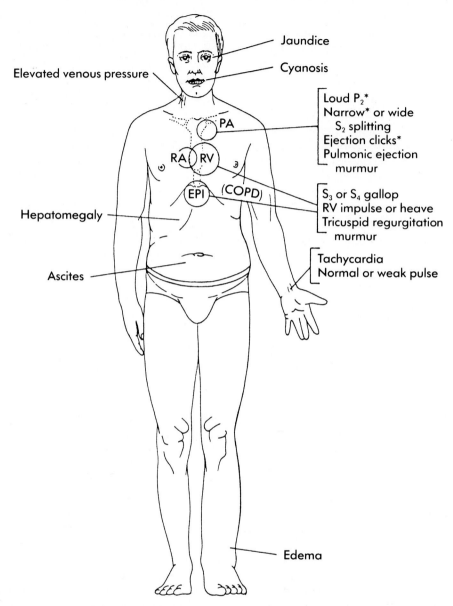

**Fig. 10-1** Common physical findings in pulmonary hypertension and cor pulmonale and locations where they are found. Asterisk indicates findings associated with milder pulmonary hypertension. Jaundice, elevated venous pressure, hepatomegaly, ascites, and massive edema are seen with frank right heart failure. Right ventricular findings are best noted in epigastrium *(EPI)* in patients with COPD. *PA,* Pulmonary area; *RV,* right ventricular area; *RA,* right atrial area. (Modified from Hill NI: *Clin Chest Med* 8:273-285, 1987.)

**Table 10-1**   Signs and Symptoms of Congestive Heart Failure

| | Right ventricular failure | Left ventricular failure |
|---|---|---|
| Signs | Weight gain<br>Dependent edema<br>Jugular venous distention<br>Heptomegaly<br>Hepatojugular reflux<br>Tachycardia<br>Increased blood pressure<br>Ascites (late) | Dry cough, worse at night (early) → moist cough; pink frothy sputum (late)<br>Moist crackles and wheezes<br>Tachypnea → Cheyne-Stokes respirations (late)<br>Tachycardia; rapid weak peripheral pulse<br>Increased blood pressure initially → drop in blood pressure as cardiac output drops (late)<br>Pulsus alternans → irregular heart rate<br>Central apneas and hypopneas (in stable, severe CHF) (White, 1985) |
| Findings on chest examination | $S_3$ gallop along lower left sternal border, increased with deep inspiration<br>Right ventricular heave | $S_3$ or summation gallop at apex<br>Left ventricular heave<br>Diffuse PMI, shifted to left |
| Symptoms | Fatigue, weakness<br>Diuresis at rest; nocturia<br>Abdominal symptoms<br>  Anorexia, nausea, vomiting<br>  Abdominal fullness, distention<br>  Constipation<br>  Liver tenderness to palpation<br>Impaired mental function | Fatigue, weakness (due to decreased cardiac output)<br>Exertional dyspnea<br>Anorexia, nausea, vomiting<br>Orthopnea, paroxysmal nocturnal dyspnea<br>Impaired cerebral function<br>  Nightmares, insomnia<br>  Confusion, memory loss (late)<br>  Anxiety, restlessness, agitation (late)<br>Palpitations, if arrhythmias present |
| Laboratory values | Increase in liver enzymes (SGOT, LDH, and bilirubin) | Values consistent with impaired renal function:<br>  Increased potassium, BUN, uric acid, creatinine<br>  Decreased sodium |
| Chest x-ray findings | Right ventricular enlargement<br>Enlarged pulmonary arteries | Cardiomegaly<br>Prominent pulmonary veins<br>Interstitial pulmonary edema (late)<br>Possible pleural effusion (late) |
| ECG findings | Nonspecific; generally not helpful<br>Changes associated with right ventricular hypertrophy may include:<br>  P-pulmonale<br>  Right axis shift of P wave and QRS complex<br>  Incomplete RBBB | Nonspecific; generally not helpful<br>Changes associated with left ventricular hypertrophy:<br>  Left axis deviation<br>  Widened QRS complexes<br>  Inverted T waves<br>Arrhythmias: atrial fibrillation<br>  PACs, PVCs may be present |

*CHF*, Congestive heart failure; *PMI*, point of maximal impulse; *SGOT*, serum glutamic-oxaloacetic transaminase; *LDH*, lactate dehydrogenase; *BUN*, blood urea nitrogen; *RBBB*, right bundle-branch block; *PACs*, premature atrial contractions; *PVCs*, premature ventricular contractions.

| To Improve Oxygenation | To Reduce Fluid Retention |
|---|---|
| Relieve bronchospasm | Reduce sodium intake |
| Enhance secretion clearance using: | Consider need for diuretic therapy |
| Bronchodilators | |
| Bronchial hygiene measures | |
| Use antibiotic therapy for infection | |
| Use low-flow oxygen if $O_2$ saturation is low | |

### Oxygen Therapy

The fundamental approach to the long-term management of cor pulmonale, with or without right ventricular failure, is to initiate low-flow oxygen therapy. This reverses the hypoxemia, which acts as the primary stimulus. Continuous (24 hour/day) low-flow oxygen is typically prescribed when:

- $PaO_2$ is persistently below 55 mm Hg or oxygen saturation is less than 85%
- $PaO_2$ is between 56 and 59 mm Hg or oxygen saturation is less than 90%, with evidence of right ventricular failure (NOTT, 1980)

The presence of right ventricular failure in a patient whose daytime $PaO_2$ is adequate (greater than 60 mm Hg) suggests nocturnal oxygen desaturation. These patients should be evaluated for the need for noctural oxygen therapy.

For both children and adults the goal of low-flow oxygen therapy is to maintain oxygen saturation above 90%. *In children with evidence of PHD, a flow rate sufficient to keep saturation between 92% and 94% is prescribed.* To compensate for the further drop in $PaO_2$ that typically occurs with sleep, a nighttime flow rate 0.5 to 1 L higher than the daytime flow rate is often required.

If patient compliance with oxygen therapy is good and $PaO_2$ is maintained above 55 mm Hg, signs and symptoms of right ventricular failure should begin to lessen in about 3 to 4 weeks.

### Sodium Restriction

■ *Dietary Measures.* A standard "no added salt" (NAS) diet is usually adequate. However, compliance with a sodium-restricted diet is often difficult, especially for older patients with diminished taste, limited energy, and well-established dietary preferences. Suggestions include the following:

- Avoid canned and convenience foods that tend to be high in sodium.
- Substitute alternative seasonings, such as lemon juice, herbs, and pepper, for salt.
- Provide simple, clearly written educational materials on low-sodium diets. The American Heart Association is an excellent resource.
- Stress foods the patient *can* eat as well as those that should be eliminated.

A balance must be struck between sodium restriction and an unacceptable loss of dietary palatability. For the malnourished patient a modest increase in diuretic dosage is often preferable to stringent dietary sodium restrictions. *The sodium content of infant formulas varies, and a lower-sodium formula (e.g., SMA) may be helpful for the infant with fluid retention.*

■ *Elimination of Other Sources.* Whenever possible substitute low-sodium medications (e.g., for an antacid, magaldrate [Riopan]) for higher-sodium preparations. Discourage the use of sodium bicarbonate to treat indigestion.

### Diuretics

Most patients with right ventricular failure also have some left ventricular failure. If right ventricular failure persists despite the measures outlined previously, diuretic therapy is usually prescribed. Diuretics are discussed in the section on the management of left ventricular failure.

### Phlebotomy

If the hematocrit remains high despite the implementation of home oxygen therapy, restoration of adequate fluid volume, and other supportive measures, phlebotomy may be required. This medical procedure is rarely done unless the hematocrit exceeds 60% to 65% when the risk for thromboembolism and heart strain is increased.

## LEFT VENTRICULAR FAILURE

Left ventricular failure in patients with chronic lung disease may occur as a progression of right ventricular failure or the effects of blood gas alterations on myocardial functioning. Generally, however, it is caused by an independent coexisting problem affecting the left side of the heart. Untreated left ventricular failure inevitably leads to right ventricular failure.

## Etiology

The two most common causes of left ventricular failure are systemic hypertension and ischemic heart disease. Systemic hypertension increases the resistance against which the left ventricle must pump. Myocardial ischemia impairs left ventricular functioning and increases the risk of failure. Contributing factors include mitral valve dysfunction and hypermetabolic states such as anemia, fever, or hyperthyroidism, which demand a compensatory increase in heart rate and cardiac output. The increased cardiac output is necessary to meet tissue oxygen requirements, but it may be just enough to precipitate overt left ventricular failure, particularly in the frail, elderly, home care patient already at risk for febrile respiratory tract infection or malnutritional anemia. Right ventricular dysfunction may also play a role in precipitating left ventricular failure, although the exact mechanisms for this are unclear.

## Assessment

Whatever the cause, a failing left ventricle cannot maintain cardiac output. This results in fatigue and weakness, especially with exercise when demand is increased. Patients often complain that their arms and legs feel like lead weights. An increase in exertional dyspnea is another early indication of left ventricular failure.

As the cardiac output drops, blood backs up into the pulmonary vascular bed, resulting in pulmonary vasocongestion. This bogginess of the pulmonary capillaries is most pronounced in dependent areas of the lungs, where it causes premature closure of the airways. This causes ventilation-perfusion inequalities and results in hypoxemia. Because a larger surface area of lung is dependent when the patient is recumbent than when the patient is sitting up, dyspnea is worse in the recumbent position.

Patients with left ventricular failure tend to prop themselves up on several pillows during the day and often sleep sitting up in a reclining chair. The approximate severity of orthopnea is assessed by asking how many pillows the patient uses at night. Paroxysmal nocturnal dyspnea usually occurs 2 to 5 hours after going to sleep and results, in part, from nocturnal reabsorption of edema. This increase in circulating blood volume causes volume overload, and the patient awakens suddenly with a smothering sensation. The patient finds relief only by sitting bolt upright in bed, dangling the legs over the edge of the bed, or getting up, perhaps to throw the window open for air. Signs and symptoms of left ventricular failure are summarized in Table 10-1.

## Nursing Interventions

The management of left ventricular failure includes treatment of the underlying cause (e.g., systemic hypertension, myocardial ischemia, or arrhythmias), rest, dietary sodium restriction, and usually digitalis and diuretic therapy. It may also include fluid restriction and vasodilators. Nursing interventions are summarized in the box on p. 172. Nurses must know the signs and symptoms of toxicity for all drugs the patient is taking and should notify the physician immediately if they occur.

## Acute Pulmonary Edema

If left ventricular failure worsens, fluid leaks into the extravascular spaces and finally into the alveolar spaces, causing pulmonary edema. Clues to incipient pulmonary edema include a dry, hacking cough, which is often worse at night, and an increase in symptoms of left ventricular failure. The signs and symptoms of frank pulmonary edema include the following:
- Marked dyspnea, tachypnea, and orthopnea
- Distended neck veins
- A moist cough with expectoration of pink, frothy sputum
- Anxiety, agitation, confusion
- Hypotension, tachycardia, and diaphoresis
- Pallor and cyanosis

It is rare for home care staff to find a patient in

# Nursing Management of Left Ventricular Failure

## REST

Rest is necessary to reduce cardiac workload.

The need for rest may mean a readjustment of the physical reconditioning program.

## SEMI-FOWLER'S POSITION FOR RELIEF OF ORTHOPNEA

Use pillows, a firm back rest cushion, or a recliner chair for adults *and an infant or car seat for young children.*

Consider a hospital bed for the patient with chronic failure and persistent orthopnea.

## SODIUM AND FLUID RESTRICTION

The patient's sodium intake should be restricted according to the severity of failure.

Fluid restriction is rarely necessary because fluid intake is often already low.

## WEIGHT REDUCTION

Because obesity adds to cardiac work, implement a planned weight reduction program for overweight patients.

## DIGITALIS THERAPY

Digitalis therapy slows the heart rate and improves ventricular contractility.

A high individual variability exists in dose requirements.

Obtain a serum level measurement to confirm that the patient is within the therapeutic range of 0.8 to 2 ng/ml.

Toxicity:

   Likely to occur at levels greater than:

   2 ng/ml in adults

   *2.2 ng/ml in infants and young children*

   Patients with chronic lung disease are at high risk for toxicity because of hypoxemia; the concurrent use of potassium-wasting diuretics, quinidine, or verapamil; medication compliance problems; renal dysfunction; electrolyte abnormalities and acid base disturbances; and advanced age.

   Signs and symptoms in the adult include anorexia, nausea, vomiting, diarrhea, visual disturbances, headache, weakness, and (later) bradycardia and arrhythmias.

   *Arrhythmias are the earliest and most reliable sign of digitalis toxicity in children.*

## DIURETIC THERAPY

Diuretic therapy relieves fluid retention.

Frequent choices include hydrochlorothiazide (Hydrodiuril) and furosemide (Lasix).

Potential adverse side effects include:

   Electrolyte disturbances, such as hypokalemia, hyponatremia, and hypochloremia

   Metabolic alkalosis, caused by bicarbonate retention as sodium and chloride are lost

   Excessive volume depletion, especially if the oral fluid intake is low, resulting in:

   Reduced cardiac output

   Fatigue and reduced activity tolerance

   Postural hypotension

Prevention of side effects includes:

   Encouraging adequate fluid intake

   Having the patient wear support hose

   Instructing the patient regarding slow, cautious position changes

## PREVENTION OF HYPOKALEMIA

Hypokalemia alters myocardial function and can precipitate digitalis toxicity with associated arrhythmias.

Patients on high-dose corticosteroid therapy are at greater risk because of the potassium-wasting effect.

Signs and symptoms include (Felver, 1991):

   Weakness; flaccid paralysis

   Postural hypotension

   Abdominal distention; diminished bowel sounds; constipation

   Polyuria; nocturia

Preventive measures include:

   Increased dietary intake of potassium-rich foods (provide list of appropriate foods)

   Potassium supplementation if serum potassium level is less than 3.5 mEq/L

   Potassium-sparing diuretics (e.g., spironolactone), but these may cause hyperkalemia

   Teaching symptoms of hypokalemia

## VASODILATOR THERAPY

Vasodilator therapy causes arteriolar vasodilation, which reduces afterload by reducing peripheral vascular resistance.

Choices may include nitrates, hydralazine (Apresoline), angiotensin-converting enzyme (ACE) inhibitors (e.g., captopril, enalapril), and calcium antagonists (e.g., nifedipine).

Potential side effects include postural hypotension.

the home in frank pulmonary edema because symptoms are so severe that patients quickly seek emergency care. If the condition is encountered, "911" or another emergency telephone number must be called, and supportive interventions must be provided until an ambulance arrives.

## CARDIAC ARRHYTHMIAS

Many arrhythmias are relatively benign and need no treatment. Others have adverse effects, and some are life threatening. When an arrhythmia causes a rapid or erratic ventricular response, the ventricular filling time is shortened and cardiac output is reduced. This can result in hypotension, weakness, light-headedness, mental confusion, and angina. Reduced cardiac output also results in a lower mixed venous oxygen tension that, in the patient with preexisting hypoxemia, lowers the $PaO_2$ even further.

Arrhythmias may originate in the sinus node or the atrial muscle (supraventricular); at or near the atrioventricular node between the atria and the ventricles (junctional); or in the ventricles. Generally, arrhythmias associated with acute respiratory failure are more likely to be atrial, whereas those associated with chronic stable COPD are more likely to be ventricular (Brashear, 1984). Arrhythmias are described in Table 10-2.

Arrhythmias probably explain most sudden, unexpected deaths in patients with pulmonary disease. Multifocal atrial tachycardia and ventricular tachycardia are frequently seen in patients with acute respiratory failure and are considered to be a poor prognostic sign.

### Etiology

Cardiac arrhythmias are most often associated with hypoxemia; acute respiratory failure; pH and electrolyte disturbances; cor pulmonale; coexisting coronary artery disease; excessive caffeine, alcohol, or nicotine intake; or side effects of medication such as digitalis, theophylline, and β-adrenergic bronchodilators. Arrhythmias, especially premature ventricular contractions (PVCs), are much more likely to occur at night in association with profound drops in noctural oxygen saturation (Sullivan, 1985; Shepard, 1985).

Coronary artery disease coexists in many patients with COPD and is associated with an increased frequency of PVCs (Shepard, 1985). Arrhythmias are triggered by myocardial ischemia. If the $PaO_2$ is already compromised, such as in lung disease, this risk is even higher. The sequelae of myocardial ischemia, myocardial infarction, or overstretching of the myocardium associated with congestive heart failure also increases the risk for subsequent arrhythmias.

High levels of stress, anxiety, and even overt panic are not uncommon in patients with chronic lung disease in response to increasing dyspnea, chest tightness, and overall functional impairment. Heightened sympathetic nervous system stimulation increases circulating catecholamines and may be enough to precipitate arrhythmias, especially if combined with further deterioration of blood gases. Transient hypoxemia in association with coughing and reflex stimuli arising from pressure receptors in the right atrium, ventricle, and pulmonary arteries may also trigger sympathetic and parasympathetic responses.

### Assessment

Although the diagnosis of arrhythmias is based on specific ECG changes, clues to their presence can readily be identified through careful observation. Home care nurses must be sufficiently skilled in cardiac assessment to recognize the presence of potentially dangerous rhythm changes and to respond accordingly. Any significant change in cardiac rate or rhythm from baseline should be reported to the physician promptly. Signs and symptoms include the following:

| Signs | Symptoms |
|---|---|
| Irregular rate or rhythm | Skipped heart beats |
| Pulse deficit | Palpitations; a "sinking feeling" |
| Weak peripheral pulse | Light-headedness |
| ECG abnormalities | Sudden-onset weakness, dyspnea, or chest pain |

### Evaluation of Blood Levels

If drug toxicity or electrolyte abnormalities are suspected, the physician should be contacted and authorization obtained to draw blood for the appropriate test. This most often is a venipuncture

**Table 10-2**   Common Arrhythmias in Patients with Chronic Lung Disease

| Arrhythmia | Characteristics | Causal associations | Clinical implications |
|---|---|---|---|
| **SUPRAVENTRICULAR ARRHYTHMIAS** | | | |
| Sinus tachycardia | Identical to normal sinus rhythm except for rate >100 bpm | Normal response to exercise, anxiety, pain, anemia, fever and other hypermetabolic states; often seen with adrenergic stimulants, anxiety, heart failure, or hypoxemia | If heart rate >140 bpm, less time available for coronary artery and left ventricular filling, and signs of myocardial ischemia or reduced cardiac output possible |
| Premature atrial contractions | Episodic, with sudden onset and resolution; rhythm regular except when PACs occur; heart rate between 60 and 100 bpm; pulse deficit possible; patient complains of "skipped beats"; results from firing of ectopic focus in atrium | Increased cardiac irritability caused by caffeine, alcohol, nicotine, or stretching of heart muscle in CHF; hypokalemia, hypoxia, hypermetabolic states, sympathomimetics, stress, anxiety, fatigue, and atrial ischemia or infarction | Usually do not need treatment; may precipitate atrial fibrillation if more than six PACs occur in 1 min; may precipitate angina or CHF |
| Atrial flutter | Rapid, regular fluttering of atria, caused by rapid firing of atrial ectopic focus; usually some degree of block, which reduces ventricular response to one half or one quarter of atrial rate; heart rate usually regular; usually asymptomatic | Congestive heart failure, acute cor pulmonale, atherosclerotic heart disease, myocardial infarction, rheumatic heart disease, thyrotoxicosis | |
| Atrial fibrillation | Disorganized quivering of atria; caused by multiple atrial ectopic foci firing at different rates; rapid, irregularly irregular rhythm at 120-200 bpm; pulse deficit | Associated with heart failure, cor pulmonale, atherosclerotic heart disease, rheumatic heart disease, digitalis toxicity, and thyrotoxicosis | If ventricular response rate is high, decreased cardiac output, weakened pulse, and possible heart failure |

*BPM*, Beats per minute; *PACs*, premature atrial contractions; *CHF*, congestive heart failure; *PVCs*, premature ventricular contractions; *CPR*, cardiopulmonary resuscitation; *DNR*, do not resuscitate; *AV*, atrioventricular; *PAT*, paroxysmal atrial tachycardia.

**Table 10-2**   Common Arrhythmias in Patients with Chronic Lung Disease—cont'd

| Arrhythmia | Characteristics | Causal associations | Clinical implications |
|---|---|---|---|
| Multifocal atrial tachycardia | Chaotic irregular rhythm with heart rate >100 bpm | Occurs most often in patients with severe pulmonary disease who are in acute respiratory failure | High mortality in association with acute respiratory failure |
| Paroxysmal atrial tachycardia | Rapid heart rate (150-250 bpm) with abrupt onset and cessation; regular rhythm | Triggered by tobacco, caffeine, alcohol, sympathomimetics, fatigue, or emotions | Rapid rate and decreased cardiac output may precipitate angina or CHF |

**VENTRICULAR ARRHYTHMIAS**

| Arrhythmia | Characteristics | Causal associations | Clinical implications |
|---|---|---|---|
| Premature ventricular contractions | Irregular rhythm with rate of 60-100 bpm; contractions originating from ectopic focus in ventricle; pulse deficit possible; may be asymptomatic or associated with palpitations; dizziness, weakness, and fatigue, if cardiac output drops | Occasional PVCs triggered by nicotine, caffeine, or lack of sleep; frequent PVCs associated with hypoxia, hypokalemia, hyperkalemia, digitalis or theophylline toxicity, heart failure, acidosis, alkalosis, and increased catecholamines; more likely to occur at night in association with severe nocturnal $O_2$ desaturation | Increased risk of ventricular fibrillation and sudden death if PVCs occur in pairs or triplets, more often than six per min, or occur on the T wave in patients with coronary heart disease |
| Ventricular tachycardia | Runs of three or more sequential PVCs; ventricular rate between 120-150 bpm; radial pulse often not detectable because of low cardiac output; patient usually highly anxious or confused | | Angina due to low cardiac output; a medical emergency: call 911 (or other emergency number) and prepare to initiate CPR |
| Ventricular fibrillation | Ineffectual, chaotic quivering of ventricles caused by stimuli from many ectopic foci | | Circulation ceases and cardiac arrest has occured; CPR initiated unless a DNR order has been written |

*Continued.*

**Table 10-2**  Common Arrhythmias in Patients with Chronic Lung Disease—cont'd

| Arrhythmia | Characteristics | Causal associations | Clinical implications |
|---|---|---|---|
| **ARRHYTHMIAS CAUSED BY DIGITALIS TOXICITY** | Slows conduction to AV node causing blocks, bradycardia; stimulates ventricular ectopic foci, causing arrhythmias; most commonly present with PVCs and ventricular tachycardia; in COPD, often see PAT with AV block, atrial tachycardia, and atrial tachycardia with block | | Toxicity assumed cause of any new arrhythmia in a patient on a digitalis preparation; hold dose; consult with physician, and obtain serum level measurement |

for serum electrolytes or drug levels, but it may include arterial puncture for arterial blood gas analysis.

### Electrocardiographic and Holter Monitoring

Electrocardiograms may be obtained in the home if the patient cannot easily be transported to the physician's office or hospital. Because of their episodic nature, however, arrhythmias often go undetected using standard ECG. Further evaluation, perhaps including Holter monitoring for a more extended period of time, may be indicated for symptomatic pulse irregularities, especially if these are associated with deterioration in cardiopulmonary or cognitive status. The patient is generally fitted with the Holter monitor in the ECG department. Home care responsibilities include supervision to ensure that (1) the monitor remains in place and (2) the patient keeps a diary of symptoms and key events such as time of arising, going to bed, and taking medications. Older monitors may require a battery change after 24 hours. Patients cannot shower or be close to electrical equipment (e.g., electrical blankets) while being monitored.

## Nursing Interventions
### Elimination of Precipitants

Elimination of the precipitants is the single most important factor in the management of patients with cardiac arrhythmias. Preventive measures include adequate oxygenation, maintenance of normal acid-base and electrolyte balance, control of heart failure, and careful monitoring of serum levels of drugs such as digitalis that tend to cause arrhythmias at toxic levels. Elimination of smoking and excessive consumption of coffee and alcohol will reduce the incidence of some arrhythmias (Table 10-2).

### Use of Nocturnal Oxygen

When associated with known or suspected severe nocturnal desaturation, nocturnal arrhythmias (usually PVCs) are usually treated with oxygen. Because these patients do not necessarily experience dyspnea at night, they may not understand the importance of using their oxygen during sleep. Home care staff need to reinforce the preventive role of oxygen.

### Treatment of Respiratory Failure

Arrhythmias precipitated by acute respiratory failure are generally treated in the hospital and respond to improved ventilation and correction of metabolic and hemodynamic abnormalities. Cardiac output can be improved by slowing the ventricular rate and restoring normal fluid volume. Tissue oxygenation can be improved by low-flow oxygen, rigorous bronchial hygiene, treatment of infection and anemia, and reduction of fever.

### Use of Antiarrhythmic Agents

Arrhythmias associated with myocardial infarction are generally treated with antiarrhythmic drugs. Examples of commonly used medications include digoxin, quinidine, disopyramide (Norpace), calcium channel-blocking agents such as verapamil and diltiazem, and procainamide.

## ANGINA AND MYOCARDIAL INFARCTION

A coexisting diagnosis of angina or a past history of myocardial infarction is not uncomon in older patients with chronic lung disease and complicates the course and treatment of the pulmonary problem.

### Etiology

Hypoxemia, anemia, hypertension, congestive heart failure, tachyarrhythmias, exercise, anxiety, and bronchodilators may all contribute to an increased frequency of angina and myocardial infarction.

### Assessment

Home care nurses must attempt to differentiate chest pain of cardiac origin (angina or myocardial infarction) from that of pulmonary, esophageal, or musculoskeletal origin. These differences are summarized in Table 1-2 (p. 23).

### Nursing Interventions
#### Angina

Angina is generally treated with nitrates, β-blocking agents, or calcium antagonists (Opie, 1987). Vasodilators such as nitroglycerin improve coronary flow. These drugs also dilate the pulmonary vessels and, in the patient with chronic lung disease, may increase pulmonary blood flow to underventilated alveoli, thereby worsening V/Q mismatching and decreasing the PaO$_2$. It is important to observe the patient for increased dyspnea, right ventricular failure, or other evidence of reduced tissue oxygenation following initiation of vasodilators. Nitrate-induced arterial hypoxemia may be prevented by the administration of nasal oxygen or an increase in the flow rate of oxygen already prescribed. Oximetry may help to identify patients for whom such an adjustment in oxygen would be helpful.

If aspirin has been prescribed to reduce the risk of thromboembolic complications, the nurse must be alert for signs of gastric irritation or bleeding. Patients with chronic lung disease are at increased risk for gastric ulcer formation, which can result from the use of unbuffered aspirin.

### Myocardial Infarction

Prompt recognition of symptoms consistent with myocardial infarction is particularly important because medications are available that can reduce the size of the infarct if treatment is initiated within a few hours. Patients with chronic lung disease may delay notifying their physician when new symptoms occur because they "don't want to bother the doctor" or think that the symptoms will go away on their own. Patients and families should be instructed to place an urgent call to the physician or call "911" (or another emergency telephone number) if severe chest pain is not relieved with three nitroglycerin tablets administered sublingually at 10-minute intervals.

### Long-Term Care for Coronary Artery Disease

The long-term care of patients with coronary artery disease should include a reduction of risk factors such as smoking, obesity, hypertension, high serum cholesterol, diabetes, and stress. The importance of dietary restriction of sodium, cholesterol, and saturated fats should be reinforced and patient education materials provided. Elevated serum cholesterol levels should be evaluated, and the results should be shared with the patient as a means of promoting compliance with therapy.

### Cardiopulmonary Resuscitation

*Cardiopulmonary resuscitation (CPR) instruction is routinely provided for parents of high-risk infants and children, especially those using home oxygen or ventilators or with tracheostomies.*

With older adults, family members who are physically and emotionally capable of performing CPR may benefit from instruction in the technique. CPR instruction is best carried out in the context of general first aid preparedness. However, hearing that a loved one is at risk for a cardiac arrest and that his or her survival may depend on the family's intervention can be frightening and may outweigh any potential benefits of such preparedness.

It is essential to determine the patient's wishes in the event of a cardiac arrest. Home care staff are in a unique position to develop the trust and rapport that such anticipatory planning requires. A "do not resuscitate" (DNR) decision requires careful consideration and discussion between the patient, the physician, family members, clergy, and key home care staff. Ethical and legal aspects of DNR issues are discussed in Chapters 23 and 24.

**REFERENCES**

Brashear RE: Arrhythmias in patients with chronic obstructive pulmonary disease, *Med Clin North Am* 68:969, 1984.

Felver L: Fluid and electrolyte balance and imbalances. In Patrick ML et al: *Medical surgical nursing: pathophysiological concepts,* ed 2, Philadelphia, 1991, JB Lippincott.

Laurent-Bopp D: Heart failure. In Patrick ML et al: *Medical surgical nursing: pathophysiological concepts,* ed 2, Philadelphia, 1991, JB Lippincott.

Nocturnal Oxygen Therapy Trial Group: Continuous or nocturnal oxygen therapy in hypoxemic chronic obstructive lung disease, *Ann Intern Med* 93:391, 1980.

Opie LH et al: *Drugs for the heart,* ed 2, New York, 1987, Grune & Stratton.

Shepard JW et al: Relationship of ventricular ectopy to nocturnal oxygen desaturation in patients with COPD, *Am J Med* 78:28, 1985.

Sullivan CE, Issa FG: Obstructive sleep apnea, *Clin Chest Med* 6:633, 1985.

White DP: Central sleep apnea, *Clin Chest Med* 6:623, 1985.

**SUGGESTED READINGS**

Hill NS: The cardiac exam in lung disease, *Clin Chest Med* 8:273, 1987.

Kersten LD: Pulmonary heart disease. In *Comprehensive respiratory nursing,* Philadelphia, 1989, WB Saunders.

Matthay RA, Berger HJ: Cardiovascular performance in chronic obstructive pulmonary diseases, *Med Clin North Am* 65:489, 1981.

Patrick ML et al, editors: Heart function. In *Medical surgical nursing: pathophysiological concepts,* ed 2, Philadelphia, 1991, JB Lippincott.

Shih HT et al: Frequency and significance of cardiac arrhythmias in chronic obstructive lung disease, *Chest* 94:44, 1988.

Underhill SL: Assessment of cardiac function. In Patrick ML et al: *Medical surgical nursing: pathophysiological concepts,* ed 2, Philadelphia, 1991, JB Lippincott.

Wiedemann HP, Matthay RA: Cor pulmonale in chronic obstructive pulmonary disease: circulatory pathophysiology and management, *Clin Chest Med* 11:523, 1990.

# CHAPTER 11

# NUTRITION

DIANA R. OPENBRIER • MARGARET M. IRWIN •
MARGARET F. GLONINGER • ANN CONDON MEYERS

Problems with nutrition and fluids are common in patients with chronic lung disease. The assessment, etiologic factors, and important nursing interventions for malnutrition, fluid problems, and obesity are discussed in this chapter.

## MALNUTRITION

Protein-calorie malnutrition is a disorder that can be caused by inadequate intake or absorption of food or an uncompensated increase in nutritional requirements. Reports suggest that malnutrition is a problem for 30% to 60% of adults with chronic obstructive lung disease (Braun, 1984). Malnutrition in this group usually takes the form of low body weight and muscle mass and loss of subcutaneous fat stores, or marasmus. *In children, protein-calorie malnutrition is often accompanied by overt vitamin deficiencies caused by malabsorption.* Malnutrition can increase the risk of infection, impair wound healing, and adversely affect the respiratory system, as summarized in Table 11-1 (Wilson, 1986; Edelman, 1986; Openbrier, 1983).

### Etiology

Children and adults with chronic lung disease may have protein-calorie deficiencies caused by anorexia, gastrointestinal disturbances, malabsorption, increased metabolic requirements, dyspnea (Rindfleisch, 1985), or fatigue. Contributing factors for each are summarized in Table 11-2. Medications commonly prescribed to treat lung disease can also affect appetite or nutritional status in a number of ways (Table 11-3).

Because patients with chronic lung disease often have a marginal nutritional balance, other factors that may influence the adequacy of dietary intake can be significant enough to cause protein-calorie deficiencies. Poorly fitting dentures and a sore mouth from dental caries and oral infections may impair dietary intake. Patients with chronic lung disease typically experience a high level of day-to-day stress associated with chronic infection and disability. There is evidence that many of these patients have higher than expected metabolic requirements.

Other factors that may inhibit the patient from maintaining a nutritionally balanced diet include lack of income to purchase nutritious food, limited access to grocery stores, and inadequate meal preparation facilities. Individuals may lack the knowledge about nutritional requirements needed to make appropriate food selections. Religious and cultural beliefs may also affect the adequacy of dietary intake.

### Assessment

Given the prevalence of nutritional problems in patients with chronic lung disease, a nutritional assessment should be performed on every respiratory patient referred for home care. The goals of

**Table 11-1**    Potential effects of malnutrition on the respiratory system

| Age group | Lung structure | Defense mechanisms | Muscle function |
|---|---|---|---|
| *Infants and children* | *Fewer cells; fewer alveoli; decreased lung size; decreased surfactant; decreased alveolar-capillary surface area* | *Decreased ciliary clearance; decreased immune function* | *Decreased growth and development; decreased strength* |
| Adults | Decreased lung size; decreased surfactant; air space enlargement; loss of septa; decreased alveolar-capillary surface area; decreased elasticity; increased air trapping | Decreased ciliary clearance; increased adherence of bacteria to airway lining; decreased immune function; decreased sighs | Decreased muscle strength caused by decreased intercostal and diaphragmatic mass |

**Table 11-2**    Potential causes of malnutrition in chronic lung disease

| Cause | Contributing factors |
|---|---|
| Anorexia | Anxiety; depression; side effects of medications; right ventricular failure; acute respiratory tract infection; abdominal fullness from air swallowing; blunted sense of taste from smoking or medication; reduced sense of smell from smoking and nutritional depletion; social isolation; unattractive, poorly presented meals |
| Gastrointestinal system disturbances | *Improper positioning and excessive rate and volume of feeding in infants;* food allergies or intolerances; reduced gastrointestinal motility from high inspiratory pressure in ventilator-dependent patients; early satiety; nausea and vomiting; indigestion caused by air swallowing with dyspnea |
| Malabsorption | Pancreatic enzyme deficiencies in cystic fibrosis, impairing absorption of protein and fat; *premature infants are unable to digest lactose and long-chain fatty acids because of insufficient lactase, bile salts, and carnitine (involved in transport of fatty acids to mitochondria, where they are metabolized)* |
| Increased metabolic requirements | Acute infection; fever; increased work of breathing in airflow obstruction and restrictive lung disease (adults with severe chronic lung disease increase energy expenditures by 30% to 50% with activity and are often unable to increase intake enough for caloric needs; ventilator dependency may increase needs by 50% to 70%); *growth and development of child;* surgery; chemotherapy, radiation therapy |
| Meal-related dyspnea and fatigue | Severe airflow obstruction; oxygen desaturation during meals; copious respiratory tract secretions; energy expended during meal preparation leaves none for eating; steroid myopathy; decreased muscle mass from nutritional depletion; *poorly established sucking reflex in premature infant (normally present after 32 to 34 weeks' gestation)* |

**Table 11-3** Potential impact of medications on dietary intake

| Medication | Effects | Nursing intervention |
|---|---|---|
| Theophylline | Anorexia and nausea with serum level in therapeutic range; vomiting with serum level in toxic range | Administer with food or antacids. Recognize changes in smoking patterns or other medications that can increase serum levels and monitor serum theophylline levels. |
| $\beta_2$-Agonists | Oral preparations may cause nausea, inhaled preparations usually do not | Use inhaled preparation instead of oral whenever possible. Use inhaled preparation 15 min before meals to decrease meal-related dyspnea. Administer oral preparation at least 1 hr after meals. |
| Prednisone | Usually increases appetite, but metabolic effect is protein catabolism; ulcerogenic | Capitalize on positive effect on appetite to improve nutritional intake while on prednisone; maintain protein intake. Avoid long-term use because of catabolic effects. Administer with food or antacids. |
| Inhaled steroids | Fungal infections of oral mucosa | Have patient rinse mouth well with water after use or use before meals so food can act as a mechanical cleanser, removing steroid residue from mucosa. |
| Antibiotics | Nausea, vomiting, diarrhea, impaired production or absorption of nutrients (e.g., vitamin K) | Check if antibiotic given with food. Administer vitamin K supplements if necessary (e.g., abnormal prothrombin time). |

this assessment are to determine the following:

- Degree of nutritional impairment
- Current body nutrient stores
- Baseline nutritional requirements
- Patient's ability to alter food intake to meet nutritional needs

The assessment should be repeated as often as necessary to evaluate the effects of the established nutritional repletion program.

### History and Physical Examination

Deficient dietary intake should be suspected if the patient has a history of nutritional problems or if the physical examination reveals signs of nutritional depletion (Table 11-4).

### Dietary History

An accurate estimate of daily nutritional intake is important. However, patient recall is notoriously inaccurate, even for foods consumed the previous day. It is preferable to determine calorie intake from ongoing records. An example of a simple food intake chart that patients can be taught to keep if nutritional intake is thought to be inadequate is presented in Fig. 11-1. Patients should maintain the food intake record for at least 1 week to ensure that any significant deficits in nutritional intake are revealed.

### Quantitative Measures

■ *Body Weight.* Body weight is the single most important indicator of nutritional status for these patients and may be the only measurement available to the home care nurse. It is important to monitor body weight in relationship to normal standards. The Metropolitan Life Insurance Company's table of normal weights is the standard commonly used (Table 11-5). The percentage ideal body weight (% IBW) compares the actual weight with the *midpoint* of the normal range. Although % IBW

**Table 11-4**   Physical abnormalities in nutritional depletion

| Location | Signs | Deficiencies |
|---|---|---|
| Hair | Alopecia | Protein-calorie |
| | Brittle | Protein-calorie |
| | Dryness | Zinc |
| | Easy pluckability | Vitamins E and A |
| Head | Temporal wasting | Protein-calorie |
| | *Soft spot that does not harden* | Vitamin D |
| Eyes | Pale conjunctiva | Iron, folate, vitamin $B_{12}$ |
| | *Bitot's spots in children* | Vitamin A |
| | Conjunctival xerosis | Vitamin A |
| Lips | Cracked, red, flaky corners | Riboflavin, niacin, iron, pyridoxine |
| Tongue | Edema | Folate, niacin |
| | Smooth tongue; atrophied taste buds | Riboflavin, iron, vitamin $B_{12}$ |
| Gums | Pale | Iron |
| | Bleeding | Vitamins K and C |
| | Inflamed; sores | Vitamin C |
| Nails | Spooning | Iron |
| | Transverse lines; ridges | Protein-calorie |

is commonly used, it is misleading because it assumes that only the midpoint is normal. A preferable measure is the minimal acceptable weight (MAW), corrected for height. This interpretation uses the *minimum* weight that is considered normal for a given height, frame, and sex. For example, the MAW for a 72-inch man with a medium frame is 157 lb. If this person's actual weight were only 148 lb, his % MAW would be:

$$\text{MAW} = \frac{\text{Actual weight}}{\begin{array}{c}\text{Lowest point}\\ \text{of standard}\end{array}} \times 100 \; or \; \frac{148 \text{ lb}}{157 \text{ lb}} \times 100$$

$$= 94\% \text{ MAW}$$

A body weight of less than 90% of MAW is indicative of clinically relevant malnutrition. For routine home care assessments, the assumption of a medium frame is probably sufficient. To be reproducible, weights should be measured (1) with the patient wearing light clothing without shoes, (2) in the early morning after voiding, (3) in a fasted state, and (4) on the same scale. Strain-gauge weight scales are generally more reliable than spring-gauge types. Because inexpensive, commercially available bathroom scales may have either a strain gauge or a spring gauge, it is important to check the label before purchasing a scale.

The most common pattern of weight change seen in chronic obstructive pulmonary disease (COPD) is a slow decline in weight or a cyclic step decline in weight, with plateau periods during which weight is stable. Sudden weight loss, such as 20 lb in 1 month, is more likely to be seen in malignancies or with rapid diuresis. Weight loss in patients with cystic fibrosis is strongly associated with respiratory tract infection.

■ *Anthropometric Measures.* Anthropometric measures such as skin-fold thickness and measurement of muscle circumference are sometimes used to assess nutritional status. These measures provide much the same type of information as body weight measurements in terms of overall nutritional status. Anthropometric measures can be useful in assessing and evaluating nutritional status in individuals

**Record What You Eat**
(one day actual, not "typical," intake)

Date _____

Weight _____

| Meal or Snack | Food/Liquid (Describe ingredients) | Amount* |
|---|---|---|
| Morning foods (note time of day) | | |
| Afternoon foods | | |
| Evening foods | | |
| Night foods | | |

*Estimate portion sizes as best you can in terms of ounces, cups, teaspoons, tablespoons, whenever possible. Otherwise, record as "small," "medium," or "large" servings. Record intake as soon as you have had something to eat or drink. Describe how food was cooked (e.g., baked chicken, fried pork chops).

**Fig. 11-1**    Sample food intake chart.

**Table 11-5** Height and weight tables for men and women*

| Feet | Inches | Centimeters | Small frame | | Medium frame | | Large frame | |
|---|---|---|---|---|---|---|---|---|
| | | | Pounds | Kilograms | Pounds | Kilograms | Pounds | Kilograms |
| **MEN (INDOOR CLOTHING)†** | | | | | | | | |
| 5 | 1 | 154.9 | 128-134 | 58.2-60.9 | 131-141 | 59.5-64.1 | 138-150 | 62.7-68.2 |
| 5 | 2 | 157.5 | 130-136 | 59.1-61.8 | 133-143 | 60.4-65.0 | 140-153 | 63.6-69.5 |
| 5 | 3 | 160.0 | 132-138 | 60.0-62.7 | 135-145 | 61.4-65.9 | 142-156 | 64.5-70.9 |
| 5 | 4 | 162.6 | 134-140 | 60.9-63.6 | 137-148 | 62.3-67.2 | 144-160 | 65.5-72.7 |
| 5 | 5 | 165.1 | 136-142 | 61.8-64.5 | 139-151 | 63.2-68.6 | 146-164 | 66.4-74.5 |
| 5 | 6 | 167.6 | 138-145 | 62.7-65.9 | 142-154 | 64.5-70.0 | 149-168 | 67.7-76.4 |
| 5 | 7 | 170.2 | 140-148 | 63.6-67.2 | 145-157 | 65.9-71.4 | 152-172 | 69.1-78.2 |
| 5 | 8 | 172.7 | 142-151 | 64.5-68.6 | 148-160 | 67.2-72.7 | 155-176 | 70.5-80.0 |
| 5 | 9 | 175.3 | 144-154 | 65.5-70.0 | 151-153 | 68.6-74.1 | 158-180 | 71.8-81.8 |
| 5 | 10 | 177.8 | 146-157 | 66.4-71.4 | 154-166 | 70.0-75.5 | 161-184 | 73.2-83.6 |
| 5 | 11 | 180.3 | 149-160 | 67.7-72.7 | 157-170 | 71.4-77.3 | 164-188 | 74.5-85.5 |
| 6 | 0 | 182.9 | 152-164 | 69.1-74.5 | 160-174 | 72.7-79.1 | 168-192 | 76.4-87.3 |
| 6 | 1 | 185.4 | 155-168 | 70.5-76.4 | 164-178 | 74.5-80.9 | 172-197 | 78.2-89.5 |
| 6 | 2 | 188.0 | 158-172 | 71.8-78.2 | 167-182 | 75.9-82.7 | 176-202 | 80.0-91.8 |
| 6 | 3 | 190.5 | 162-176 | 73.6-80.0 | 171-187 | 77.7-85.0 | 181-207 | 82.3-94.1 |

## WOMEN (INDOOR CLOTHING)‡

| | | | 102-111 | 46.4-50.0 | 109-121 | 49.5-55.0 | 118-131 | 53.6-59.5 |
|---|---|---|---|---|---|---|---|---|
| 4 | 9 | 144.8 | 102-111 | 46.4-50.0 | 109-121 | 49.5-55.0 | 118-131 | 53.6-59.5 |
| 4 | 10 | 147.3 | 103-113 | 46.8-51.4 | 111-123 | 50.0-55.9 | 120-134 | 54.5-60.9 |
| 4 | 11 | 149.9 | 104-115 | 47.3-52.3 | 113-126 | 51.4-57.2 | 122-137 | 55.5-62.3 |
| 5 | 0 | 152.4 | 106-118 | 48.2-53.6 | 115-129 | 52.3-58.6 | 125-140 | 56.8-63.6 |
| 5 | 1 | 154.9 | 108-121 | 49.1-55.0 | 118-132 | 53.6-60.0 | 128-143 | 58.2-65.0 |
| 5 | 2 | 157.5 | 111-124 | 50.5-56.4 | 121-135 | 55.0-61.4 | 131-147 | 59.5-66.8 |
| 5 | 3 | 160.0 | 114-127 | 51.8-57.7 | 124-138 | 56.4-62.7 | 134-151 | 60.9-68.6 |
| 5 | 4 | 162.6 | 117-130 | 53.2-59.0 | 127-141 | 57.7-64.1 | 137-155 | 62.3-70.5 |
| 5 | 5 | 165.1 | 120-133 | 54.5-60.5 | 130-144 | 59.0-65.5 | 140-159 | 63.6-72.3 |
| 5 | 6 | 167.6 | 123-136 | 55.9-61.8 | 133-147 | 60.5-66.8 | 143-163 | 65.0-74.1 |
| 5 | 7 | 170.2 | 126-139 | 57.3-63.2 | 136-150 | 61.8-68.2 | 146-167 | 66.4-75.9 |
| 5 | 8 | 172.7 | 129-142 | 58.6-64.5 | 139-153 | 63.2-69.5 | 149-170 | 67.7-77.3 |
| 5 | 9 | 175.3 | 132-145 | 60.0-65.9 | 142-156 | 64.6-70.9 | 152-173 | 69.1-78.6 |
| 5 | 10 | 177.8 | 135-148 | 61.4-67.3 | 145-159 | 65.9-72.3 | 155-176 | 70.5-80.0 |
| 5 | 11 | 180.3 | 138-151 | 62.7-73.6 | 148-162 | 67.3-73.6 | 158-179 | 71.8-81.4 |

Basic data from Society of Actuaries and Association of Life Insurance Medical Directors of America: *Build study, 1979,* New York, 1980, Copyright 1983, Metropolitan Life Insurance Company.

*This table corrects the 1983 Metropolitan tables to height without shoe heels.

†Weight includes 5 lb for clothing.

‡Weight includes 3 lb for clothing.

**Table 11-6**    Common laboratory measures of nutritional status

| Test | Normal value | Comments |
| --- | --- | --- |
| Serum albumin | 3.5-5.5 g/dl | Low in malnutrition; most important test for protein-calorie deficiency; also reduced in liver disease |
| Creatinine height index | See Comments column | Measure of skeletal protein; requires 24-hr urine specimen; helpful when weight fluctuations caused by fluid loss or nutrition confuse clinical picture; most useful to monitor patient changes in muscle mass rather than comparison with any "normal" values |
| Total lymphocyte count | 1500-4000/μl | Measure of cellular immunity; low in diseases affecting cellular immunity such as HIV infection; low in protein-calorie deficiency |
| Serum transferrin | 200-400 mg/dl | Serum globulin that binds and transports iron; low in malnutrition |
| Serum vitamin A Serum vitamin E | 300-650 μg/L 5-20 μg/L | Fat-soluble vitamins poorly absorbed in cystic fibrosis; water-soluble supplements often required; dose based on serum level |

who cannot be easily weighed in the home.

■ TRICEPS SKIN-FOLD THICKNESS. Skin-fold thickness measurements provide an estimate of fat stores. Although the measurements may be made at any body site, the triceps skin-fold (TSF) thickness test is most commonly used and is based on the average of three measurements made at the midpoint of the upper arm with a skin-fold thickness caliper. The individual who makes the measurements must use consistent and proper technique.

■ MIDARM MUSCLE CIRCUMFERENCE. Midarm muscle circumference (MAC) measurements give an estimate of muscle size. The measurement is made at the midpoint of the upper arm between the acromion process of the scapula and the olecranon process of the ulna. Some authors report muscle surface area instead of MAC; however, both measurements provide information about muscle stores.

■ *Biochemical Measurements.* Biochemical measurements can be used to assess nutritional status. As increasing numbers of seriously ill patients receive care at home, these measures may be used more frequently by the home care nurse in the future. These measurements are necessary for the assessment of visceral nutrient stores and vitamin and trace element status. Such assessment parameters are used in more seriously ill patients and patients receiving highly invasive home nutritional therapy, such as total parenteral nutrition. Laboratory measurements used to evaluate nutritional status are summarized in Table 11-6.

**Functional Assessment**

A functional assessment in combination with the nutritional assessment is a useful way to determine nutritional adequacy and the effectiveness of interventions. Any measurement can be used that depicts changes in functional ability over time. In adults the functional assessment might include the following:

• Maximal inspiratory pressures
• Maximal expiratory pressures
• Hand-grip strength
• Ambulation (12-minute walk)
• General ability to perform activities of daily living
• Exacerbation incidence
• Hospitalization incidence

### Evaluation of the Nutritional Program

*In infants and children, advancement on the growth chart and the accomplishment of normal developmental tasks are associated with adequate dietary intake (see Chapter 3).* The efficacy of nutritional interventions for the adult is based on the degree to which nutritional goals have been met. These may include an increase (or decrease) in weight in terms of percentage MAW, an improvement in maximum inspiratory and expiratory pressures, and other functional measures. Adults can be expected to gain no more than about 2 lb lean mass per week. Weight gain at a greater rate should raise the suspicion of fluid retention. Noticeable improvement in the patient's ability to perform activities of daily living usually provides sufficient motivation to continue with nutritional support measures.

In patients with initial visceral protein depletion or problems with malabsorption, the evaluation should include periodic repetition of biochemical measurements.

## Nursing Interventions
### Goals for Nutritional Repletion

Specific nutritional interventions can be used individually or in combination, depending on the goals for nutritional repletion. These goals, based on the patient's disease, functional status, and baseline nutritional status, include the following:

- Prevention of nutritional depletion
- Maintenance of nutritional status
- Nutritional repletion

The specific dietary plan based on the nutritional goal should specify when interventions will be implemented, how serial evaluations will be performed, and when the goal should be realized. Unmet goals require reevaluation of the nutritional care plan. To be most effective, plans need to include patient and caregiver counseling and multiple strategies to increase caloric and protein intake.

Nutritional counseling should include patient education about the elements of a balanced diet, including the four basic food groups, and information on specific measures to manage typical symptoms associated with nutritional depletion. Specific suggestions for improving the nutritional status of patients with chronic lung disease are summarized in Table 11-7.

### Increasing Caloric Intake

Caloric intake should be based on needs for weight gain and growth.

*Infants. Infants without lung disease require 100 to 150 Kcal/kg of body weight for normal growth. The caloric intake must be increased by 150% to 200% for catch-up growth of infants with cystic fibrosis or other chronic lung diseases.*

*Children. Children with cystic fibrosis require 130% to 150% of the normal caloric intake, usually taken with pancreatic enzymes to enhance absorption.*

*Adults. Adults with COPD need from 45 to 75 Kcal/kg of body weight to gain weight.*

■ ***Oral Food Supplements*** (Table 11-8)

■ COMPLETE FORMULATIONS. Complete formulations are products that can be used in place of meals. They are usually liquid supplements made from blenderized natural foods. These products provide calories, protein, fat, vitamins, and minerals in fairly complex forms that can be digested when the gastrointestinal tract is functioning normally. Some of the calorically dense preparations may cause diarrhea, and a more isosmotic product should be used instead. Complete formulations may be more palatable if semifrozen or heated.

■ MODULAR PRODUCTS. Modular diets are formulations composed of single nutrients. Most are bland powders that can be mixed with the normal diet to increase fat, carbohydrate, or protein content. Glucose polymers are the most common type and can be used to increase carbohydrate content. An example is Polycose powder, which can be added to any kind of diet without changing the taste of the food. Glucose polymers are often prescribed for patients with cystic fibrosis or COPD.

■ DISEASE-SPECIFIC FORMULAS. Disease-specific formulas have become accepted modes of nutritional therapy for patients with renal or hepatic failure. A formulation that is specific for patients with pulmonary disease has also been marketed

**Table 11-7**   Interventions for problems affecting dietary intake

| Symptom | Approach for patient |
|---|---|
| Anorexia | Check with physician about possible adjustments in medications that may cause anorexia, such as theophylline and antibiotics.<br>Encourage patient to eat even if appetite is poor because appetite usually improves with improved nutritional status.<br>Encourage patient to try a glass of wine ½ hr before meals.<br>Prepare aromatic foods such as fried onions or fresh baked bread.<br>Have high-calorie foods readily available for snacks.<br>Encourage bedtime snacks.<br>Rely on favorite foods.<br>Avoid huge portions of food, which may only overwhelm the patient.<br>Eat small portions of food more frequently.<br>Serve attractive meals.<br>Make the meal an enjoyable event.<br>Exercise 2 hr after a meal.<br>Rely on calorie-dense foods. |
| Early satiety | Eat high-calorie foods first.<br>Limit liquids until the end of the meal or drink fluids between meals.<br>Eat small amounts often. |
| Dyspnea | Rest before meal.<br>Use bronchodilators or a caffeine drink ½ to 1 hr before meals.<br>Implement secretion clearance strategies, if indicated, at least 1 hr before meal to allow for rest before eating. A hot drink may facilitate secretion clearance.<br>Eat in a leisurely manner. Try soft music and a pleasant atmosphere. Practice relaxation techniques before eating to reduce anxiety and wheezing.<br>Eat in a sitting position with the feet and elbows supported (tripod position).<br>If dyspnea increases during the meal, rest for a short period while using pursed lip breathing until breathlessness subsides. Use pursed lip breathing between bites if breathlessness is severe.<br>Use oxygen with meals if prescribed. Evaluate oxygen desaturation with meals with pulse oximeter and adjust flow rate of oxygen if necessary.<br>Consider possible effect of high CHO intake on $CO_2$ production for patients who retain $CO_2$, and alter diet if indicated. |
| Fatigue | Prepare meals several hours before eating, then rest to conserve energy for meal.<br>Prepare large amounts of food, then package food into serving sizes and freeze for later use.<br>Use easy to prepare meals such as frozen or canned foods when tired.<br>Use community agency meals such as Meals on Wheels.<br>*Give toddlers and preschool age children finger foods that are easy to chew so that they can pace their meal.*<br>Eat slowly and use foods that are easy to chew and digest.<br>Use tripod position.<br>*Infants with marginal sucking musculature should be fed with a soft pliable nipple, preferably with a cross-cut opening.* |

**Table 11-7**   Interventions for problems affecting dietary intake—cont'd

| Symptom | Approach for patient |
| --- | --- |
| Depression | Make meals a pleasant experience.<br>Encourage exercise.<br>Encourage socialization.<br>Refer patient for treatment if depression is significant. |
| Anxiety | Make meals enjoyable.<br>Avoid stressful discussions during meals.<br>Practice relaxation before meal.<br>Rest before meal.<br>Watch favorite TV show while eating.<br>Refer patient for treatment if anxiety is significant. |
| Taste changes | Eat foods that taste good.<br>Keep mouth moist to improve taste bud sensitivity.<br>Suck on a sour candy or eat a pickle ½ hr before meal to stimulate taste.<br>Keep nostrils clear so sense of smell is enhanced.<br>Clean teeth or dentures before meals. |
| Dry mouth | Consume enough fluids to prevent dehydration.<br>Adjust medication schedule to limit dry mouth before meals.<br>Suck on a sour candy or eat a pickle ½ hr before meal to stimulate salivation.<br>Humidify oxygen if flow rate is over 4 L/min. |
| Bloating | Eat small frequent meals and stop eating when uncomfortable.<br>Avoid rushed meals and relax before eating.<br>Use controlled pursed lip breathing to prevent air swallowing.<br>Prevent constipation.<br>Avoid gas-forming foods that cause bloating.<br>*Position infant so that esophagus is higher than stomach during feeding.*<br>*Most bottle feedings should take between 10 and 20 min.* |
| Food aversion | Avoid foods that are disliked.<br>Substitute different types of food that are high in calories.<br>Do not mix disliked food into other foods. |
| Nausea and vomiting | Check with physician about adjusting medications if indicated.<br>Avoid foods that are unappetizing and highly spiced.<br>Seek medical advice for other possible causes. |
| Diarrhea | Avoid hypertonic liquids.<br>Avoid highly spiced foods.<br>Seek medical advice. |
| Constipation | Implement a regular exercise program.<br>Increase dietary fiber.<br>Ask physician about stool softeners. |
| Chewing problems | Facilitate proper dental care.<br>Refit dentures if loose.<br>Eat soft foods or liquids. |

*Continued.*

**Table 11-7** Interventions for problems affecting dietary intake—cont'd

| Symptom | Approach for patient |
|---|---|
| Lack of meal socialization | Encourage participation in community center meal programs.<br>Encourage asking friend to lunch or dinner.<br>If eating alone, make the occasion enjoyable by watching favorite TV program or reading. |
| Lack of meal preparation facilities | Refer to community meal facility or arrange home delivery of meals.<br>Plan meals that are easily prepared with available facilities. |
| Lack of support system | Arrange for grocery delivery.<br>Arrange for someone to prepare meals.<br>Arrange for community meal delivery.<br>Evaluate for alternative living site. |
| Financial constraints | Refer for financial assistance through food stamp program, community meal assistance, or other program.<br>Discuss inexpensive but nutritious foods and cost-saving measures such as bulk food purchases and food banks. |

**Table 11-8** Enteral nutritional supplementation

| Type | Form | Indications | Caloric content | | | Density (Kcal/ml) |
|---|---|---|---|---|---|---|
| | | | Protein (%) | Fat (%) | CHO (%) | |
| Complete formulations<br>High density (e.g., Ensure, Sustacal, Instant Breakfast*) | Liquid | When balanced diet in liquid form required<br>Replaces or supplements solid food | 10-16 | 32-40 | 45-53 | 1.5-2.0 |
| Isotonic (e.g., Isocal) | Liquid | Less sweet and isosmotic; often used for cancer patients | 14-15 | 31-40 | 45-55 | 1-2.0 |
| Modular diets (Polycose) | Powder | When increased amounts of a specific nutrient required | — | — | 100 | (8 Kcal/teaspoon) |
| Disease-specific formulas (Pulmocare) | Liquid | To reduce $CO_2$ production | 17 | 55 | 28 | 1.5 |

*A good food supplement that is the least expensive of the formulations.

(Table 11-8). The rationale for the pulmonary formula is to reduce the dietary carbohydrate in an effort to reduce $CO_2$ production. Because there is little indication that nutritionally caused $CO_2$ production is a problem in patients with stable chronic lung disease and because the efficacy of the formula has not been well studied, the cost is probably not justified in most instances. However, the special pulmonary formula may be beneficial for patients with acute respiratory failure or chronic $CO_2$ retention. Generally, such high-fat diets should not be advocated because they increase the risk of cardiovascular disease.

The decision to use dietary supplements is based on patient preference and the failure of noncommercial supplements, such as milkshakes and eggnogs, to achieve nutritional goals. Many supplements such as Ensure, Sustacal, or Instant Breakfast are available in grocery stores. Third-party payors usually do not reimburse for nutritional supplements unless they are used as meal replacements.

■ *Other Approaches with Oral Intake.* Other measures that may be used to increase oral intake include mixing a favorite ice cream with a carbonated drink, eating a snack 1 to 2 hours before bedtime, and taking advantage of the "hungry time" of the day to eat the biggest meal. Using calorically dense foods such as butter, mayonnaise, peanut butter, cream cheese, and dried fruit and reducing intake of empty-calorie drinks such as water, coffee, or tea with meals may enhance nutritional intake without increasing the volume consumed. Good dental hygiene to enhance taste may also help to stimulate the appetite. If the diet does not include appropriate servings of the four basic types of food, vitamin and mineral supplements may be indicated.

■ COMBINING ORAL SUPPLEMENTS WITH ORAL FEEDING. The combination of oral supplements with a normal diet may be the best way to increase caloric intake. However, some patients simply substitute supplements for meals and little is gained. When taken too close to mealtime, supplements often reduce hunger. It is better to add the supplement 1 hour after meals, allowing a longer time for feelings of hunger to return before the next main meal. If the patient rarely eats breakfast, an early morning supplement may be appropriate. Late night supplements are also helpful.

A common problem of long-term supplementation involves "taste fatigue." Patients quickly grow tired of three vanilla milkshakes each day. Taste fatigue may be prevented by rotating the flavors of the food supplements. Modular products that can be added to table foods to increase caloric intake can also help to prevent supplement taste fatigue. Excessive use of glucose polymers should be avoided because increased glucose intake enhances sodium absorption and can precipitate heart failure. Thus, when carbohydrate intake is increased significantly, expecially in a fragile elderly patient, care must be taken to limit sodium intake and observe for signs of fluid retention. Excessive CHO intake can also precipitate increased $CO_2$ production as noted earlier.

### Infant Feedings

*Infant formulas are prescribed according to the gestational age and the condition of the gastrointestinal tract. The concentration and volume of the formula are important considerations. Full-strength formula generally contains 20 calories/oz or 0.67 calories/cc. Caloric density can be increased to 24 calories/oz but should rarely exceed 30 calories/oz. The recipe for making 24 to 27 calories/oz formula is presented in Table 11-9.*

*Infants have a small gastric capacity. The total volume of a tube feeding that can be tolerated may limit the number of calories received. When a desired volume is reached, the concentration of the feeding may be increased in quarterly increments for 3 to 5 days until full strength is reached.*

*The volume and the concentration of a feeding should never be changed at the same time. If complications such as osmotic diarrhea or cramps occur, it will be impossible to know if they were caused by the volume or the concentration.*

■ *Feeding Progression.* Some infants or young children who have not been fed by mouth and who

**Table 11-9** Increasing the caloric content of formulas

| Type of formula | Recipe |
| --- | --- |
| *24 calories/oz* | *Decrease the amount of water added to the formula: 13 oz concentrate with 13 oz of water = 20 cal/oz; 13 oz concentrate with 9 oz of water = 24 cal/oz.* |
| *Increase caloric concentration without increased osmolarity* | *Add prescribed amounts of medium-chain triglycerides (MCT oil) or a glucose polymer (Polycose). By adding 15 ml of MCT oil or 6 ml of liquid Polycose to each 4-oz formula portion of a 24-calories/oz formula, the concentration would be increased to 27 calories/oz.* |
| | *Vegetable oil can be substituted for MCT oil when the infant is 4 to 6 mo for considerable cost savings.* |
| | *If there is concern that the infant may aspirate because of a swallowing disorder or gastroesophageal reflux, oil should not be added to the formula.* |

*have had much adverse oral stimuli have difficulty with the progression of normal feeding. For example, infants who are fed only by gastrostomy may refuse oral feeding (bottle or solids). A plan devised by the team caring for the child (parents, nurses, occupational therapist, nutritionist, and physician) can be helpful in addressing the problem.*

### Invasive Nutritional Support

The overall goal of invasive nutritional support is the prevention or treatment of severe malnutrition. Invasive nutritional support may be considered as an alternative or supplement to oral intake in the following patients:

- Those who are temporarily unable to consume adequate calories by mouth (e.g., those with

bronchopulmonary dysplasia and some ventilator-dependent patients)
- Those who are chronically unable to maintain an adequate oral intake (e.g., those with cystic fibrosis or emphysema). Patients waiting for lung transplant may require invasive nutritional support to improve their operative risk.
- Those who have poor gastrointestinal function (e.g., cystic fibrosis patients with recurrent bowel obstruction)

Factors that must be considered in planning invasive nutritional interventions are the following:

*Physiologic factors*
- Gastrointestinal tract function
- Associated risks and complications of intervention
- Disease process
- Nutrient requirements
- Degree of nutritional debility

*Psychosocial factors*
- Financial resources
- Family support and technical assistance available
- Self-care capabilities
- Type of equipment available
- Patient body image concerns

■ *Delivery Options for Invasive Nutritional Interventions.* The indications for use and the advantages and disadvantages of some enteral and parenteral access devices are summarized in Table 11-10. Enteral tube feeding is less expensive and usually poses fewer risks to the patient than parenteral feeding. It should be noted, however, that the risk of tube feeding aspiration has special significance for pulmonary patients. Individuals with a disease such as cystic fibrosis who have severe gastrointestinal digestive and absorptive dysfunction may require parenteral nutrition periodically.

Quality of life issues and patient preference also play a role in selecting the mode of nutritional access. *Some patients, especially adolescents, have a strong aversion to being fed through a tube but are willing to receive intravenous therapy.* Some individuals may feel less disfigured with a gas-

**Table 11-10**  Enteral and parenteral access methods and devices

| Method/device | Indications | Advantages | Disadvantages |
|---|---|---|---|
| Nasogastric tube | | | |
|   Large-bore polyvinyl tube | Short-term feeding of less than 7 days | Easy insertion; inexpensive; patency easily maintained | Increased risk of aspiration and gastroesophageal reflux |
|   Small-bore, polyurethane or silicone tubes | Short- or long-term feeding | Reduced risk of aspiration and reflux; do not cause esophagitis; reduced mucosal injury; more comfortable for patient | Expensive; potentially more difficult insertion; tendency to become clogged because of small lumen |
| Nasojejunal or nasoduodenal | Long- or short-term feeding in patients with increased risk for aspiration (e.g., gastric retention, history of gastroesophageal reflux) | Low risk for aspiration; may allow increased feeding volumes; flexibility in patient positioning during feeding | Placement and confirmation of tube placement more difficult |
| Gastrostomy tube | Long-term feeding | Rarely becomes plugged; easy insertion and removal; does not interfere with sputum clearance and patient ability to cough and expectorate; tube presence not obvious | Requires endoscopic or surgical procedure for insertion; risk for local skin irritation or infection; risk for peritonitis with placement; improper tube position can cause ulceration or gastric outlet obstruction |
| Peripheral vein cannulation | Short-term peripheral feeding; supplementation of oral or enteral tube feeding | Low technical risk; low septic risk | Limited caloric intake because of low calorie content of peripheral fluids; high risk for phlebitis |
| Long-term central venous access devices | Long-term central feeding | | |
|   Indwelling Silastic catheter (e.g., Hickman) | | Relatively low risk for sepsis | Requires surgical procedure and skill to insert; potential for catheter breakage or thrombosis at tip; daily irrigation required |

*Continued.*

**Table 11-10**  Enteral and parenteral access methods and devices—cont'd

| Method/device | Indications | Advantages | Disadvantages |
|---|---|---|---|
| Subcutaneous injection port (e.g., Porta-Cath) | | Decreased need for heparinization, care, and dressings; decreased overall infection rate with intermittent use; decreased alteration in body image | Patient discomfort with port access; surgical procedure to insert; potential for thrombosis at tip |
| Peripherally inserted central catheter (PICC) | | Less risk with insertion and care; does not require surgical procedure for insertion; provides long-term alternative for peripheral access | Difficult to place in some patients; daily care required |

trostomy tube than with a nasogastric tube that can be seen coming out of the nose. Some may prefer to insert and remove a nasogastric tube periodically for feeding, rather than have any feeding device constantly in place. *For infants receiving night feedings, this technique may be indicated to decrease continuous nasal, esophageal, and gastric irritation.*

The feeding schedule should disrupt usual activities of daily living as little as possible. If the patient does well with gravity drip feedings, they can be administered periodically throughout the day while the patient is watching TV or performing other sedentary activities. Some patients prefer to receive tube feedings during the night while sleeping. Others may not tolerate nighttime feedings because sleep is disrupted by pump alarms, discomfort with feedings, fear of accidental tube dislodgment, or the need to keep the head elevated to prevent aspiration. For nutritional support to improve or enhance a patient's quality of life, it should be compatible with the life-style of the patient.

■ *Initiating Feedings.* To avoid potential gastrointestinal complications, enteral tube feedings should be started at a slow rate and isosmotic strength, then increased gradually. The patient's response to the feeding should be monitored throughout the process of rate advancement. If gastric retention, loose stools suggestive of dumping, abdominal cramping, or bloating develops, the last tolerated flow rate should be resumed. In our experience most patients can tolerate a rapid increase in feeding rate (e.g., 50 ml increase every 2 hours). This also permits the use of gravity drip rather than pump control. Gravity drip is less costly and provides more flexibility for the patient in the home. We have found that a feeding rate of 175 ml/hr can be well approximated using gravity drip.

■ *Parenteral Nutrition.* Parenteral nutrition in the home may be administered continuously or intermittently. Intermittent administration allows the patient to engage in normal activities of daily living without being attached to intravenous equipment.

Intravenous solutions of 5% dextrose may be given at a steady flow rate over relatively short periods of time (e.g., 1 L over 8 hours = 125 ml/ hr). At the end of the infusion the solution can be discontinued and the intravenous catheter capped. However, total parenteral nutrition (TPN) with concentrated dextrose solutions (e.g., greater than 15% dextrose) must be administered continuously or in a cyclic schedule that mimics normal changes in blood glucose occurring during and after meals.

In a cyclic schedule the flow rate is initiated slowly and advanced gradually to a peak rate that is maintained for a length of time. The flow rate is then gradually reduced over the final few hours of the infusion until it is discontinued. Pumps with the capability for such programming are available. In this way the individual can adjust to gradual changes in blood glucose, and hyperglycemia or rebound hypoglycemia are avoided. An example of a cyclic schedule for total parenteral nutrition is shown in the following:

Total volume to be infused: 2000 ml
Desired time of infusion: 10 hours

| Hour | Flow Rate | Volume Infused |
|------|-----------|----------------|
| 1 | 100 ml/hr | 100 ml |
| 2-8 | 250 ml/hr | 1850 ml |
| 9 | 100 ml/hr | 1950 ml |
| 10 | 50 ml/hr | 2000 ml |

The IV is discontinued at the end of the tenth hour. The following are critical periods in the cyclic schedule.

■ TIME OF MAXIMUM FLOW RATE. At the time of maximum flow rate, it is important to observe the patient for signs of hyperglycemia (thirst, polyuria, hunger). If hyperglycemia occurs, the patient may require a longer total feeding time with a slower maximum flow rate, the addition of insulin to the nutritional solution, or both.

■ TIME OF FLOW RATE REDUCTION. At the time of flow rate reduction (the ninth to eleventh hour in the preceding example), the patient should be observed for signs of rebound hypoglycemia (pallor, diaphoresis, nervousness, tremor, hunger, slurred speech, confusion). If this occurs, the pa-

tient will require a flow rate reduction in smaller increments over a longer period. Generally, flow rates are reduced by appoximately 50% per hour, and the TPN can be discontinued when flow rates are reduced to 50 to 75 ml/hr. *Generally, flow rates for children are one quarter of the maximum rate for 1 hour, one half of the maximum rate for 1 hour, and maximum flow until the last 2 hours. They are then tapered in reverse.*

Most patients need to void during feedings with high infusion rates. A glucometer can be used for accurate and reliable monitoring of urine glucose levels with home TPN.

■ ***Treatment Complications.*** Enteral and parenteral nutrition are associated with a variety of potential infectious, technical, and metabolic complications and gastrointestinal dysfunctions. These complications are summarized in Table 11-11.

## FLUIDS

Nutritional repletion, especially with invasive nutritional therapy, can cause problems that may affect fluid balance. Pulmonary patients with heart failure are at risk for problems with fluid overload. Dehydration may also occur in adults and children with chronic lung disease.

### Etiology

The etiologic factors of fluid retention are discussed in Chapter 10. Dehydration occurs when fluid intake is less than fluid loss. When the patient is dehydrated, plasma electrolyte and protein levels are higher, increasing plasma osmolarity and causing fluid to move from the interstitial space. This compensatory effect can maintain blood volume only temporarily. As blood volume is decreased, a compensatory reduction in cardiac output occurs. The patient becomes easily fatigued and less able to exercise. Postural hypotension and tachycardia may occur, and the hematocrit is increased. Pulmonary secretions become thicker and more tenacious and are more difficult to expectorate.

Potential causes of dehydration in patients

**Table 11-11**  Complications of invasive nutrition

| Complication | Therapy type | Causes | Prevention/intervention |
|---|---|---|---|
| **INFECTION** | | | |
| Catheter-related sepsis | Parenteral | Catheter contamination or colonization | Aseptic technique in catheter care and catheter removal; antibiotic therapy to sterilize catheter (usually only done with long-term catheter use) |
| Aspiration pneumonia | Enteral tube | Use of PVC tube; keeping gastro-esophageal junction open; regurgitation of feeding | Use Silastic or polyurethane tube; transpyloric tube placement to reduce risk; keep head elevated during and 30 min after feedings |
| **METABOLIC** | | | |
| Hyperglycemia | Parenteral/enteral | Excessive CHO intake; too rapid feeding rate; insufficient insulin response; chromium deficiency | Gradual initiation of feeding; appropriate CHO intake; insulin administration as needed |
| Hypoglycemia | Parenteral/enteral | Sudden or too rapid cessation of feeding (more common with parenteral), causing "rebound" | Continuous feeding rate or gradual tapering to stop feeding |
| Electrolyte imbalances (K, Na, Cl, Ca, Mg, $PO_4$) | Parenteral/enteral | Inadequate mineral intake; unrecognized mineral losses; insufficient supplementation | Provide minimum daily requirement of minerals; monitor serum electrolytes; assess patient for mineral status and potential losses or increased requirements, and replace minerals to meet needs |
| Essential fatty acid deficiency | Parenteral/enteral (defined formula or elemental products) | Inadequate essential fatty acid intake | Provide fat intake regularly to meet requirement |
| **GASTROINTESTINAL TRACT** | | | |
| Gastric retention | Enteral | Bolus or too high a volume of feeding; reduced gastrointestinal motility | Check gastric aspirates and if greater than 100 ml hold feeding or decrease feeding rate; transpyloric tube administration of metoclopramide to increase motility |

**Table 11-11** Complications of invasive nutrition—cont'd

| Complication | Therapy type | Causes | Prevention/intervention |
|---|---|---|---|
| Diarrhea | Enteral | Too rapid feeding and dumping | Slow initiation of rate<br>Rate as tolerated |
| | | Hyperosmolar feeding | Begin with isotonic feedings, increase only as tolerated |
| | | Fat malabsorption (e.g., cystic fibrosis) | Pancreatic enzymes for cystic fibrosis; provide medium chain triglyceride oil |
| | | Lactose intolerance | Use lactose-free fluids |
| | | Antibiotic therapy | Replace gut bacteria with yogurt or lactobacillus; control diarrhea with medication (e.g., Kaopectate, Imodium, Pepto Bismol); addition of fiber |
| Constipation | Enteral | Prolonged tube feeding with low fiber content | Use fiber-containing product |

with chronic lung disease are summarized in the following:

| Reduced Fluid Intake | Increased Fluid Loss |
|---|---|
| Inability to communicate thirst (infants) | Diuretic therapy |
| | Fever |
| | Diarrhea |
| Blunted awareness of thirst (elderly adults) | Excessive sodium loss associated with diaphoresis (increased risk in cystic fibrosis) |
| Anorexia | |
| Early satiety | |
| Inconvenience of frequent urination | |

## Assessment

The assessment of fluid retention and dehydration is discussed in Chapters 2, 3, and 10.

## Nursing Interventions

Nutritional therapy in individuals with fluid overload must be planned with attention to fluid volume, and the choice of nutritional products must include attention to sodium content. Other specific interventions for fluid retention are discussed in Chapter 10.

The primary approach to the patient with dehydration is to replenish fluids. If the symptoms of fluid loss are acute, parenteral fluid supplementation may be necessary. It is important to treat the cause of dehydration (e.g., fever or diarrhea). The nurse should also be alert to signs and symptoms of dehydration in patients receiving long-term diuretic therapy and contact the physician if they occur.

## OBESITY

Obesity is defined as excessive body fat or as body weight in excess of metabolic needs. Extreme obesity can result in a restrictive impairment of lung function. The incidence of obesity in chronic lung disease has not been well studied. However, it is known that patients with chronic bronchitis tend to be overweight. Obesity adds greatly to the work of breathing, predisposes the patient to obstructive sleep apnea, and is a distinguishing feature of obesity hypoventilation syndrome. Marked increases in energy costs are associated with increased body weight. These energy costs may be so great for the obese patient with chronic lung disease that only minimal physical exercise is possible.

### Etiology

The causes of obesity are being widely studied. The "fat cell theory" purports that the number of fat cells, established in utero during the last trimester of pregnancy and through adolescence, results in obese people having more fat cells than slim people. No more fat cells are made beyond adolescence. Future weight gain or loss then occurs only by a change in the volume of lipid in these fat cells.

### Assessment

An actual weight of more than 120% *maximal* acceptable weight suggests clinically significant obesity. The actual weight should be divided by the highest weight for height within the normal range on the height and weight table (Table 11-5).

### Nursing Interventions

Weight control is a matter of energy balance. When weight is stable, the caloric intake is balanced by the energy output. To lose weight, one must reduce caloric intake or increase energy expenditures by exercise or activity.

Therapeutic reduction diets assist the patient to lose weight safely. A sensible long-range diet that includes all essential nutrients and minerals should be planned. Diets that severely restrict any nutrient should be avoided. The appropriate diet can be chosen after an assessment of individual habits and needs. Formal programs such as Weight Watchers are often successful and provide group support

when the patient is well enough to leave the home. The patient, home care dietitian, nurse, and physician must work together to select the most appropriate program.

Starvation diets are generally not advocated because they cause rapid depletion of glycogen stores, the burning of fat, and subsequent acidosis. Starvation diets also cause potassium deficiency that may precipitate cardiac arrhythmias. The "advantages" of starvation diets include loss of appetite in 7 days, rapid initial weight loss, and control of compulsive eating. The appropriate weight reduction diet can be chosen after an assessment of individual habits and needs.

### REFERENCES

Braun SR et al: The prevalence and determinants of nutritional changes in chronic obstructive pulmonary disease, *Chest* 86:558, 1984.

Edelman NH, Rucker RB, Peary HH: NIH workshop summary: nutrition and the respiratory system, *Am Rev Respir Dis* 134:347, 1986.

Openbrier DR et al: Nutritional status and lung function in patients with emphysema and chronic bronchitis, *Chest* 83:17, 1983.

Rindfleish S, Zwillich CW: The interaction of dyspnea, oxygen desaturation and caloric consumption in COPD, *Am Rev Respir Dis* 13:4:A164, 1985.

Wilson DO et al: Nutritional intervention in malnourished emphysema patients, *Am Rev Respir Dis* 134:672, 1986.

### SUGGESTED READINGS

Donahoe M, Rogers RM: Nutritional assessment and support in chronic obstructive pulmonary disease, *Clin Chest Med* 11:487, 1990.

Irwin MM, Openbrier DR: A delicate balance: strategies for feeding ventilated COPD patients, *Am J Nurs* 85:274, 1985.

Krey SH, Murray RL: Dynamics of nutritional support, Norwalk, Conn, 1986, Appleton & Lange.

Ramsey BW et al: Nutritional assessment and management in cystic fibrosis: a consensus report, *Am J Clin Nutr* 55:108, 1992.

# CHAPTER 12

# SLEEP DISTURBANCE

GWENDOLYN J. McDONALD

Sleep disturbance is common in patients with chronic lung disease, is associated with a wide range of physiologic and psychologic factors, and has a significant adverse effect on functional activity. Primary sleep disorders, especially sleep apnea syndrome, occur in children and adults and may coexist with chronic lung disease. The etiologic factors, assessment, and management of sleep problems are presented in this chapter.

## NORMAL SLEEP

To understand sleep problems that may affect the patient with chronic lung disease, it is necessary to review normal sleep patterns.

### Sleep Stages

#### Non–Rapid Eye Movement Sleep

Sleep is divided into two phases: non–rapid eye movement (NREM) and rapid eye movement (REM) (Table 12-1). NREM (quiet) sleep occupies about 80% of sleep time and is the major phase during the early part of the night. It consists of four stages. Slow-wave delta sleep (stages III and IV) is thought to be important for tissue regeneration and repair. Disruption of NREM sleep causes patients to wake feeling unrefreshed. Severe disturbance of restorative stage IV sleep can result in chronic sleep deprivation with fatigue, morning headache, visual disturbance, intellectual impairment, poor concentration, apathy, depression, or musculoskeletal coordination problems.

During normal NREM sleep, skeletal muscle tone is reduced and the basal metabolic rate is reduced by 10% to 20%. In addition, $PaCO_2$ increases and $O_2$ saturation drops slightly as the result of such factors as a modest increase in ventilation-perfusion mismatching as the patient's position changes from upright to supine, changes in respiratory drive during sleep, and hypoventilation associated with deep sleep. Reduced tone of the upper airway and tongue muscles can predispose susceptible individuals to upper airway obstruction (Krieger, 1985).

### Rapid Eye Movement Sleep

The first episode of REM sleep occurs 45 to 120 minutes after the onset of sleep. As the night progresses, however, REM periods grow longer and occur closer together, resulting in a predominance of REM sleep during the second half of the night. REM sleep has two stages: tonic and phasic. During the tonic stage there are reduced tone of intercostal and upper airway muscles and profound flaccidity or "paralysis" of skeletal muscles. The phasic stage is characterized by increased sympathetic nervous system output, a highly irregular breathing pattern, and bursts of rapid eye movements. An increase in heart rate, blood pressure, muscle twitches, and penile erections also occurs during phasic REM sleep. Although diaphragmatic activity is increased in REM sleep, it is slightly dyssynchronous and therefore less efficient. In ad-

**Table 12-1** Sleep stages

| Stage | Sleep time (%) | Characteristics | Respiratory pattern |
|---|---|---|---|
| **NREM** | | | |
| I | 5-10 | Drowsiness | Variable depth; frequent sighs, in association with arousals; apneas, hypoventilation, or decreased respiratory rate often follows sighs |
| II | 50-60 | Light sleep | |
| III | 10-20 | Deep sleep | Regular rhythm; progressively more shallow depth as sleep deepens; marked reduction in sigh frequency |
| IV | 10-20 *(less in older adults)* | Deepest sleep | |
| **REM** | 20-25 *(50% in infants)* | Dream sleep; two phases: tonic and phasic | Highly irregular respirations; brief apneas and hypopneas |

dition, diaphragmatic excursion is periodically inhibited, predisposing the patient to periods of apnea or hypopnea (Bixler, 1987). Small decreases in $O_2$ saturation are normal during REM sleep, and the electroencephalographic (EEG) pattern is similar to a waking pattern. This is the dream phase of sleep and is considered important for learning and memory. REM deprivation has been shown to increase anxiety, irritability, appetite, and difficulty in concentrating.

### Sleep Requirements

Daily sleep requirements can vary widely between individuals and with age. A newborn typically needs about 18 hours of sleep a day, compared with 6 to 8 hours for an adult. Daytime naps are usual for young children, but they are also a normal part of the circadian sleep-rest cycle for many adults.

### Characteristics of "Good Sleep"

The defining characteristics of "good normal sleep" are as follows:
- Falling asleep within a half hour of turning out the light
- Sleeping through the night without interruptions
- Waking at a normal time of the morning feeling refreshed
- Remaining awake and alert during the day

### Apneas and Arousals During Sleep

People of all ages experience brief (less than 15 seconds), occasional (less than 8 to 12 an hour) apneas at sleep onset and during REM sleep (Strohl, 1986). These are typically followed by arousals, transient changes to a light sleep stage, or a wakeful EEG pattern.

### Snoring

Snoring is most common in overweight adults, older adults, and males and is enhanced by alcohol and hypnotic drugs. Potential harmful effects include cardiac dysfunction, systemic hypertension (Partinen, 1983), and sleep disturbance of the bed partner. *Snoring in children is abnormal and is usually caused by increased tonsillar or adenoidal tissue.*

### Factors Affecting Sleep

Sleep patterns in health are influenced by many factors. These are listed and described in the box on p. 201.

## GENERAL SLEEP PROBLEMS
### Insomnia

Insomnia is the most common of the sleep disorders in all populations and is more prevalent in women and the elderly. It affects 40% of people over 50 years of age. It most often is manifested as difficulty in falling asleep (early insomnia) but

## Factors Influencing Sleep Patterns

### AGE

Newborns: 50% of sleep time spent in REM sleep

With increasing age:

Reduced or absent stage IV sleep

Increased frequency of awakenings; earlier final wakening

Increased myoclonus

Reduced total sleep time

More periodic breathing; more frequent apneas; more frequent episodes of $O_2$ desaturation

Postmenopausal women:

Snore more

More easily awakened by noises

### GENDER

Snoring and oxygen desaturation more common in adult males

### BODY TEMPERATURE

Time of lowest body temperature ($\pm 4$ AM):

Correlates with greatest frequency of REM

Occurs approximately 2 hr before arousal from sleep (temperature nadir most likely predicts "larks" versus "owls")

Higher mean body temperatures associated with wakefulness (Vitiello, 1986)

### ENVIRONMENTAL EFFECTS

Disturbed sleep from noise, changes in lighting, ventilation, or room temperature, especially in the elderly

### STRESS, MOOD DISORDERS

Stress: increases NREM sleep requirements

Anxiety: increases sympathetic arousal → early, middle, and late insomnia

Depression:

Middle and late insomnia, restless sleep

Increased daytime sleep → vicious cycle of increased nocturnal insomnia

### EXERCISE

Regular daytime exercise reduces stage I, enhances deep sleep

Late evening exercise → sympathetic arousal, delayed stage I

Erratic daytime rest and activity pattern → insomnia, especially in the elderly (Kales, 1987)

### DIETARY HABITS

Large meals or stimulants (e.g., coffee) at bedtime → delay of sleep onset

Alcohol: may enhance sleep onset but increases frequency of nocturnal awakenings

### EXCESSIVE DAYTIME NAPPING

Interferes with nighttime sleep (Kales, 1987)

### BIOCHEMICAL/HORMONAL EFFECTS

Circadian changes in autonomic nervous system stimulation (reduced adrenergic secretion and increased vagal tone at night) → airway narrowing → impaired nocturnal ventilation, especially in individuals with asthma

Testosterone may potentiate sleep apnea

### DRUG EFFECTS

Stimulants (e.g., theophylline, oral β-agonists, caffeine, cigarettes) impair sleep

Barbiturates:

Suppress REM sleep

Rebound effect when discontinued → nightmares

Sedatives, narcotics, anxiolytics, alcohol increase frequency and duration of apneas in those who snore, are obese, or experience obstructive sleep apnea may also include middle insomnia (restless sleep, frequent nocturnal wakenings) or late insomnia (a final wakening much too early in the morning). The normal sleep-wake cycle may shift, with wakefulness occurring far into the night, followed by extreme difficulty in getting up in the morning.

Restless leg syndrome is a familial disorder characterized by periodic jerking leg movements (nocturnal myoclonus) that disrupt sleep and can cause injuries. Restless legs in a patient with COPD may reflect a worsening blood gas status.

Sleep deprivation is the inevitable result of prolonged sleep disturbance caused by insomnia or other problems. Symptoms (Lee, 1991) and physiologic effects are listed in the following:

| Symptoms | Physiologic Effect |
|---|---|
| Fatigue | Reduced hypoxic and hypercapneic ventilatory drive |
| Impaired memory and attention span | |
| Reduced coordination | Increased apnea frequency |
| Confusion and illusions, with severe deprivation | In chronic obstructive pulmonary disease, small though significant reductions in forced expiratory volume in 1 second ($FEV_1$) and forced vital capacity (FVC) (Phillips, 1987) |

### Hypersomnolence

Hypersomnolence may represent a true increase in the amount of sleep during a 24-hour period. More often, however, it is present only during the day (daytime somnolence) as a result of sleep deprivation caused by insomnia.

## SLEEP PROBLEMS IN CHRONIC LUNG DISEASE
### Chronic Obstructive Pulmonary Disease

The prevalence of sleep disturbance in chronic obstructive pulmonary disease (COPD) is high, affecting more than 50% of patients with chronic bronchitis (Kinsman, 1983). This most often is manifested as insomnia. However, nocturnal desaturation is a major contributing factor to sleep disturbance in COPD. In the hypoxemic individual a normal, sleep-related drop in $PaO_2$ can significantly compromise oxygenation. This problem is compounded in a subset of patients (typically those with chronic bronchitis or hypercapnia) who desaturate during REM sleep. Nocturnal desaturation is assumed to be the result of both reduced hypoxic ventilatory drive and the normal loss of upper airway muscle tone that occurs during REM sleep. It is associated with an increase in life-threatening arrhythmias. Long-term effects include increased pulmonary vascular resistance and pulmonary artery pressure, secondary polycythemia, and pulmonary heart disease.

Individuals without daytime hypoxemia are unlikely to experience profound hypoxemia during sleep unless they have a sleep apnea syndrome.

### Kyphoscoliosis

Patients with kyphoscoliosis spend proportionally more time in stage I sleep. They may have Cheyne-Stokes respirations or obstructive apneas. Prolonged central apneas occurring primarily during REM sleep result in severe desaturation and may eventually lead to pulmonary heart disease. In the face of severe thoracic cage abnormalities, patients must work harder to achieve adequate ventilation, especially at night. They eventually become sleep deprived, developing residual muscle fatigue and daytime hypoventilation.

### Interstitial Lung Disease

Patients with interstitial lung disease have a rapid shallow breathing pattern and chronic hypocapnia. This increase in respiratory drive is needed for an adequate $PaO_2$ in the face of markedly reduced lung volumes. In these individuals sleep is characterized by more arousals, sleep stage changes, and sleep fragmentation than in normal individuals (Kryger, 1985; Perez-Padilla, 1985). Oxygen desaturation may occur with hypoventilation during REM sleep. Overall, however, patients maintain their usual rapid shallow respiratory pattern during sleep and have relatively few apneas.

### Factors Contributing to Sleep Disturbance

Factors contributing to sleep impairment in patients with chronic respiratory problems are presented in Table 12-2.

**Table 12-2**   Factors contributing to sleep impairment in patients with chronic lung disease

| Factor | Possible mechanisms |
|---|---|
| Hypoxemia | Stimulates nocturnal arousals, especially with REM-associated desaturations<br>Arousals lead to sleep deprivation and fatigue on awakening |
| Limited sleep positions | Positional increase in dyspnea associated with localized $\dot{V}/\dot{Q}$ abnormalities or orthopnea limits options for sleep positions and results in arousal if an uncomfortable position is assumed during sleep |
| Lack of exercise (e.g., due to exertional dyspnea, loss of motivation) | Insufficient exercise inhibits deep sleep |
| Respiratory symptoms (dyspnea, wheeze, cough, congestion) | Nocturnal cough or wheezing common in asthma. Possible mechanisms:<br>    Decreased nocturnal catecholamine output<br>    Increased mediator release<br>    Increased parasympathetic tone<br>    Inhalation of cooler, drier air at night<br>    *Gastroesophageal reflux (common in children)*<br>    Impaired nocturnal mucociliary clearance<br>Nocturnal symptoms interrupt sleep and lead to daytime somnolence and fatigue<br>Sleep deprivation leads to decreased ventilatory drive, which may worsen blood gas abnormalities |
| Medication side effects | Methylxanthines lead to increased stage I sleep and sleep fragmentation<br>β-Adrenergics lead to increased sympathetic nervous system stimulation<br>Diuretics cause nocturia |
| Mood disturbance (anxiety, depression) | Cause early, middle, or late insomnia and frequent awakenings<br>Loss of energy and engagement with life leads to daytime sleeping and worsened nocturnal insomnia |
| Sensory deprivation of homebound elderly who live alone | Boredom leads to daytime napping |
| Coexisting illness | Often have associated nocturnal symptoms:<br>    Pain (e.g., due to arthritis, steroid-related compression fractures)<br>    Paroxysmal nocturnal dyspnea, nocturia, orthopnea due to left ventricular failure<br>    Central or obstructive sleep apnea<br>    Increase in gastroesophageal reflux in flat position, associated with hiatus hernia<br>    Nocturnal myoclonus due to restless leg syndrome or worsening blood gas status |

## ASSESSMENT OF SLEEP DISTURBANCE
### Sleep History

Sleep disturbance is best evaluated by taking an in-depth sleep history. Components include the following:

- Description of a typical 24-hour period of sleep and rest
- Emotional factors, medications, and changes in cardiopulmonary status that may contribute to sleep disturbance
- Specific information regarding snoring, nocturnal restlessness, and other symptoms of obstructive sleep apnea

Use of a sleep questionnaire (Fig. 12-1) may facilitate the gathering of pertinent information and, if left for the patient to complete between home care visits, will minimize interview time.

### Oxygen Saturation Monitoring

If sleep disturbance is believed to be due to nocturnal desaturation, the patient may need to be referred to a sleep laboratory or hospitalized briefly for a more comprehensive evaluation, including nighttime oxygen saturation monitoring. Objective data on nocturnal saturation can also be obtained in the home using a portable oximeter with printout capabilities. However, sensors are easily dislodged with movement during sleep. Careful attachment of finger probes, use of newer probes that permit greater movement, and nocturnal observation by a spouse or caregiver improve the accuracy of the data. A Holter monitor may help identify changes in heart rate and rhythm suggestive of apneas and is easier to keep in place.

## NURSING INTERVENTIONS
### Implementing "Granny" Instructions

The management of mild, nonspecific sleep disturbances is largely based on common sense. These "granny" instructions constitute a folklore of home remedies for insomnia, and many have been subsequently supported by research.

- Exercise regularly (but not at bedtime).
- Maintain a regular sleep and wake schedule.
- Limit daytime naps.
- Reduce overall stress; reduce stressful activities, especially before sleep.
- Avoid cigarettes, alcohol, and stimulants (e.g., caffeine) during evening.
- Drink warm milk and honey or herbal tea or eat a light protein and carbohydrate snack at bedtime (high-protein foods release tryptophan, which has mild sedative properties).
- Practice relaxation techniques at bedtime, including pursed lip breathing, visualization, and "counting sheep."
- Create a quiet, peaceful environment.
- Encourage a gentle bedtime backrub.
- If not contraindicated, take acetylsalicylic acid (aspirin), 10 grains, which releases tryptophan (Hauri, 1978) and is effective in some patients.

### Reducing Respiratory Symptoms

For nocturnal cough and sputum, encourage the use of an inhaled bronchodilator and controlled cough at bedtime, adding other bronchial hygiene measures (e.g., chest physical therapy) as indicated. This clears airways before sleep, reducing the volume of secretions that would otherwise accumulate during the night.

For nocturnal wheezing, inhaled bronchodilators should be used at bedtime and with every wheeze-related wakening. Inhaled steroids, 4 to 8 puffs bid, may also be used. If wheezing continues, a long-acting oral bronchodilator is usually added at bedtime. A $\beta$-agonist with a low side effect profile is usually preferable to theophylline. However, if theophylline is used, the bedtime dose may need to be increased slightly because of lower nocturnal theophylline absorption. Some patients set an alarm so they can take medication or clear secretions during the night rather than waiting to waken in distress.

### Nocturnal Oxygen Therapy

Nocturnal oxygen is indicated when sleep disruption is due to hypoxemia. Criteria for its use are presented in Table 12-3. Benefits include the following:

- Fewer nocturnal hypoxemic episodes
- Reduced risk of arrhythmias

## Sleep History Questionnaire

A. *Getting to sleep*

   1. What time do you usually turn out the light at night to go to sleep? _____

   2. How long does it typically take you to fall asleep? _____

   3. Do you take any medication to help you sleep?    Y     N
      If yes, describe _____

   4. Do you try other methods to help you get to sleep?    Y     N
      If yes, describe _____

   5. How much of the following beverages do you drink in the evening?
      Coffee _____
      Tea _____
      Cola drinks _____
      Chocolate drinks _____
      Alcohol _____

   6. How many ounces of fluids (any kind) do you usually drink betwen 6 PM and midnight?
      _____

B. *Staying Asleep*

   1. How often do you wake up during the night on most nights? _____

   2. How long does it usually take you to go back to sleep if you waken during the night?
      _____

   3. What seems to waken you at night? (Check all that apply)
      a. Need to urinate      _____
      b. More short of breath      _____
      c. Coughing or wheezing      _____
      d. Upset stomach, heartburn      _____
      e. Other (describe)      _____
      f. Don't know      _____

C. *Snoring*   (important to ask both patient and bed partner)

   1. Do you snore a lot at night?    Y     N

**Fig. 12-1**   Sleep history questionnaire.      *Continued.*

**Sleep History Questionnaire, cont'd**

D. *Oxygen Therapy:*    If you are using oxygen therapy at home,

    1. Do you sleep with your oxygen on at night?        Y        N
       If yes, what liter flow do you use? _____
       Do the nasal prongs usually stay in place?        Y        N

    2. Do you wake up often with headaches?        Y        N

E. *Waking Up*

    1. What time do you wake up most mornings? _____

    2. What time do you get up? _____

    3. Do you feel rested when you waken?        Y        N

F. *Daytime Sleep*

    1. Do you often feel tired or sleepy during the day?        Y        N

    2. Do you take naps during the day?        Y        N
       If yes, when? _____
       How long do you nap? _____

G. Overall how would you rate the quality of your sleep?    (Check one)

       a. Excellent; I sleep like a log        _____
       b. Good; I sleep well most of the time        _____
       c. Fair; I have good nights and bad nights        _____
       d. Poor; my sleep is restless much of the time        _____
       e. Terrible; I hardly sleep at all        _____

**Fig. 12-1, cont'd.**    Sleep history questionnaire.

- Lower pulmonary artery pressure, less polycythemia, and better control of pulmonary heart disease
- Increased total sleep time and increased REM sleep
- Improvement in the quality of sleep
- Alleviation of early morning headaches

## Treating Congestive Heart Failure

More aggressive treatment of heart failure is indicated when orthopnea, paroxysmal nocturnal dyspnea, or frequent wakenings for urination disturb sleep. Interventions include the following:

- Adjustment of diuretic dose or dosing time
- Greater dietary sodium restriction

**Table 12-3**   Criteria for use of nocturnal oxygen therapy

| Criterion | Interventions |
|---|---|
| A. Adults: | |
| Stable daytime $Pao_2$ <55 mm Hg *or* Oxygen saturation <85% | Implement continuous $O_2$ therapy, including at night. Patient may need a higher flow rate at night to compensate for nocturnal hypoventilation and increased $\dot{V}/\dot{Q}$ mismatch. |
| *Children:* | |
| *Saturation <90%* | |
| B. Daytime $Pao_2$ of 56 to 59 mm Hg or saturation of 89% to 90%, combined with complaints of disturbed sleep, early morning headaches, or evidence of pulmonary heart disease | Evaluate for nocturnal oxygen desaturation. If present, initiate nocturnal $O_2$, but only if $O_2$ does not induce or increase frequency or duration of apneas, nocturnal hypercapnia, or early morning headaches. |

- Elevation of head using foam wedges, a hospital bed, or comfortable recliner
- Nocturnal or continuous $O_2$ therapy

## Readjusting Medication Regimen

Avoid evening administration of diuretics. Experiment with different dosing times for bronchodilators (e.g., change theophylline administration times from 9 AM and 9 PM to 6 AM and 6 PM). Eliminate the bedtime dose altogether. Substitute an inhaled for an oral bronchodilator.

## Treating Depression and Anxiety; Reducing Stress

Interventions to treat depression and anxiety and to reduce stress include the following:
- Counseling; relaxation techniques
- Tricyclic antidepressant therapy (Chapter 17)
  Initial side effects of tricyclic agents, administered at bedtime, include sleepiness.
  Later improvements in depression and anxiety correct the underlying, mood-related sleep disturbance.

## Nocturnal Mechanical Ventilation

Nocturnal ventilation may be indicated for the patient with severe kyphoscoliosis or neuromuscular disease who is experiencing nocturnal hypoventilation and apnea. Ventilatory assistance allows respiratory muscle rest, thereby reducing respiratory muscle fatigue and daytime respiratory failure (Kryger, 1985). Newer, less invasive methods for nocturnal ventilation (e.g., Nasal BiPap) are often adequate (Waldhorn, 1992).

## Sedatives and Hypnotics

Barbiturates and sedatives disrupt normal sleep patterns and increase the risk of respiratory depression. They are not recommended.

## SLEEP APNEA SYNDROME

Sleep apnea syndrome is a phenomenon characterized by frequent (up to 120 times an hour) and often prolonged (up to 140 seconds) episodes of apnea occurring during sleep. Apneic episodes can result from either central or obstructive events or from a combination of both. They occur more often during NREM sleep but result in more severe oxygen desaturation when they occur during REM sleep.

## Types of Apneas

Sleep apnea syndrome affects 1% to 4% of adults. Apneas may be obstructive, central, or mixed. Obstructive or mixed apneas are more common than central. The incidence in young men is at least double that in young women; following

**Apnea type**

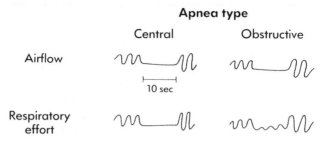

Fig. 12-2   Relationship between airflow and respiratory effort in both central and obstructive apnea. Respiratory effort is measured using a strain gauge or esophageal balloon. (From White DP: *Clin Chest Med* 6:623, 1985.)

menopause the incidence is about equal (Bliwise, 1987). Apneas meet diagnostic criteria for sleep apnea syndrome if the following criteria apply (Strohl, 1986; White, 1985):

- Last more than 15 seconds
- Occur at least five times per hour or thirty times per night in young adults; more than fifteen times per hour in older adults
- Are associated with severe oxygen desaturation, symptoms of hypoxia, or excessive daytime somnolence

**Obstructive Sleep Apnea**

During an episode of obstructive sleep apnea (OSA) the patient actively struggles to breathe, but flaccid or redundant tissue obstructs the oropharyngeal airway and prevents inspiratory airflow (Fig. 12-2). As hypoxemia worsens, the patient arouses just enough to restore oropharyngeal muscle tone. The airway bursts open with loud snorts, breathing resumes, and oxygen saturation returns to normal. Sleep arousals, although present as often as 500 times a night, only occasionally cause the patient to be aware of "waking up." However, apneas are so frequent during NREM sleep that patients typically never reach either deep or REM sleep stages. This causes severe sleep disruption and deprivation.

People with milder OSA tend to experience hypopneas or obstructive episodes mostly at sleep onset and during REM sleep, but preserve deep sleep. Thus they have less daytime somnolence and may be harder to identify. The total number of apneas is often less (10 to 20 an hour) and desaturation is milder. Sleep deprivation increases the frequency and severity of apneas.

An association between systemic hypertension and sleep apnea syndrome has been noted in middle-aged and older men, suggesting that sleep apnea should be considered in the differential diagnosis of hypertension (Fletcher, 1985).

**Central Sleep Apnea**

Central sleep apnea is a relatively rare central nervous system problem involving impaired motor output from the medullary respiratory center. Respiratory efforts are absent during the apneic episode, but some degree of obstructed ventilatory effort usually follows (Fig. 12-2). It is more common in the elderly.

Obesity hypoventilation syndrome (OHS) is characterized by morbid obesity and profound daytime hypercapnia. The increased work of breathing caused by obesity, combined with a blunted respiratory drive, causes severe hypoventilation with hypoxemia and $CO_2$ narcosis. Should the patient with OHS have sleep apnea as well, the sedative effect of hypercapnia combined with apnea-induced chronic sleep deprivation may cause the individual to fall asleep without warning and at inappropriate times. Arousal occurs when $PaO_2$ reaches a critical low level. A normal pattern of sleep stages is never achieved, and the patient remains chronically sleep deprived.

## Pathophysiologic Effects of Apneas

The pathophysiologic effects of apneas include the following:

- Bradycardia during the obstruction; reflex tachycardia when ventilation resumes
- Increase in pulmonary artery and systolic blood pressure, which is more severe with obstructive (as compared with central) apneas
- Profound recurrent drops in oxygen saturation (e.g., to 50%) during REM sleep
- High risk of cardiac arrhythmias associated with severe desaturation episodes or concomitant heart disease
- Increased $PaCO_2$ in association with drops in $PaO_2$ may cause complaints of morning headache (assumed to be due to hypercapnia-induced cerebral vascular dilation)
- Eventually, right ventricular failure resulting from frequent and profound hypoxemic episodes, especially if daytime hypoxemia is also present; abnormalities of right-sided hemodynamics greatly exaggerated when sleep apnea coexists with chronic lung disease (Fletcher, 1987)

## Etiology

### Obstructive Sleep Apnea

The etiologic factors of obstructive sleep apnea include the following:

- Reduced pharyngeal diameter: *seen in children with enlarged tonsilar tissue;* in people with excess or redundant oropharyngeal tissue, acromegaly, or an unusually large tongue or small lower jaw; and in obese men with short squat necks; in predisposed obese individuals, simple head flexion can result in oropharyngeal obstruction
- Nasal obstruction (e.g., caused by deviated nasal septum) in which the large negative oropharyngeal pressures that must be generated to overcome the obstruction lead to airway collapse
- Reduced oropharyngeal muscle tone during sleep
- Poor neuromuscular coordination
- Thyroid deficiency

■ ***Role of Obesity.*** Most patients with OSA are only moderately overweight. However, the role of obesity in OSA is unclear. By increasing fatty deposition in the neck, obesity predisposes the individual to upper airway obstruction. It is also possible that the physiologic effects of hypoventilation alter hypothalamic pituitary function in such a way that weight loss is difficult, or that increasingly sedentary behavior associated with sleep deprivation predisposes an individual to weight gain (Sullivan, 1985). Thus moderate obesity may be an effect of hypoventilation, rather than its cause, and may be difficult to control until apneas are well controlled.

### Central Sleep Apnea

The etiologic factors of central sleep apnea are unclear, but they are thought to include both genetic differences in respiratory drive and hormonal factors. Normal drops in hypoxic and hypercapneic ventilatory drives during sleep may potentiate central apneas, especially in men with naturally blunted drives. Some hypoxic, hypercapneic patients with COPD develop central apneas with the use of nocturnal oxygen. Other influencing factors include the following:

- Stable, severe congestive heart failure
- Disorders involving compromised neurologic output to respiratory muscles (e.g., polio, spinal cord injuries)
- Nasal obstruction (e.g., resulting from colds, allergic rhinitis, or deviated nasal septum)
- Central nervous system depressants

## Assessment

Symptoms of obstructive and central sleep apnea are summarized in the box on p. 210. A thorough sleep history is the first step in assessment. Input from the spouse or parent is particularly important in characterizing snoring and apnea patterns.

If symptoms of sleep apnea are present and include impaired daytime function (e.g., falling asleep in potentially dangerous situations), a full nocturnal sleep study (nocturnal polysomnography) is indicated.

Less expensive daytime sleep studies identify

---

### Symptoms of Sleep Apneas

**OBSTRUCTIVE SLEEP APNEA—MILD**

Long periods of heavy snoring, with apneas occurring only when patient is in supine position

Sudden wakening, choking, and severe dyspnea associated with apneas during REM (complaints of sleep disturbance and night choking)

Daytime somnolence if apneas become more frequent

**OBSTRUCTIVE SLEEP APNEA—MODERATE TO SEVERE**

Snoring, punctuated by periods of silence, then loud, stertorous respirations as breathing resumes (70% have snored since childhood)

Wild, thrashing movements

Profound daytime somnolence caused by long-term deprivation of deep and REM sleep; interferes with work and increases risk for motor vehicle accidents

Early morning headaches, irritability

Impaired concentration, short-term memory deficits

Profuse nocturnal sweating

Nocturnal angina

Impotence

Mild systemic hypertension (a common feature)

**CENTRAL SLEEP APNEA**

Insomnia and disrupted sleep: frequent wakenings with sudden, severe, transient dyspnea; often confused with orthopnea or paroxysmal nocturnal dyspnea caused by left ventricular failure

Depression

Decreased libido

Individual typically of normal body weight

---

most patients with significant sleep apnea, but the incidence of false-negative results is higher. Daytime studies usually involve 3 to 4 hours of monitored sleep following a 24-hour period of sleep deprivation. It is important that patients assume a variety of body positions during the study so that positional increases in apnea frequency (usually in the supine position) are identified. Patients may

have difficulty staying awake for 24 hours and, if not sufficiently sleep deprived, may not reach REM sleep during the study. Thus some daytime studies miss that sleep period during which the most severe sleep disturbances tend to occur.

## Nursing Interventions

The specific treatment of choice for sleep apnea in the adult depends on both the type of apnea (central, obstructive, or mixed) and the severity of the problem. Patients with moderate to severe symptomatic apnea need treatment; patients with mild to moderate apnea may not or may do well with relatively benign and noninvasive measures. Many of the more aggressive treatments for sleep apnea have proved disappointing. The home care nurse's role in managing the patient with a primary sleep disorder is to review and reinforce the importance of preventive measures and prescribed medications, instruct the patient and family in the use of special equipment, and assess the response to therapy.

### Obstructive Sleep Apnea

The following are recommendations for the management of OSA.

1. Treat the underlying problem: surgical correction of upper airway obstruction caused by problems such as a deviated nasal septum, nasal polyps, or enlarged tonsils or adenoids is often helpful.

2. Instruct the patient to avoid alcohol and sedative-hypnotics.

3. Position training: Patients should avoid sleeping in a flat supine position because this permits the tongue to fall back into the pharynx, worsening obstruction. Suggestions include having the patient sleep in a chair or sewing tennis balls into the back of a nightshirt so that the patient cannot comfortably lie on his or her back.

4. Weight loss: Even modest (5% to 10%) weight loss may reduce symptoms. Compliance with a weight loss program is often poor but may be improved as a result of nasal continuous positive airway pressure (CPAP) treatment, which often increases energy and motivation.

5. CPAP: Nasal CPAP is the most common treat-

ment for symptomatic obstructive sleep apnea that has not responded to preventive measures. Placed snugly over the nose, the CPAP mask delivers positive pressure to the oropharynx during sleep, preventing upper airway collapse by counteracting the high suction pressures created during inspiration. The use of nasal CPAP is discussed in Chapter 14.

6. Tracheostomy: Tracheostomy results in dramatic improvement in daytime somnolence, cardiopulmonary symptoms, and mental function, although coexisting central apneas may persist. It is the treatment of choice for severe, life-threatening obstructive sleep apnea that has not responded to nasal CPAP. It may be the only effective treatment for patients who also have significant chronic lung disease (Fletcher, 1987). Indications include the following (Guilleminault, 1981):

- Disabling daytime somnolence
- Life-threatening cardiac arrhythmias occurring during hypoxemic phases
- More than 60 apnea episodes of at least 10 seconds duration per hour
- Sleep desaturation below 40%
- No improvement with less invasive measures

7. Medications: Protriptyline is a nonsedating tricyclic antidepressant that reduces the frequency and duration of OSA in some patients, typically those with mild apnea. Patients generally start with 5 mg at bedtime, increasing slowly to a maximum dose of 30 mg. Anticholinergic side effects may limit tolerance of the drug for some patients. A 2-week trial is needed to evaluate the medication's efficacy. Medroxyprogesterone may help in a subset of patients with more severe awake hypoxemia and hypercapnia, but overall it has proved disappointing. Theophylline is a respiratory stimulant that reduces the frequency of coexisting central apneas in people with OSA; however, it does not reduce the frequency or duration of obstructive events or the degree of desaturation and it may even potentiate upper airway occlusion during sleep. It may be useful in patients with COPD because of its bronchodilating properties but is not indicated for the treatment of OSA in a non-COPD population (Espinoza, 1987).

8. Orthodontic devices: These are often uncomfortable and only partially effective in reducing the frequency of obstructions.

9. Other surgical interventions: Procedures such as uvulopalatopharyngoplasty (UPPP) increase airway diameter by removing redundant oropharyngeal tissue but have limited success, and postoperative scarring may actually worsen airway narrowing, resulting in speech or swallowing problems. Efficacy of mandibular advancement is also variable.

### Central Sleep Apnea

The following are recommendations for the management of central sleep apnea:

1. Treat the underlying problem.

2. Encourage weight loss, if the patient is obese.

3. Medications: Acetazolamide, a carbonic anhydrase inhibitor, produces a metabolic acidosis that acts as a respiratory stimulant. The usual dose is 250 mg qid. Although it reduces the frequency of central apneas, patients often develop obstructive apnea after a few weeks of therapy. It is *not* recommended for patients with coexisting COPD because it will worsen acidosis.

Medroxyprogesterone is a hormone with respiratory-stimulating properties used to treat patients with obesity hypoventilation syndrome. The usual dose is 20 mg tid. It is not helpful in COPD because patients cannot increase ventilation in response to increased respiratory drive.

4. Low-flow oxygen therapy is occasionally helpful but requires a sleep study to identify those likely to benefit.

5. Mechanical ventilation using a rocking bed, negative-pressure ventilator (e.g., chest cuirass), tracheostomy with positive-pressure ventilation, and diaphragmatic pacing may help but are invasive and indicated only for severe disease.

### Patient Support Groups

A national support group for people with sleep apnea, called AWAKE (Alert, Well, and Keeping Energetic), has chapters in many cities. Information about AWAKE can be obtained from the American Sleep Apnea Association, P.O. Box 3893, Charlottesville, VA 22908.

## APNEA IN CHILDREN

*Irregular breathing patterns, brief respiratory pauses, and paradoxic breathing during REM sleep are common and normal in infants up to 6 months of age. Infants also frequently develop apnea and bradycardia during feedings, probably because of difficulties in coordinating sucking and swallowing with breathing. Prolonged apneas, however, are life threatening whether they occur during sleep or wakefulness, and they require evaluation and treatment.*

### Etiology

*The most common cause of OSA in children is hypertrophied tonsils or adenoids, although a variety of other problems may be implicated. OSA is more common in older children.*

*Potential causes of apnea in infants and young children include anatomic facial or airway abnormalities; infections, including sepsis, meningitis, upper and lower respiratory tract infections; CNS disorders (tumors, seizures, sedative overdose); congenital heart disorders; electrolyte disturbances; trauma including hypothermia or hyperthermia; inborn errors of metabolism; anemia or cardiopulmonary or neurologic immaturity in the preterm infant; gastroesophageal reflux; hypoxia associated with chronic respiratory diseases such as bronchopulmonary dysplasia; and abnormalities of ventilatory control such as Ondine's curse (Ariagno, 1985).*

*Ondine's curse is a disorder of central control in which breathing stops as soon as the infant falls asleep. The underlying mechanism is primary alveolar hypoventilation resulting from reduced respiratory center responsiveness to $CO_2$.*

*When no specific cause for apnea can be identified, the term "apparent life-threatening event" (ALTE) is used. Fifty percent of apneic infants fall into this category. ALTE is defined as "an unexplained episode of cessation of breathing for 20 seconds or longer, or a shorter respiratory pause associated with bradycardia, cyanosis, pallor and/ or marked hypotonia" (National Institutes of Health, 1987). When apneas are severe enough to require frequent cardiopulmonary resuscitation or vigorous stimulation, the risk of sudden death is increased.*

### Assessment

*In children the severity of sleep apnea is judged more by associated bradycardia, oxygen desaturation, and the need for stimulation to restart breathing than by the actual number of apneic episodes. Typical symptoms of OSA in children include the following:*

- *Heavy snoring interspersed with pauses and respiratory snorts*
- *Profuse night sweats, disrupted sleep*
- *Parasomnias such as nightmares, night terrors, enuresis, and sleep walking*
- *Morning headaches*
- *Daytime sleepiness, tiredness, and fatigue*
- *Hyperactivity, asocial or inappropriate behavior, poor school performance*
- *Failure to thrive*
- *Eventually, pulmonary hypertension and pulmonary heart disease*

### Nursing Interventions

*1. Treat the underlying cause: Surgery is usually indicated for any child with enlarged tonsils or adenoids who snores. Removing enlarged tissue relieves the airway obstruction.*

*2. Respiratory stimulants: Methylxanthines (e.g., theophylline, aminophylline, or caffeine) are often used to reduce the frequency and severity of apneic events in preterm infants. Side effects (hyperactivity, impaired sleep, tachycardia, or vomiting) suggest the need to reduce the dose. The slower clearance in premature infants increases risk of theophylline toxicity. To reduce the risk of toxicity, the serum level should be maintained between 8 and 12 µg/ml.*

*3. Home apnea cardiac monitoring: Monitoring of apnea and bradycardia is the intervention most often used for the management of infant apneas (Ariagno, 1985). Specific indications, however, re-*

*main controversial. As with all "high-tech" interventions, an acceptable cost-to-benefit ratio must be demonstrated and the psychosocial impact on the family carefully evaluated. Currently the use of monitoring is medically indicated for the following categories of children (National Institutes of Health, 1987):*

- *Infants who have experienced an apparent life-threatening apneic event that required vigorous stimulation or resuscitation*
- *Siblings of two or more sudden infant death syndrome (SIDS) victims*
- *Some symptomatic premature infants, as an alternative to prolonged hospitalization*
- *Infants with conditions such as central hypoventilation*

*Monitoring is usually continued until the infant has been free of symptomatic apneas for 2 to 3 months and has demonstrated the ability to tolerate stress (e.g., an upper respiratory tract infection or symptoms associated with immunization) without an apneic episode. The typical duration is 5 to 9 months. Holter monitoring may also be used to determine whether cardiac arrhythmias coexist, either independently or in association with sleep apnea desaturation.*

*In the event of an apneic episode, the infant should be aroused by physical stimulation. If respirations are not restored, mouth-to-mouth resuscitation should be instituted, with cardiac resuscitation if necessary.*

*Reassurance and training of the family in the use of the monitor and cardiopulmonary resuscitation are of paramount importance. Most parents are initially fearful, but with support they become confident in their ability to react appropriately to the alarm. Parents are instructed to record the following:*

- *The child's behavior during the alarm*
- *The type of alarm (apnea, bradycardia, or both)*
- *The child's response to interventions*

*4. Mechanical supports: Nasal CPAP is often used for children with sleep apnea syndrome.*

*Phrenic nerve electrostimulation may be indicated for some children with spinal cord injuries.*

*5. Tracheostomy: Tracheostomy is indicated for children with severe impairment of ventilatory control.*

## PARASOMNIAS

*Parasomnias are more prevalent in children than adults and include sleepwalking, night terrors, nightmares, and enuresis (Kales, 1987). Sleepwalking affects as many as 15% of children. Sleepwalking and night terrors occur mostly during stages III and IV of sleep, are usually seen in older children with a positive family history, and are considered maturational problems of impaired arousal. Symptoms usually disappear by late adolescence, and treatment consists primarily of protection against injury.*

*Nightmares occur in both children and adults during REM sleep. The prevalence in children is greatest from 3 to 8 years of age, when the child's fantasy life is most active.*

*Enuresis affects 10% to 15% of children between 3 and 12 years of age, occurs most often during the first third of the night, and is primarily associated with a small functional bladder capacity.*

**REFERENCES**

Ariagno RL, Guilleminault C: Apnea during sleep in the pediatric patient, *Clin Chest Med* 6:679, 1985.

Bixler EO, Vela-Bueno A: Normal sleep: physiological, behavioral and clinical correlates, *Psychiatr Ann* 17:437, 1987.

Bliwise DL et al: Risk factors for sleep disordered breathing in heterogeneous geriatric populations, *J Am Geriatr Soc* 35:132, 1987.

Espinoza H et al: The effect of aminophylline on sleep and sleep-disordered breathing in patients with obstructive sleep apnea syndrome, *Am Rev Respir Dis* 136:80, 1987.

Fletcher EC et al: Undiagnosed sleep apnea in patients with essential hypertension, *Ann Intern Med* 103:190, 1985.

Fletcher EC et al: Long term cardiopulmonary sequelae in patients with sleep apnea and chronic lung disease, *Am Rev Respir Dis* 135:525, 1987.

Guilleminault C et al: Obstructive sleep apnea syndrome and tracheostomy: long-term follow-up experience, *Arch Intern Med* 141:985, 1981.

Hauri PJ, Silberfarb PM: The effects of aspirin on the sleep of insomniacs, *Sleep Res* 7:100, 1978 (abstract).

Kales A, Soldatos CR, Kales JD: Sleep disorders: insomnia, sleepwalking, night terrors, nightmares, and enuresis, *Ann Intern Med* 106:582, 1987.

Kinsman RA et al: Symptoms and experiences in chronic bronchitis and emphysema, *Chest* 83:755, 1983.

Krieger J: Breathing during sleep in normal subjects, *Clin Chest Med* 6:577, 1985.

Kryger MH: Sleep in restrictive lung disorders, *Clin Chest Med* 6:675, 1985.

Lee KA: Sensory overload, sensory deprivation and sleep deprivation. In Patrick ML et al, editors: *Medical surgical nursing: pathophysiological concepts,* ed 2, Philadelphia, 1991, JB Lippincott.

National Institutes of Health: Consensus statement: NIH consensus development conference on infantile apnea and home monitoring, *Pediatrics* 79:292, 1987.

Partinen M et al: Snoring and hypertension: a cross-sectional study on 12,808 Finns aged 24-65 years, *Sleep Res* 12:273, 1983.

Perez-Padilla R et al: Breathing during sleep in patients with interstitial lung disease, *Am Rev Respir Dis* 132:224. 1985.

Phillips BA, Cooper KR, Burke TV: The effect of sleep loss on breathing in chronic obstructive pulmonary disease, *Chest* 91:29, 1987.

Strohl KP, Cherniak NS, Gothe B. Physiologic basis for therapy of sleep apnea, *Am Rev Respir Dis* 134:791, 1986.

Sullivan CE, Issa FG: Obstructive sleep apnea, *Clin Chest Med* 6:633, 1985.

Vitiello M: Circadian temperature rhythm in young and old men, *Neurobiol Aging* 7:97, 1986.

Waldhorn RE: Nocturnal nasal intermittent positive pressure ventilation with bi-level positive airway pressure (BiPAP) in respiratory failure, *Chest* 101:516, 1992.

White DP: Central sleep apnea, *Clin Chest Med* 6:623, 1985.

## SUGGESTED READINGS

Kryger MH: Symposium on sleep disorders, *Clin Chest Med* 6:1, 1985.

Martin RJ: The sleep-related worsening of lower airways obstruction: understanding and intervention, *Med Clin North Am* 74:701, 1990.

Strohl KP, Cherniack NS, Gothe B: Physiologic basis of therapy for sleep apnea, *Am Rev Respir Dis* 134:791, 1986.

White DP: Obstructive sleep apnea, *Hosp Pract* 27:57, 1992.

# CHAPTER 13

# Associated Problems

JOAN TURNER

Patients with chronic lung disease frequently develop problems with other body systems. These include gastrointestinal complaints (gaseousness, gastroesophageal reflux, gastritis, peptic ulcer disease, and constipation), urinary and fecal incontinence, and rib and vertebral fractures. The etiologic factors, assessment, and nursing care of each are presented in this chapter.

## GASEOUSNESS

Gaseousness is defined as the accumulation of excessive gastrointestinal gas. Upper (burping, eructation) and lower (flatulence) gastrointestinal gaseousness are common complaints of the home care patient.

## Etiology

The possible etiologic factors of gastrointestinal gaseousness and flatulence are summarized in the following.

### Gastrointestinal Gaseousness

*Aerophagia (air swallowing)*
- Aerophagia is probably the main source of gas in the esophagus and stomach.
- It is often the result of nervous tension; predisposed individuals can swallow enough air to cause gastric distention.
- Patients with chronic lung disease may gulp and swallow air when they feel excessively short of breath, use their metered-dose inhalers, or use oxygen.

*Eating and drinking*
- Normally a bolus of air of approximately 2 to 3 ml accompanies each swallow of food.
- About two or three times more air is swallowed with liquids than with solid food because air is trapped between the upper lip and the surface of the liquid.
- Air swallowing increases with gulping, with rapid eating, and in the supine position.

*Digestion*
- Bowel gas (e.g. hydrogen, carbon dioxide, and, for some, methane) is produced by bacterial fermentation of food substances in the ileum and colon.
- The volume produced depends on the type and amount of bowel flora present and the type of food ingested.
- Flatulence typically begins about 1 hour after eating and lasts about 20 minutes.

*Bowel flora*
- Increased bacterial and yeast organisms and abnormal anaerobic intestinal flora enhance fermentation and cause flatus.
- Bowel flora are altered by gastrointestinal infections and antibiotic therapy.

*Gaseous foods*
- Foods that are high in cellulose fiber provide more substrate for bacterial fermentation. Examples include navy, soy, and lima beans; cabbage; onions; broccoli; cauliflower; peas; brussels sprouts; kohlrabi; radishes; cucumbers; and celery.

- The ingestion of inadequately cooked starch also increases the amount of carbon dioxide and hydrogen that is produced during digestion.

*Gastrointestinal disease*

- Peptic ulcer disease, hiatal hernia, gallbladder disease, and irritable bowel syndromes may be associated with increased gaseousness (Roth, 1985).

*Altered bowel peristalsis*

- Increased peristalsis results from dietary bulk, laxative use, and irritable bowel problems.
- Decreased bowel peristalsis may be caused by inadequate dietary fiber, advanced age, a sedentary life-style, right ventricular failure, and medications such as narcotic, anticholinergic, and antidepressant agents.

*Malabsorption problems*

- In cystic fibrosis the pancreatic enzyme deficiencies cause malabsorption of fats and proteins, increasing the amount of food substrate available for bacterial fermentation.
- In lactase deficiencies lactose is retained in the colon, causing increased production of carbon dioxide.

## Assessment

The assessment of gastrointestinal gaseousness and flatulence is based primarily on the patient history and an understanding of factors that may produce the symptom.

## Nursing Interventions
### Strategies to Prevent Gaseousness

Strategies that may prevent gaseousness include the reduction of air swallowing, avoidance of gas-forming foods and beverages, reduction of nervous tension, and consultation with the physician on the treatment of underlying problems such as constipation, heart failure, malabsorption and gastrointestinal disease. The following are recommendations for preventing gaseousness.

*Reduce air swallowing*

- Make meals a relaxed occasion; eat and chew slowly.
- Avoid excessively large meals or eat the main meal early in the day.
- Eat in the upright position.
- Do not drink liquids with meals.
- Avoid excessive salivation and the associated urge to swallow by avoiding gum chewing and smoking, repairing ill-fitting dentures, and treating oral lesions.
- Review the patient's metered-dose inhaler technique. If patient swallows air with use of the inhaler, advise the patient to keep his or her mouth open after inhalation. This makes it difficult to swallow air.
- Encourage a more relaxed respiratory pattern, using pursed lip breathing as an alternative to air gulping with increased dyspnea.

*Avoid gas-forming foods*

- Maintain a balanced fiber diet and cook foods properly.
- Omit foods that are known to produce excessive gas. If offending foods are unknown, try eliminating one possible food at a time to determine the cause of excessive gas.
- If lactose intolerance is suspected, try decreasing the dietary intake of lactose or use lactase supplements.

*Reduce nervous tension*

- Compassionate home care personnel may relieve patient anxiety by allowing the patient to discuss fears and concerns and by being available when the patient needs help.
- Relaxation techniques, psychotherapy, and antianxiety medications may facilitate a more relaxed state, thereby reducing associated air swallowing.

### Strategies to Relieve Discomfort from Gaseousness

The following strategies may relieve discomfort from excessive gas:

- Massage the abdomen while walking to stimulate the passage of gas.
- Assume the knee-chest position and rock forward and backward slowly.
- Apply heat to the abdomen.

- Take a warm, relaxing bath.
- Avoid lying down or sitting in a slumped position after meals when gas can be trapped above the liquid overlying the gastroesophageal junction and passed into the bowel.
- Avoid tight-fitting clothes.
- Use a rectal tube if discomfort cannot be relieved by the above measures.
- As a last resort, try a 1-pint lukewarm tap water enema.

## GASTROESOPHAGEAL REFLUX

Gastroesophageal reflux (GER) is defined as a backward flow of the contents of the stomach into the esophagus that can cause inflammation of the esophagus (reflux esophagitis). Other problems that occur as a result of reflux are contact of refluxed material with the airways and significant loss of calories in infants (Orenstein, 1991). Approximately 75% of patients with asthma have GER, and 40% have reflux esophagitis (Sontag, 1991). Gastrointestinal reflux occurs more often in patients with cystic fibrosis as compared with normal controls (Scott, 1985) *and may be a contributing factor in children with recurrent pulmonary infection* (Chen, 1991).

### Etiology

GER occurs primarily because of a reduction in the tone of the lower esophageal sphincter, allowing gastric contents to enter the esophagus (Orenstein, 1991). Damage to the mucosa of the esophagus is more likely to occur if reflux is more frequent, if clearance from the esophagus is impaired, and if the gastric contents are more noxious.

Complex interactions between GER and the respiratory system may cause respiratory disorders and aggravate reflux. Gastric reflux may cause respiratory disease by three main mechanisms: (1) aspiration of gastric contents; (2) stimulation of nerve endings in the airways and esophagus; and (3) the direct effects of inflammation or the release of chemical mediators (Orenstein, 1991). These factors cause narrowing of the airways from the secretion of mucus, edema of the airway mucosa, and contraction of muscles in the wall of the airways. Vagally mediated reflex mechanisms induced by acid infusions in the esophagus and microaspiration of acid reflux cause increased airway resistance in patients with asthma (Sontag, 1991). A causal relationship between GER and nonallergic asthma was documented in one study in which pulmonary symptoms and expiratory flow rates improved after treatment of GER (Larrain, 1991). Even though a high incidence of GER has been documented in patients with COPD (Ducolone, 1987), a relationship between GER and lung function has not been demonstrated in this population (Orr, 1992). The possible relationship between GER and respiratory disorders is summarized in the box on p. 218.

### Assessment

The symptoms of GER include both pulmonary and gastrointestinal manifestations and are summarized below.

### Symptoms of GER

*Infants and children*
  *Protracted vomiting*
  *Gagging, regurgitation, and mouthing and swallowing of stomach contents (rumination)*
  *Nocturnal wheezing, coughing, or both*
  *Hematemesis*
  *Failure to thrive*
  *Recurrent bronchitis and pneumonia*
Adults
  Pulmonary manifestations
    Early morning hoarseness
    Nocturnal or early morning wheezing, cough, or both
    Ache or lump at base of neck
    Nocturnal dyspnea
    Laryngeal stridor
    Bronchitis
  Gastrointestinal manifestations
    Heartburn that usually occurs approximately 1 hour after meals
    Regurgitation of fluid into the mouth at night

## Relationship Between Reflux and Respiratory Tract Disorders

**RESPIRATORY TRACT DISORDERS CAUSED BY REFLUX**

Macroaspiration (usually occurs only in patients with altered levels of consciousness) leading to:
Mechanical obstruction of airway lumen
Chemical pneumonitis
Reflex closure of airways
Loss of surfactant
Epithelial damage
Pulmonary edema
Pulmonary hemorrhage
Hypoxemia
Microaspiration leading to:
Possible nonspecific lower respiratory tract disease
*Possible apnea (especially infants in their first 6 months of life)*
Reflux without aspiration may stimulate afferent nerves in the esophagus causing:
Reflex bronchospasm
Reflex laryngospasm (obstructive apnea, stridor)
Reflex central responses (central apnea, bradycardia)

**RESPIRATORY TRACT DISORDERS (ACTIVITES AND THERAPIES) CAUSING REFLUX**

Thoracoabdominal pressure relationships
Forced expiration (cough, wheeze) increases abdominal pressure
Forced inspiration (stridor, hiccups) enhances negative intrathoracic pressure

Lower esophageal sphincter incompetence
Relaxation of lower esophageal sphincter with deep inspiration when diaphragmatic contraction inhibited (may occur with mechanical ventilation and hiatal hernia)
Smoking: relaxes lower esophageal sphincter tone and increases frequency of reflux, probably because of action of nicotine, stimulation of adrenergic nervous system, or both; *passive smoking may have similar effects in children*
Drugs: theophylline and caffeine, which relax lower esophageal sphincter and stimulate gastric acid secretion; isoproterenol, metaproterenol, carbuterol, and terbutaline, which may also relax sphincter tone
Nasogastric tube: reduces lower esophageal sphincter pressure (stomach may not be able to stretch fast enough to accommodate rapid high-pressure tube feedings)
Volume and noxiousness of gastric contents
Gravity
Supine, supine-seated positions and head-down positions worsen GER (Orenstein, 1991)
Chest physiotherapy increases GER with head-dependent positions and possibly with forced expiration and cough maneuvers
Mechanical ventilation: tracheal intubation may impair upper airway reflexes and lead to aspiration by inhibiting upper esophageal sphincter opening during swallowing; supine position increases reflux and slows gastric emptying

Modified from Orenstein SR: *Curr Probl Pediatr* 21:193, 1991.

or when bending over (Secretions may be seen on the pillow in the morning.)
Painful swallowing (odynophagia)
Difficulty swallowing solid foods (dysphagia)
Hemorrhage of coffee ground–like material or bright red blood; may be the first symptom of GER

Sudden presence in the mouth of clear salty fluid thought to be salivary gland secretions (water brash)

### Diagnosis of Gastroesophageal Reflux

The relief of symptoms in response to antireflux therapy is considered presumptive evidence for GER. If empiric antireflux therapy does not relieve the symptoms, intraluminal esophageal pH monitoring is considered to be the gold standard for the diagnosis of GER. Other diagnostic procedures include radiographic imaging, acid perfusion tests, endoscopy, esophageal biopsy, and esophageal manometry.

## Nursing Interventions

The following are recommended measures for the treatment of the individual with GER:

*Positioning (Orenstein, 1991)*
- Stand or sit upright while awake.
- Elevate head of bed or sleep prone. The prone position is preferable to the supine recumbent position for all ages; *position infants upright after feeding.*
- Fast before chest physiotherapy if head-down position is required. Consider pretreatment with antacids.
- Consider prone position for ventilator-dependent patients.

*Dietary measures*
- Promote weight loss if the patient is overweight. Avoid large meals.
- Reduce dietary fat, chocolate, caffeine, and alcohol.
- Avoid hot liquids and citrus juices during periods of exacerbation of symptoms. *Infant formulas may be thickened by adding 2 tablespoons of rice cereal per 4 ounces of formula (Orenstein, 1988).*
- Eat and take medications in an upright position. Do not lie down directly after meals. Fast several hours before going to bed.

*Miscellaneous measures*
- Use measures to control cough.
- Avoid tight-fitting clothes that increase abdominal pressure.
- Stop smoking. Avoid exposure to secondhand smoke.

*Medications*
- Medications include the following:
    Antacids
        Administer 30 ml/hr for adults *(0.5 to 1 ml/kg 3 to 8 times daily for children)*

during exacerbations to neutralize acidity.
    Alternate magnesium hydroxide with aluminum hydroxide preparations to prevent diarrhea and constipation.
$H_2$-receptor antagonists
    Administer ranitidine, 300 mg, at dinnertime or 150 mg bid *(2 mg/kg tid for children).*
Proton pump inhibitor
    Administer omeprazole, an inhibitor of basal and stimulated gastric secretions.
Cholinergic agents
    Bethanechol chloride, 10 to 20 mg for adults *(0.1 to 0.3 mg/kg tid or qid for children),* with meals may increase motility and improve gastric emptying.
Gastrointestinal stimulants
    Metoclopramide, 10 to 20 mg/day adults *(0.1 mg/kg qid children),* stimulates intestinal smooth muscle and may increase the rate of gastric emptying.
Barrier therapy
    Sucralfate 1 to 4 g qid on an empty stomach in adults *(1 g in a 5- to 15-ml solution qid [slurry] for children),* protects against acid, pepsin, and bile salts.

*Surgery*
- Surgery is advocated for patients who do not respond to medical management.

## GASTRITIS AND PEPTIC ULCER DISEASE

Gastritis is defined as inflammation of the stomach. Peptic ulcer disease is a defect in the mucous lining of the esophagus, stomach, or duodenum from the action of gastric acid. The risk for duodenal and gastric ulcers is significantly increased in the presence of chronic gastritis (Sipponen, 1990). Up to 30% of patients with chronic lung disease develop peptic ulcers (Soll, 1989), whereas approximately 10% of the population in general develops gastric or duodenal ulcers (Miller, 1991). Associations have been shown between increased bronchial secretions, reduced expiratory airflow, and peptic ulcers (Soll, 1989). Stress gastritis (inflammation of the stomach in response to stress) occurs in response to shock, significant trauma, organ failure, and sepsis, among other things. Respiratory failure is an important risk factor for gastric injury and bleeding associated with organ failure because of decreased oxygenation of the gastric mucosa (Miller, 1991).

### Etiology

Mucous secretions play a significant role in protecting the gastric mucosa. Chronic gastritis alters mucous secretions and damages the gastric epithelium, increasing the likelihood of ulceration (Jamieson, 1991). Genetic factors may play a role in the relationship between chronic lung disease and peptic ulcers in that patients with $\alpha$-1-antitrypsin deficiency have a one and a half to three times greater risk for peptic ulcers than the general population. This is probably because of a lack of protease inhibitors (Soll, 1989). Patients with chronic lung disease are treated with medications known to cause gastric injury. Doses equivalent to 10 mg prednisone a day or more for over 6 months are associated with gastric injury. An even greater risk is associated with the use of alcohol and nonsteroidal antiinflammatory drugs, including acetylsalicylic acid, indomethacin, ibuprofen, and phenylbutazone. These drugs increase the permeability of the gastric epithelium to acid, causing cellular damage (Miller, 1991). Caffeine and theophylline may also cause epigastric distress. Smoking, a cause of chronic lung disease, is an additional risk factor for ulcer disease. Smoking increases acid secretions, decreases secretion of pancreatic bicarbonate, retards healing, and promotes the recurrence of ulcers (Soll, 1989).

Infection with the gram-negative organism *Helicobacter pylori* has been associated with gastritis (Soll, 1992) and may be related to the development of peptic ulcer disease. More research needs to be carried out, however, before a cause and effect relationship can be clearly established.

### Assessment

Common complaints include a sensation of exaggerated hunger, fullness, or gaseous distress, epigastric pain or retrosternal burning, nausea or vomiting, and anorexia. Right lower quadrant abdominal pain or midepigastric pain radiating to the shoulder and hematemesis or melena may indicate perforation of an ulcer. A significant number of patients with gastritis and ulcers may not have symptoms. Gastrointestinal radiography and endoscopy may be necessary to establish a diagnosis.

### Nursing Interventions

The home care nurse should consult with the physician about prophylaxis with antacids or $H_2$-receptor antagonists such as cimetidine in patients who require long-term nonsteroidal antiinflammatory drugs, particularly if there is a history of gastric ulcer disease. Some physicians also advocate prophylactic therapy for patients who require long-term corticosteroid therapy, although the risk of corticosteroid-induced gastric disease is low. Patients should be advised to stop smoking and avoid medications, foods, and fluids that aggravate gastric symptoms.

Patients are often treated with hydrogen receptor antagonists (cimetidine, ranitidine, and famotidine), omeprazole, antacids, and other therapies discussed in the section on GER. Because cimetidine reduces hepatic clearance of theophylline, serum theophylline levels should be monitored if patients receiving theophylline are treated with cimetidine.

## CONSTIPATION

Constipation is defined in three ways: (1) as a reduced frequency of bowel movements compared with what is considered to be normal; (2) as the lack of urge to move the bowels; and (3) as difficulty in passing the stool. Constipation is a frequent complaint of patients with chronic lung disease. In patients with cystic fibrosis, it may signal the onset of meconium ileus equivalent.

Fecal impaction (hard stool in the rectum or colon) is common in the homebound patient and the elderly. It may be caused by anorectal disease, tumor, neurogenic disease of the colon, excessive use of bulk laxatives, antacids, low-residue diets, starvation, colonic stasis from drugs such as opiates, or prolonged bed rest or immobility. The rectal ampulla becomes distended with feces, thereby decreasing muscular tone and reducing the urge to defecate. Sometimes fecal fluid leaks around the impacted stool, causing "paradoxic diarrhea." Pressure necrosis of the bowel mucosa can also occur, leading to ulceration of the wall of the rectum.

## Etiology

Constipation may be caused by several factors (Table 13-1). Normally, food particles and secretions are mixed in the small intestine. The resultant solution (chyme) is passed into the colon where water and electrolytes are absorbed and the stool is stored until defecation takes place. During defecation the normal person takes a deep breath, the diaphragm descends, and the abdominal muscles contract, thereby increasing intraabdominal pressure and forcing the stool from the rectum so it

**Table 13-1**   Possible causes of constipation

| Cause | Comments |
|---|---|
| Muscle weakness | Flattened diaphragm and weakened abdominal muscles in COPD cause difficulty in generating adequate intraabdominal pressure to pass the stool. In neuromuscular disease, there may be difficulty in closing glottis sufficiently to increase intraabdominal pressure to pass the stool. |
| Drugs | Opiate analgesics such as codeine that may be prescribed for dyspnea and pain or cough control depress bowel motility. |
| Sedentary life-style | A sedentary life-style promotes constipation, whereas regular exercise stimulates stool elimination. Chronic respiratory failure and heart failure cause a more sedentary life-style, which can lead to constipation. |
| Lack of dietary bulk | Dietary fiber enhances the fecal mass in the large intestine and stimulates bowel motility by increasing the water content of the stool and acting as a source of carbon for bacterial growth. Constipation is more likely if the diet does not contain adequate nonabsorbable bulk. If the patient has sores in the mouth, poor dentition, or poorly fitting or no dentures, food with adequate fiber cannot be properly chewed. |
| Dehydration | Adequate fluid intake is necessary to prevent hard, dry stools. |
| Psychologic factors | Constipation may occur in depression, but the etiologic factors are unclear. Excessively anxious patients may have irritable bowel syndrome characterized by alternating constipation and diarrhea. Some patients may think that a daily bowel movement is essential; if they miss one, they think that they are constipated. Some patients consider stools dirty and may suppress the urge for a bowel movement, particularly if they do not have privacy or if they think that others are aware that they are going to the bathroom to move their bowels. |
| Miscellaneous causes | Lack of convenient access to toilet facilities may cause constipation. Lack of privacy can contribute to constipation. Excessive breathlessness when ambulating to toilet facilities or as a result of a bowel movement can inhibit stooling and promote constipation. High spinal cord transection with an intact isolated cord below the lesion leads to decreased resting colonic activity, promoting constipation. |

can be expelled. The external anal sphincter is voluntarily controlled by the conscious mind. Very often conceptions about what constitutes "normal" bowel habits develop during childhood and persist throughout the adult years. It is usual to have three to twelve bowel movements each week with an average daily weight of 200 g or less (Knauer, 1992).

### Assessment

The assessment of constipation is based primarily on the patient history and an understanding of factors that may cause the symptom. Persistent constipation without a known cause, abdominal pain, and distention may indicate diseases that require further workup. All patients with such symptoms should be referred to their physician without delay.

### Nursing Interventions

Strategies for nursing care of the patient with constipation are presented in Table 13-2. Laxatives that may be prescribed for the patient with chronic lung disease are listed in Table 13-3. The nurse should consult with the physician and dietitian to resolve problems with constipation.

## URINARY AND FECAL INCONTINENCE

Urinary and fecal incontinence is defined as an inability to control the passage of urine and feces. When patients with chronic obstructive pulmonary disease become acutely short of breath or cough excessively hard, they often complain of urinary incontinence and, less frequently, of fecal incontinence. Patients with chronic neuromuscular diseases and spinal cord injuries may also have incontinence, depending on the level of the lesion.

### Etiology
#### Increased Use of Abdominal Muscles

Usually the incontinence occurs during periods of acute resiratory tract obstruction or when there is a need to suddenly increase activity. At these times patients increase their respiratory effort to maintain gas exchange in the lungs and the delivery of oxygen to the body. Intraabdominal pressure rises with the increased contraction of the abdominal muscles, particularly during exhalation. Increased pressure may be exerted against the bladder so that it empties involuntarily, and stool that is stored in the rectum may be pushed past the anal sphincter.

#### Other Factors

Other factors that may cause urinary and fecal incontinence include the following:
- Childbearing with subsequent weakness of perineal muscles
- Age-related loss of muscle tone causing relaxation of sphincters (especially in postmenopausal women)
- Neuromuscular disease, stroke, and spinal cord injury
- Myopathy
- Urinary tract infection
- Partial urethral obstruction, prostatic hypertrophy, and prostatectomy

### Assessment

The assessment of urinary and fecal incontinence is based on the history and an understanding of factors that may cause the symptom. It is important to ask patients whether the problem exists because many patients are too embarrassed to bring it up.

### Nursing Interventions

The following strategies may help the patient with urinary and fecal incontinence:
- Have the patient empty the bowels and bladder before anticipated activity.
- Have the patient use inhaled bronchodilators 15 minutes before anticipated activity.
- Promote regular bowel elimination.
- Promote energy conservation measures (see Chapter 8).
- Have the patient try perineal muscle exercises if muscle weakness is a possible cause of urinary incontinence.

**Table 13-2** Nursing care of the patient with constipation

| Strategy | Comments |
|---|---|
| Eliminate cause | Change or reduce doses of drugs that promote constipation if possible (e.g., alternate doses of constipating aluminum hydroxide antacids with magnesium hydroxide preparations if antacids are necessary). |
| Maintain adequate fluids | Usually six to eight large glasses of liquids, such as water and juice, each day helps to promote normal bowel functioning. Sometimes drinking one glass of hot water or one cup of coffee ½ hour before breakfast each day enhances stooling. |
| Maintain adequate dietary fiber | Adequate dietary fiber requirements consist of approximately 30 g of fiber every day. Dietary fiber increases the transit time of the stool, increases bulk, and eases the elimination of the feces by two primary mechanisms: (1) by acting as a sponge for water, thereby increasing the water content of the feces, and (2) by acting as a source of carbon for bacterial growth, thereby increasing fecal matter. Vegetables, fruit, and whole-grain cereals are fiber-containing foods. Approximately 800 g of fruit and vegetables are necessary every day for normal bowel functioning (approximately four pieces of fresh fruit and one large salad). About 6 g of bran, a concentrated form of dietary fiber, increases the bulk and softens the stool and can be added to cereals and baked goods. Excessive bran consumption causes bowel irritation and results in flatulence and diarrhea. |
| Bowel training | Help the patient set aside regular and sufficient time for a bowel movement, preferably after a meal (especially breakfast). Encourage the patient to relax as much as possible and not feel rushed. Reading or meditating during time set aside for the bowel movement may promote relaxation. A squatting position, if tolerated, promotes stooling. Have the patient use a footstool so that the thighs can be flexed against the abdomen if possible. The patient can strain gently to promote the bowel movement but should not strain excessively. If there are no results after about 10 minutes, the patient should stop the effort and try again after the following meal or the next morning after breakfast. |
| Other strategies | Hypoxemic patients should always use oxygen when ambulating to the bathroom and during the bowel movement. It is important for the patient to have privacy when moving the bowels. A bedside commode may be beneficial for extremely dyspneic patients. |
| Laxatives | If the above strategies are unsuccessful, it may be necessary to ask the physician about a prescription for laxatives (Table 13-3). If possible, patients should be encouraged to avoid chronic use of laxatives because they interfere with normal bowel motility and reflexes. Despite this, many patients with chronic lung disease require laxatives to promote bowel functioning. |
| Enemas | Fleet enemas (disposable 118 ml enema containing sodium biphosphate and sodium phosphate) can be effective if necessary. Plain warm tap water (irritating), 500 to 1000 ml, or warm physiologic saline solution (nonirritating), 500 to 2000 ml, may also be effective. Enemas are generally not advocated unless all other actions have failed. |

*Continued.*

**Table 13-2**    Nursing care of the patient with constipation—cont'd

| Strategy | Comments |
| --- | --- |
| Fecal impaction | If the fecal mass is not excessively hard, it may be removed by a 60 ml oil retention enema followed by one or more warm saline enemas. If the feces are hard, it may be necessary to dilate the anus manually and remove the fecal particles. |
| Avoid oral use of mineral oil | Oral administration of mineral oil should be avoided because of the risk of aspiration pneumonia and interference with absorption of fat-soluble vitamins in the intestine. |

**Table 13-3**    Laxatives that may be prescribed for the patient with chronic lung disease

| Laxative | Comments |
| --- | --- |
| Bulk-forming mucilaginous colloids (Metamucil, Konsyl) | Generally safe for long-term use; slight danger of asthmatic response in patients sensitive to psyllium seed from which these laxatives made; usually not recommended for children; average adult dose: 1 heaping teaspoon in water or juice twice daily after breakfast and before supper; drink a full glass of water with all bulk-forming laxatives to prevent gastrointestinal obstruction; preparations containing large amounts of sodium should not be used if edema is a problem |
| Stimulant or irritant laxatives | |
| Stool softeners (Colace) | Interfere with sodium resorption in the bowel, causing increased water content of feces; may also have irritant action on wall of bowel; doses range from 50 to 350 mg/day |
| Glycerin suppositories | Lubricate hard feces and stimulate retrocolic reflex; one suppository generally acts within 30 min of rectal insertion |
| Anthraquinone (Senokot) | Extract of senna fruit; counteracts opiate-induced constipation; advocated for adults and children; also combination preparation with stool softener; prepared as syrup, tablet, or granule; see package insert for dosages |
| Contact laxative (Dulcolax) | Promotes peristalsis by acting directly on mucosa of large intestine; prepared as tablet and suppository; see package insert for dosages |
| Osmotic laxatives (Milk of Magnesia) | Most commonly used osmotic laxative; acts by osmotic properties in lumen of bowel; usual doses: 15 to 30 ml at bedtime for adults and *0.5 ml/kg for children* |
| Prunes | Contain dehydroxyphenylisatin; one 150 to 200 ml glass of prune juice or a dish of stewed prunes before breakfast every day promotes normal bowel functioning (recipe for stewed prunes: cook dried prunes with water and black molasses, and add lemon juice to taste; eat four or five stewed prunes every day as needed) |
| *Malt suprex* | *Add to formula for infant less than 1 year of age; prescription dosage according to body weight* |
| *Light Karo syrup* | *Add 1 tablespoon to 8 oz of formula for infants over 1 year of age* |
| *Unprocessed bran* | *Add to cooked food of older children; titrate dosage up to 2 teaspoons per day* |

- Advocate the use of incontinence pads or absorbent disposable panties.
- If the patient has symptoms of urinary tract infection, check with the physician about appropriate medications.
- Check with the physician about the appropriateness of surgery if urinary incontinence is uncontrollable or, for men, use of a condom catheter and leg bag.

Urinary incontinence guidelines are available free of charge from the Agency for Health Care Policy and Research (AHCPR) by writing to: AHCPR Publications Clearinghouse, P.O. Box 8547, Silver Spring, MD 20907 (phone: 800-358-9295).

# RIB AND VERTEBRAL FRACTURES

Rib and vertebral fractures occur most frequently in patients with chronic lung disease who have developed osteoporosis. Osteoporosis or reduced bone density enhances the tendency to fracture. It occurs most often in women approximately 10 years after menopause. It may also occur in younger women with estrogen deficiencies and in older men. Fractures secondary to osteoporosis usually involve vertebrae between T6 and L3.

Rib fractures can be caused by severe coughing and vigorous chest percussion. Rib fractures caused by coughing most often occur between the insertion and origin of respiratory muscles. Vertebral fractures may be caused by bending, lifting objects, or sudden twisting in susceptible patients. These fractures cause severe pain that can limit functional activity more than the lung disease itself.

## Etiology of Osteoporosis

Several factors contribute to the development of osteoporosis.

### Long-Term Corticosteroid Therapy

Patients of all ages who have received oral corticosteroid therapy for several months may develop stress or pathologic fractures of the lateral ribs and the lower thoracic and upper lumbar vertebrae, in particular. These bones have a trabecular or meshwork structure that seems to be adversely affected most frequently by corticosteroids. Corticosteroid therapy causes less calcium to be absorbed in the intestine and more to be secreted by the kidneys. Parathyroid hormone secretion stimulates the activity of osteoclasts (cells that absorb and remove bone), resulting in decreased formation and increased reabsorption of bone. Corticosteroids may also inhibit the action of osteoblasts (cells associated with bone production) (Haynes, 1990).

One recent study documented reduced bone density in patients with asthma who were treated with corticosteroids (Packe, 1992). One group took inhaled beclomethasone dipropionate in usual doses (1000 to 2000 μg daily) for 1 year with occasional courses of systemic corticosteroids; another took high doses of inhaled corticosteroids and low doses of prednisolone each day (7 mg a day on average); and a third group did not require oral or inhaled corticosteroids. Vertebral bone density was reduced in both groups of patients who were treated with corticosteroids, predisposing them to fractures. Another study documented increased bone resorption and inhibited bone formation after 2 and 4 weeks of prednisolone therapy in doses of 20 mg/day in patients with COPD (Morrison, 1992). These studies show that patients receiving inhaled corticosteroids and short courses of systemic corticosteroids may also be at risk for fractures.

### Other Factors

Other factors that may contribute to the development of osteoporosis include:

- Bone loss with aging
- Genetic predisposition (Northern European and Oriental women are at higher risk)
- Menopause or reduced estrogen levels
- Calcium regulation problems or low lifetime dietary calcium
- Immobilization (There is a 0.9% loss of mineral content in the lumbar spine vertebrae each week when young people are on bed rest [Raiz, 1987].)
- Cigarette smoking and high alcohol and caffeine (more than five cups of coffee daily) intake
- High dietary protein and phosphate, which may cause calcium loss

- Excessive vitamin A and D intake, which may stimulate bone resorption
- Metastatic carcinoma

### Assessment
#### Signs and Symptoms of Vertebral Fractures

The signs and symptoms of vertebral fractures include the following:
- Back pain: may be mild to severe
- Loss of height: common with collapse of vertebrae
- Radiographic evidence of fracture

#### Signs and Symptoms of Rib Fractures

The signs and symptoms of rib fractures include the following:
- Pain that is aggravated by coughing, deep breathing, twisting, or turning
- Point tenderness on palpation
- Radiographic evidence of fracture

### Nursing Interventions
#### Prevention of Fractures

It is important to recognize when patients are at risk for osteoporosis and fractures and to take preventive action. No treatment can effectively reverse osteoporosis once it is present, and fractures are painful and heal slowly. The following are recommendations for the prevention of fractures:
- Menopausal women should take estrogen therapy unless there is a history of breast or endometrial cancer or thromboembolic disease.
- Eat a well-balanced diet. Maintain dietary calcium at approximately 1000 to 1500 mg/day.
- Avoid excessive caffeine and alcohol and *stop smoking!*
- Maintain daily exercise programs as tolerated to prevent loss of bone mass.
- Use long-term corticosteroid therapy only if there is no alternative. If oral steroid therapy is necessary, try to maintain the lowest possible daily dosage (prednisone 15 mg/day or less) or alternate day therapy. Use aerosolized steroids with spacer devices as much as possible to reduce the need for systemic preparations.

- Avoid excessively rigorous chest physical therapy. Substitute PEP therapy for patients at high risk for fractures who require chest percussion.
- Maintain a safe environment. Avoid the use of throw rugs. Use handrails, a rubber mat in the tub to prevent slipping, and other measures to prevent accidents.

### Management of Rib and Vertebral Compression Fractures

Rib and vertebral compression fractures generally heal slowly, even with supportive care. Pain control and secretion clearance are the primary management problems in the patient with chronic lung disease.

■ *Pain Control*

■ ANALGESICS. Generally narcotic analgesics are required initially. Narcotics, especially codeine, also relieve coughing. Nonnarcotic preparations may be adequate later when the pain is less intense.

■ TRANSCUTANEOUS STIMULATION. Transcutaneous electrical stimulation may effectively relieve discomfort for some patients by blocking the perception of pain.

■ MOIST HEAT. Local application of moist heat may relieve discomfort, particularly if there is associated muscle spasm.

■ SUPPORT. Back braces or corsets may be prescribed for support when there are vertebral fractures. However, many chronic lung disease patients cannot tolerate braces or corsets because of a sensation of suffocation from pressure on the chest and abdomen. Rib belts for rib fractures should be used only during coughing. They cause pressure on the chest and interfere with deep breathing, predisposing the patient to secretion retention and atelectasis. Patients can often find positions of comfort with adequate armrests and pillows.

■ ENERGY CONSERVATION MEASURES. The convenient organization of necessities for activities of daily living can prevent pain from unnecessary activity. Place necessary items at counter level to avoid bending or reaching. Use a raised toilet seat to reduce the effort of getting on and off the toilet.

■ *Secretion Clearance.* Patients tend to avoid deep breathing and coughing because of pain from rib or vertebral fractures. It is important to maintain bronchial hygiene without causing pain whenever possible.

- Use bronchodilators regularly.
- Observe for signs of respiratory tract infection and start antibiotic therapies early.
- Teach abdominal breathing techniques to facilitate deep breathing.
- Teach controlled coughing with adequate support for painful areas using pillows or a rib belt.
- Use PEP therapy in lieu of chest physical therapy.

### REFERENCES

Chen PH, Chang MH, Shun-Chien H: Gastroesophageal reflux in children with chronic recurrent bronchopulmonary infection, *J Pediatr Gastroenterol Nutr* 13:16, 1991.

Ducolone A et al: Gastroesophageal reflux in patients with asthma and chronic bronchitis, *Am Rev Respir Dis* 135:327, 1987.

Haynes RC Jr: Adrenocorticotropic hormone: adrenocortical steroids and their synthetic analogs—inhibitors of inhibitors of the synthesis and actions of adrenocortical hormones. In Gilman AG et al: *Goodman and Gilman's the pharmacological basis of therapeutics*, ed 8, New York, 1990, Pergamon Press.

Jamieson JR, Hinder RA: Chronic gastritis, *Surg Ann* 23:13, 1991.

Knauer CM, Silverman S: Alimentary tract and liver. In Schroeder SA et al: *Current medical diagnosis and treatment*, Norwalk, Conn, 1992, Appleton & Lange.

Larrain A et al: Medical and surgical treatment of nonallergic asthma associated with gastroesophageal reflux, *Chest* 99:1330, 1991.

Miller TA et al: Stress erosive gastritis, *Curr Probl Surg* 28:453, 1991.

Morrison D et al: Bone turnover during short course prednisolone treatment in patients with chronic obstructive airways disease, *Thorax* 47:418, 1992.

Orenstein S, Orenstein D: Gastroesophageal reflux and respiratory disease in children, *J Pediatr* 112, 1988.

Orenstein SR: Gastroesophageal reflux, *Curr Probl Pediatr* 21:193, 1991.

Orr WC et al: Esophageal function and gastroesophageal reflux during sleep and waking in patients with chronic obstructive pulmonary disease, *Chest* 101:1521, 1992.

Packe GE et al: Bone density in asthmatic patients taking high dose inhaled beclomethasone dipropionate and intermittent systemic corticosteroids, *Thorax* 47:414, 1992.

Raiz LG: Osteoporosis. In Stein JH: *Internal medicine*, Boston, 1987, Little, Brown.

Roth JLA: Gaseousness. In Edward BJ, editor: *Bockus gastoenterology*, ed 4, 1985, WB Saunders.

Scott RB, O'Laughlin EV, Gall DG: Gastroesophageal reflux in patients with cystic fibrosis, *J Pediatr* 106:223, 1985.

Sipponen P et al: Cumulative 10-year risk of symptomatic duodenal and gastric ulcer in patients with or without chronic gastritis, *Scand J Gastroenterol* 25:966, 1990.

Soll AH: Duodenal ulcer and drug therapy. In Sleisenger MH, Fordtran JS, editors: *Gastrointestinal disease*, Philadelphia, 1989, WB Saunders.

Soll AH: Gastritis. In Wyngaarden JB, Smith LH, Bennett JC, editors: *Cecil textbook of medicine*, Philadelphia, 1992, WB Saunders.

Sontag SJ: Gut feelings about asthma, *Chest* 99:1321, 1991 (editorial).

### SUGGESTED READINGS

Agency for Health Care Policy and Research: *Urinary incontinence guidelines*, 1992, The Agency.

Orenstein SR: Gastroesophageal reflux, *Curr Probl Pediatr* 21:193, 1991.

# HOME CARE EQUIPMENT

## GUIDELINES FOR THE SELECTION OF AN EQUIPMENT VENDOR

A decision to implement a treatment requiring home respiratory equipment or oxygen is often made as a result of information obtained during home visits. When this happens, it is usually the home care nurse who selects the vendor and initiates the equipment referral. Home care staff must be familiar with each of the vendors in the community so that referrals are made only to reputable, reliable vendors who are committed to high-quality patient care and service.

Careful selection of vendors is especially important for home oxygen therapy because of the vendor's frequent contact with patients and because of the ramifications if oxygen equipment is poorly maintained and malfunctions. Patients may also occasionally encounter a vendor who attempts to substitute a less expensive system in order to maximize profits. In some communities tank oxygen is supplied by welding companies who may have little understanding of the needs of a chronically ill, homebound patient.

The accreditation process for vendors of medical equipment, administered by the Joint Commission on Accreditation of Healthcare Organizations (JCAHO), will help to ensure minimum levels of safety and reliability of vendors. Legal precedents exist that could hold a home care agency responsible for referring a patient to an unreputable vendor. Thus use of JCAHO-accredited vendors may also provide the agency some legal protection.

The following guidelines suggest criteria for the selection of a respiratory equipment vendor:

1. Provides a full line of oxygen and other respiratory equipment so that choices are based on patient need rather than equipment availability
2. Maintains equipment properly; is able to check the accuracy of equipment using liter meters for flow rates, oxygen analyzers for $F_{IO_2}$, etc.
3. Has a nurse or respiratory therapist on staff to instruct patients in the use of equipment, periodically assess patient compliance and

response, and report untoward changes to the physician; ideally, has an oximeter with which oxygen saturation can be checked

4. Employs delivery personnel who are honest, reliable, courteous, and caring
5. Has a consistent, reliable schedule for routine deliveries
6. Credits the patient for unused oxygen when tanks are refilled
7. Provides 24-hour emergency service
8. Accepts third-party coverage for oxygen and submits insurance claims for the patient; may ask for payment of the patient's portion of the bill, but does not demand full reimbursement on delivery; within reason, does not charge extra for stairs, mileage, or odd-hour deliveries
9. Provides for purchase as well as rental of equipment for non-Medicare patients; if equipment is purchased, provides both a warranty and an affordable servicing policy
10. Has a system of regular review to identify patients whose costs or usage are unusually high or low, and to reevaluate the appropriateness of the equipment being used

# CHAPTER 14

# RESPIRATORY THERAPY DEVICES

KATHRYN A. KANDAL

Patients with chronic lung disease are treated with many types of respiratory therapy devices. Much of the equipment developed to administer respiratory care in the hospital setting has been adapted for use in the home. A description of the various devices, indications, contraindications or side effects, and techniques for use and care are presented in this chapter.

## AEROSOL DELIVERY DEVICES
### Principles of Aerosol Therapy

Aerosol therapy involves the administration of medication and bland solutions such as saline solution or water to the respiratory tract. A variety of factors, described in the following sections, govern the effectiveness of aerosol delivery.

### Particle Size

The size of the particles produced for aerosolization are measured by their mass median aerodynamic diameter (MMAD). Aerosol devices should deliver particles less than 5 $\mu$m for therapeutic effectiveness. The depth to which the aerosol is inhaled depends primarily on the MMAD as described in the following:

| MMAD | Deposition |
|------|-----------|
| Greater than 5 $\mu$m | Oropharynx |
| 2 to 5 $\mu$m | Airways |
| 0.8 to 3 $\mu$m | Lung parenchyma |
| Less than 0.8 $\mu$m | Not deposited, exhaled |

### Diameter of Airways

Less aerosol is delivered to the lower respiratory tract if the airways are narrow or obstructed by secretions. This is a particular problem in *children because they have small airways* and in adults who have obstructive lung disease.

### Pattern of Inhalation

Particles are generally delivered more effectively if they are inhaled slowly at an inspiratory flow rate of approximately 0.5 L/sec with a large breath (approximately to inspiratory capacity). A breath hold of 10 seconds at the end of the inspiration facilitates deposition of the aerosol particles in the respiratory tree (Dolovich, 1991).

### Types of Devices
#### Metered Dose Inhalers

Metered dose inhalers (MDIs) are pressurized canisters of medication with freon propellants (chlorofluorocarbons [CFC]) that generate an aerosol bolus of medication for inhalation (Fig. 14-1). They come with a mouthpiece that fits into the nipple of the canister. The mouthpiece has a cap that protects it when it is not being used. MDIs are activated by hand, requiring coordination of the activation with inspiration. A device is available that permits hand activation by patients with arthritis (VentEase, Glaxo). Approximately 80% of the aerosol from an MDI is deposited on the mu-

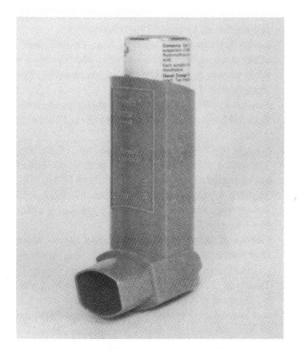

**Fig. 14-1** Metered dose inhaler. (From Kacmarek RM, Hess D: *Respir Care* 36:952, 1991.)

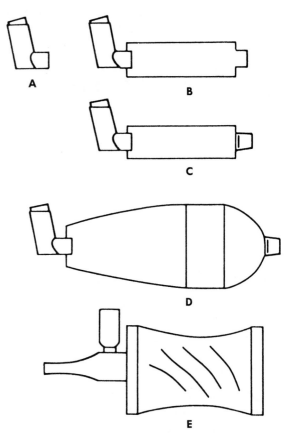

**Fig. 14-2** Schematics of metered dose inhaler spacer systems: **A,** actuator alone; **B,** open-end straight tube; **C,** aerochamber; **D,** Nebuhaler; and **E,** InspirEase. (From Kim CS, Eldridge MA, Sackner MA: *Am Rev Respir Dis* 135:157, 1987.)

cous membranes of the oropharynx and the stomach, 5% to 10% is exhaled, 5% to 10% is deposited in the device itself, and only 9% to 11% reaches the lower respiratory tract (Kacmarek, 1991).

MDIs may also be used with auxiliary spacer devices or holding chambers that eliminate the need for coordinated activation and reduce deposition of the aerosol particles on the mucous membranes of the oropharynx (Fig. 14-2). The spacer is a chamber that attaches to the nipple of the MDI. When the MDI is actuated, the aerosol is suspended within the spacer, allowing the patient to inhale out of sequence with the activation. The spacer also facilitates evaporation of the aerosol particles as they move through the chamber, thus decreasing the size of the particles. This reduces deposition on the oropharynx and facilitates deeper penetra-

tion in the airways. Spacers are manufactured in several shapes, from tubes to pear-shaped cones to collapsible bags, and are available from pharmacies with a prescription.

### Dry-Powder Inhalers

Dry-powder inhalers (DPIs) are breath-activated devices that contain powdered preparations of medications for inhalation. They do not contain CFCs, and because they are activated by inhaling, they may be easier to operate and more effective for

**Rotahaler**

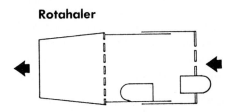

**Fig. 14-3** One commmercially available single-dose dry powder inhaler. (From Newman SP: *Respir Care* 36:939, 1991.)

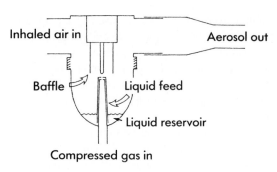

**Fig. 14-4** Design of typical small-volume jet nebulizer. (From Newman SP: *Respir Care* 36:939, 1991.)

patients with poor MDI technique. (Kacmarek, 1992). A single-dose dry-powder inhaler (Rotahaler) is available in the United States for albuterol and beclomethasone dipropionate (Fig. 14-3). A multidose device (Turbuhaler) is available in Europe for terbutaline sulfate.

### Nebulizers

Nebulizers are handheld devices attached to electrical or battery-operated air compressors or cylinders of compressed air or oxygen that generate pressure for continuous aerosolization of medication for inhalation. Nebulizers are used with masks or mouthpieces. There are two types of nebulizers: jet nebulizers and ultrasonic nebulizers.

■ *Jet Nebulizers.* Jet nebulizers are available in small- and large-volume sizes (Fig. 14-4). They operate on the Bernoulli principle in which compressed gas (from an electric compressor, air, or oxygen cylinder) passes through a constriction called a Venturi, creating an area of low pressure that draws a solution up a small tube. The airstream causes the solution to be fragmented into droplets. Small-volume nebulizers are used for the delivery of aerosolized medications. In contrast to the MDI, approximately 66% of the aerosol generated by a small-volume nebulizer is deposited on the baffles of the nebulizer itself, 8% to 12% reaches the lower

respiratory tract, and about 20% is exhaled. Only about 2% of the particles are absorbed in the mucosa of the mouth or stomach (Kacmarek, 1991).

■ *Ultrasonic Nebulizers.* Ultrasonic nebulizers transform alternating current (AC) into ultrasonic sound waves. The transmission of the waves to a piezoelectric ceramic disk or quartz crystal causes the solution to aerosolize. The size of the aerosol droplets is related to the ultrasonic frequency. These nebulizers function most effectively with water and tend to have a larger droplet size than jet nebulizers (Newman, 1991). Between 3 and 6 ml of solution is aerosolized per minute. Ultrasonic nebulizers are generally used to deliver bland aerosols, although some designed to deliver medication are now available.

## Indications for Use
### Aerosolized Medications

Aerosol therapy facilitates the delivery of medication directly to the respiratory tract. Therefore much less medication is absorbed systemically compared with parenteral or oral administration, significantly reducing side effects. Inhaled bronchodilators are first-line therapy for patients with obstructive disease (see Chapter 6). Aerosolized corticosteroids and mast cell inhibitors (cromolyn sodium) are first-line therapy for most patients with asthma. Aerosol devices are used less commonly to deliver medication for treatment and prophylaxis for parenchymal diseases such as *Pneumocystis carinii* pneumonia. In certain situations they are used to deliver aerosolized mucolytics (Aitken, 1992) and antibiotics to treat cystic fibrosis (Hodson, 1988).

The advantages of the various types of devices are summarized in Table 14-1. The MDI with or without the spacer is the best way to deliver aerosolized medication (American Association for Respiratory Care Consensus Conference, 1991). Patients who are unable to activate the MDI, who cannot take deep breaths, or who require high doses of medication that are not convenient to deliver with the MDI or not available in MDI form may benefit from nebulizer therapy.

### Bland Aerosols

Bland aerosols, such as normal saline solution and sterile water, can be generated by large-volume jet nebulizers or ultrasonic nebulizers. Large-volume jet nebulizers that are powered by air compressors can be used to humidify airways of patients with tracheostomy tubes and may prevent crusting and obstruction from secretions (see Chapter 16). Ultrasonic nebulizers are also used to induce sputum for diagnostic purposes.

## Disadvantages and Side Effects of Aerosol Therapy
### Aerosolized Medications

The disadvantages of the various devices are also summarized in Table 14-1. A high percentage of the aerosol is deposited on the walls of all current devices, thus reducing the efficiency of delivery. A significant amount of medication is also lost during exhalation. Some nebulizers are equipped with a finger-control attachment that allows the mist of medication to be released only when the opening is occluded. This facilitates aerosolization only during inhalation, conserving medication that would be wasted during exhalation. It also increases the time needed to inhale all the medication.

### Bland Aerosols

The side effects of bland aerosol therapy include bronchospasm from hypotonicity of nebulized water, infection from contaminated aerosol solutions or equipment, airway obstruction from swelling or retained secretions, and *systemic fluid overload. The last is a particular problem in infants.*

## Use and Care of Aerosol Delivery Devices
### Metered Dose Inhaler

The proper technique for use of the MDI is summarized in Table 14-2. The only maintenance the MDI requires is for the plastic mouthpiece to be washed with soap and water every few days to prevent the orifice from becoming occluded. Sometimes it is difficult for the patient to tell when the canister is empty and needs replacement. This is easily done by placing it in a bowl of water. If it sinks it is full, and if it floats on the top of the water it is empty (Fig. 14-5).

Patients should be advised to check their MDIs carefully before inhaling from them to ensure that the cap has been removed from the mouthpiece and that no foreign objects are lodged in the mouthpiece. There are reports of people who have inhaled the MDI cap (Li, 1991) and a coin and a capsule from an MDI (Schultz, 1991).

Canisters should be warmed to near body temperature if they are used in cold environments. Particle size is larger at lower temperatures (0° to 21° C, 32° to 69.8° F), thus inhibiting effective inhalation (Wilson, 1991).

### Metered Dose Inhaler with Spacer

The spacer is attached to the nipple of the MDI (Fig. 14-2). The patient activates the MDI one time. The aerosol particles enter the spacer where they are suspended; the patient then inhales from the mouthpiece of the spacer. Generally, no special technique is required for use of the MDI with a spacer; however, the MDI must be shaken before activation. Two reservoir bag spacer devices, the InspirEase and the Reservoir Aerosol Delivery Sys-

**Table 14-1**   Advantages and disadvantages of aerosol delivery devices

| Device | Advantages | Disadvantages |
|---|---|---|
| Metered dose inhaler (MDI) | Small, easily carried in pocket; easily cleaned; provides rapid, reliable dose with activation of device; cost effective; may be used "in-line" with ventilators | Requires good hand coordination and synchronization with inspiration; requires 4- to 10-sec breath hold for deposition of particles after inhalation; *difficult for child of less than 10 years of age;* considerable (60% to 80%) deposition of particles on oropharynx, depending on technique, thus increasing risk of side effects of medication; requires chlorofluorocarbon (CFC) propellants |
| MDI with spacer | May produce better deposition of aerosol than MDI without spacer; useful when patient cannot coordinate actuation of MDI with inspiration; *may be effective for children between 3 and 10 years of age; mask attachment is available with some spacers for children under 3 years of age;* reduced oropharyngeal deposition of aerosol, reducing side effects | Bulky; more complicated to clean; added expense |
| Nebulizer | Allows for longer, slower treatments; can be used for medications unavailable in MDI; easier device for poorly coordinated patients; easier for weak and debilitated patients; may be used with tracheostomy collar for patients with tracheostomy tubes and to deliver "in-line" medications for ventilator-dependent patients; cumulative dose larger than MDI | Unsuitable for "pocket" use; expensive; more complicated cleaning; increased risk of contamination; low lung deposition when breathing is shallow; waste of medication during exhalation unless a finger control attachment is used |
| Dry-powder inhaler (DPI) | Easy administration; does not require CFC propellants | Requires higher inspiratory flow rate than MDI or nebulizer, thus may be ineffective for patients who are too ill or too weak to generate adequate inspiratory pressure; many drugs unavailable in DPI; difficult to deliver high doses of medication; may have heavy oropharyngeal deposition causing irritation and cough; powder may clump in high humidity; single-dose DPI cannot be tipped after capsule is loaded |

**Table 14-2**  Optimal use of metered dose inhaler

| Technique | Rationale |
|---|---|
| Shake canister. | Shaking mixes active medication into diluent. |
| Position inhaler upside down and about 1 inch in front of open mouth. (If patient finds this too difficult, position inhaler between teeth, preferably keeping lips open.) | Activation in front of mouth causes peripheral medication to be deposited outside mouth where it is not absorbed, rather than on oral mucosa where it can be absorbed or swallowed. This also allows particles to evaporate as they move toward the pharynx, thereby decreasing particle size and facilitating deeper penetration. |
| Begin a slow deep breath coordinated with one activation of MDI. (Alternatively, one can activate MDI, followed immediatley by slow, deep breath.) | Activation during early inhalation allows medication to flow smoothly into airways with breath. When activation is late or early, medication is deposited primarily in oropharynx. Slow inhalation reduces particle velocity and impaction on upper airway walls, facilitating deposition in smaller airways. |
| Hold breath for up to 10 sec or as long as possible. | Breath holding allows suspended medication to settle on airways, thus enhancing deposition. |
| Exhale slowly using pursed lip breathing technique. | Slow pursed lip breathing reduces expiratory airflow, minimizing small airway collapse and facilitating full exhalation. |
| Wait 3 to 5 min, then repeat inhalation with second puff. Subsequent puffs may be taken as necessary (up to 20* puffs of β-agonist in 10- to 20-min period (American Association for Respiratory Care Consensus Conference, 1991). | Waiting period allows bronchodilation from first puff so that subsequent puffs penetrate deeper into airways, facilitating increased bronchodilation. |
| Rinse mouth with water or mouthwash. | Rinsing minimizes side effects from oropharyngeal deposition. |
| Cough. | Coughing mobilizes secretions. |

*This amount is controversial. The usual dose is 4 puffs for adults.

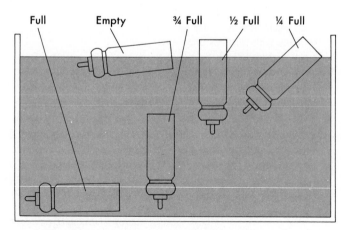

**Fig. 14-5**  How to tell whether a "spray inhaler" is full or empty.

tem, are fitted with a flow indicator whistle that makes a sound when the inspiratory flow rate exceeds 0.3 L/sec. This encourages the patient to breathe in at a rate that reduces air turbulence and promotes more effective inhalation of the aerosol. Patients should inhale slowly enough so that the whistle does not make a sound. Some medications (e.g., Azmacort) come with a built-in spacer. Spacer devices should be washed regularly in warm soapy water (if not contraindicated by manufacturer's instructions) or replaced periodically according to manufacturer's recommendations.

### Dry-Powder Inhaler

■ *Single-Dose Dispenser.* The patient should be instructed to assemble the single-dose DPI and the medication capsule according to the manufacturer's instructions, exhale to the end of a normal breath, close lips around the mouthpiece, and breathe in rapidly (more than 60 L/min) (Kacmarek, 1991). This process should be repeated until the medication capsule is empty. It is not necessary to hold the breath after each inhalation. The mouth should be rinsed after use, particularly if the medication is a corticosteroid. DPIs are cleaned by disassembling the parts, washing them in warm, soapy water, and allowing them to air dry. They should be completely dry before use because any moisture causes the powder to clump.

■ *Multidose Dispenser.* Multidose dispensers are prefilled with multiple doses of medication and do not require assembly with medication capsules. They are disposable and are discarded when empty.

### Patient Instructions for Home Nebulizer Treatments

■ *Preparation of Medication.* Medications for nebulization are generally available in two forms. Some medications are premixed with physiologic saline solution in individual dose packets or ampules, whereas others are prepared in multidose vials. Multidose vials are less expensive. If multidose vials of medication are used, the patient must be taught to measure the prescribed dose and mix it with the appropriate amount of diluent. Most undiluted bronchodilators come in 10 and 30 ml vials with a dropper. The dropper may be graduated with usual dosages. However, patients usually find it easier to count the drops than to measure the volume of solution on the dropper. The measurement of the medication must be accurate within one drop of the prescribed amount. If patients are unable to use the dropper, a tuberculin syringe can be marked with tape or a marking pen at the appropriate volume. If the patient is visually impaired or otherwise unable to measure the dose accurately, a supply of premixed syringes can be prepared by the nurse and stored in the refrigerator. Eventually someone else will need to assume the responsibility for this task or the patient will need to switch to ampules.

If the patient's hands shake, the nebulizer cup can be placed inside a container that is taped to the counter or table, leaving both of the patient's hands free to measure the medication. One hand can then be used to steady the other.

■ *Diluent.* Whenever aerosolized medications are delivered via nebulizer, it is important to discuss with the physician or pharmacist what type of diluent should be used. Normal saline solution is the recommended diluent for nebulized bronchodilators. Distilled water and tap water are irritating and may be contaminated with microorganisms. However, some medications such as pentamidine must be diluted with distilled water because of the physical properties of the medication. Sterile solutions are preferred, but clean solutions may be acceptable if they are prepared and stored in a way that prevents bacterial growth.

Sterile saline solution and water are available in 5 and 10 ml unit dose vials. These are the easiest and safest diluents for patients to use but are relatively expensive. They are available in boxes of 250 from pharmacies and some home care vendors. Some brands have tops that allow patients to use one vial for two treatments. Homemade solutions are cheaper and relatively easy to prepare. If the homemade solutions are stored properly, they are a safe substitute for the sterile unit dose vials. A formula for normal saline is to add 9 g or 1½ teaspoons of salt to 1 L of distilled water. Unsterile distilled water is inexpensive and can be purchased from grocery and drug stores. Water and saline solution can be sterilized in the following way:

1. Boil a small, clean jar and the lid in water for 10 minutes.
2. Remove the jar and the lid from the boiling water with tongs and place on a clean surface to cool. Alternatively, pour the water out, using the lid of the pan to prevent the jar from falling out, and allow the jar and lid to cool until they can be removed from the pan without touching the inside of the cap or jar.
3. Pour saline solution or distilled water into the jar, place the lid on the jar without tightening it, and place the jar and solution back in the pan of water. The water level should reach the middle of the jar.
4. Bring the water to a boil. Let the water cool, and remove the jar of solution from the pan.
5. Secure the lid tightly and store the jar of solution in the refrigerator. If any is left over after 2 days, it should be boiled again before it is used. The patient should be instructed never to pour any solution back into the jar if too much has been poured out or if solution is left over.

As a general rule, tap water should not be used in aerosol treatments because it may contain minerals, bacteria, and molds. However, some patients will take treatments only if the preparation is made as simple as possible. The use of tap water as a diluent may significantly increase compliance for such individuals. When patients live in unhygienic circumstances, fresh tap water is preferable to saline solution or distilled water that is not prepared or stored properly. The water purification systems of most urban communities keep bacterial counts to a harmless level, and if the mesh filter is removed from the faucet, the major source of potential bacterial contamination will be eliminated.

■ *Taking the Nebulizer Treatment.* The following describes the correct steps for taking a nebulizer treatment:

1. Select a comfortable area in the home where the unit can be placed and the treatment can be taken without interruption.
2. Plug the compressor in the electrical outlet (some have adaptors so that they can be plugged into automobile cigarette lighters). A two-prong plug adaptor will be necessary if the outlet is not grounded (lacks three prongs).
3. Use the machine as often as ordered by the physician. Treatments should be timed to precede meals or chest physical therapy. It may also be helpful to schedule treatments approximately 45 minutes before activities that require exertion.
4. Sit upright in a relaxed and comfortable position for treatments.
5. Assemble the nebulizer parts.
6. Fill the nebulizer cup with the prescribed amount of medication solution. Do not overfill.
7. Attach the tubing to the nebulizer and to the air compressor.
8. Turn on the machine and observe it for mist. Close lips around the mouthpiece. Take care not to occlude the mouthpiece with teeth or tongue. Take a slow, deep breath through the mouth, hold the breath for a few seconds, and then exhale slowly through pursed lips or through the mouthpiece if the unit has an exhalation valve.
9. Continue inhaling the mist from the nebulizer until the medication in the nebulizer cup is gone, usually 10 to 20 minutes. If dizziness, light-headedness, or excessive fatigue occurs, turn the nebulizer off and rest until the sensation has subsided. The treatment can then be resumed.
10. Turn the machine off when the treatment is completed. Use the controlled cough technique to raise any secretions loosened during the treatment.
11. Separate the nebulizer parts, rinse them in warm water, and let them air dry, covered with a clean towel, until it is time to assemble them for the next treatment.

The nebulizer can be set up and filled with medication at bedtime if the patient awakens at night feeling short of breath and needs a treatment in a hurry.

■ *Maintenance of the Nebulizer and Compressor.* The compressor filters should be changed regularly according to the manufacturer's recommendations. The outside of the compressor should be wiped periodically with a moist cloth to keep it clean.

Bacteria grow well in warm, dark, moist environments. Therefore it is essential that all nebulizers be disinfected regularly to prevent respiratory tract infections from contaminated equipment. Chemical disinfectants that are mixed with water are available from home care equipment vendors. White vinegar and water can also be used as a disinfectant solution. The vinegar solution is made by mixing one part white distilled vinegar and two parts tap water. This solution is generally discarded after each use.

The nebulizer parts should be cleaned three times each week (or every other day). A protocol for cleaning of the nebulizer is as follows:

1. Disassemble the nebulizer parts and wash them thoroughly with warm water and liquid detergent. It is not necessary to clean the tubing unless it is soiled.
2. Rinse the parts in warm tap water.
3. Cover the nebulizer parts completely with disinfectant solution. Soak the parts as directed by the manufacturer for commercial solutions and for 30 minutes if vinegar is used.
4. Rinse thoroughly with tap water, shake off excess moisture, and air dry on a clean towel. If the tubing is cleaned, dry the inside by attaching it to the compressor so that air can blow through it. Store in a clean, dry place until needed. Equipment should not be placed in plastic bags for storage until completely dry.

A simpler method—washing the nebulizer parts in warm soapy water, then rinsing in clear water three times each week—may suffice in place of the soak in disinfectant solution (Dettenmeier, 1985). As long as the parts are kept clean and *dry* when not in use, bacteria are unlikely to grow.

### Bland Aerosol Treatment

Patient instructions for a bland aerosol treatment with a large-volume jet nebulizer are as follows:

1. Fill nebulizer cup with approximately 500 ml of sterile (or home-sterilized) distilled water. Prefilled nebulizer cups are available and significantly reduce the risk of infection.
2. Attach large-bore tubing and aerosol mask.
3. Turn on unit. Place mask on face or tracheostomy opening.
4. Breathe mist through open mouth or tracheostomy tube for 15 to 20 minutes.
5. Cough or perform chest physical therapy if indicated.
6. Notify physician if chest tightness, increased coughing, or wheezing occurs.

Disposable masks, large-bore tubing, and prefilled nebulizers are usually provided and replaced by the home care equipment company. However, if necessary, the tracheostomy mask or face mask may be washed with warm soapy water, rinsed, and allowed to air dry. Large-bore tubing should be washed in warm soapy water, rinsed, twirled to remove excess moisture, and hung to dry.

### Aerosol Pentamidine

Pentamidine is effectively delivered to the lung parenchyma via aerosol in concentrations 10 to 100 times higher than with intravenous dosage (Matthys, 1991). Because it has a half-life of 1 month, it can be administered monthly with a standard dosage of 300 mg in 6 ml of distilled water. Aerosolized pentamidine must be inhaled with a mouthpiece because the nose acts as an effective filter. If a mask must be used, the patient should wear a noseclip.

Standard compressors and nebulizers are not used for aerosol pentamidine. An air compressor with a 50 lb per square inch (psi) capacity is required with a nebulizer (e.g., ISO-NEB, Hudson Respiratory Care, Inc., Temecula, Calif., and Res-

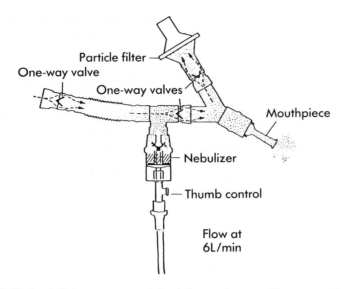

**Fig. 14-6**   Baffled nebulizing system used for delivery of pentamidine aerosol in Respirgard II nebulizing system. One-way valves reduce number of large particles delivered to patient. Thumb control is not standard, but its use would allow driving gas to bypass nebulizer if not occluded during cough or rest periods, thus obviating discharge of aerosol into atmosphere at such times. (From Fallat RF, Kandal K: *Respir Care* 36:1008, 1991.)

pirgard II, Marquest Medical Products, Inc., Englewood, Colo.) designed to maximize the output of particles in the 0.5 to 1.5 μm range (Fig. 14-6). The nebulizer also is equipped with baffles to deflect large particles that increase airway irritation. One-way valves and a submicron filter on the expiratory side of the nebulizer prevent pentamidine from being exhaled into the atmosphere, where others can be exposed.

■ *Taking a Pentamidine Treatment.* The following describes the correct steps for taking a pentamidine treatment:

1. Assemble the nebulizer circuit, 10 ml syringe, needle, sterile water, and pentamidine.
2. Prepare pentamidine solution by injecting 6 ml sterile water into the pentamidine vial and allowing the powder to dissolve.
3. Place pentamidine solution into nebulizer cup. Attach tubing to compressor outlet.

4. Turn on compressor and adjust pressure so that manometer reads 23 to 25 psi.
5. Place mouthpiece between teeth and close lips around mouthpiece. Breathe in and out of mouth without removing mouthpiece from mouth. Breathe with a slow, deep-breathing pattern. Every five breaths, exhale completely and breathe in slowly to inspiratory capacity to deliver the aerosol to the apices of the lungs.
6. Continue breathing pattern until all the medication has been used.
7. Discard the pentamidine nebulizer after the treatment is completed. Pentamidine nebulizers cannot be reused because the medication occludes the small-bore openings.

■ *Side Effects of Aerosol Pentamidine.* Systemic side effects have not been reported in patients receiving aerosol pentamidine (Matthys, 1991).

Side effects caused by the aerosol include the following:

- Coughing and bronchospasm
- Increased salivation
- Bad taste
- Throat irritation
- Fatigue

Coughing and bronchospasm are the most common side effects and may be relieved by pretreatment with an aerosolized bronchodilator administered by an MDI or nebulizer. The same nebulizer *cannot* be used for pretreatment with a bronchodilator and the pentamidine.

### Special Aerosol Delivery Techniques for Children

■ *Metered Dose Inhaler. Use a spacer for all children between 3 to 10 years of age. Use a spacer with mask for children under 3 years of age.*

■ *Nebulizer. Nebulizers may be used for children less than 10 years of age. Generally, a pediatric aerosol mask is used, but if the child objects to the mask, simply directing the mist close to the* child's mouth and nose will deliver an adequate dose of medication.

## ENVIRONMENTAL AIR SYSTEMS

Several types of equipment are available to purify, filter, and humidify the ambient environment in the home. A brief description of the various devices and their potential benefits and limitations are presented in Table 14-3.

## HUMIDIFIERS

Commercially available room humidifiers and vaporizers do not significantly increase the relative humidity of the environment. If they are used, however, the water should be changed daily and the water reservoir washed with soap and water before refilling. Heated room humidifiers are not recommended because of the potential for burns.

Ultrasonic nebulizers are not effective in increasing the relative humidity of a room because they do not disperse water vapor. Rather, they disperse particulate water that settles on room surfaces.

**Table 14-3**   Environmental air systems

| Type of device | Potential benefits | Limitations |
| --- | --- | --- |
| Air purifiers (screen collects large particles; ionizing wires and plates attract smaller particles by magnetism) | Remove high percentage of dust, smoke, pollen, bacteria, and mold spores from air | Must be meticulously maintained to prevent sparking or arcing, which produces irritating ozone; must be capable of three to seven changes of air per hour in area to be filtered; relatively expensive and may not be covered by insurance |
| Ionizers | Electrical devices that generate negative ions to which positively charged particles are attracted; heavier particles settle on room surfaces | Probably not beneficial |
| Air conditioners | Provide comfort for patients in hot climates | Reservoirs for bacteria and molds; require meticulous cleaning; drastic changes in temperature may induce bronchospasm |

## INCENTIVE SPIROMETRY

Incentive spirometers are devices that encourage deep-breathing exercises through maximal sustained inspiration. Examples include the Tri-Flo and the Voldyne.

### Indications

Incentive spirometers may be used to improve ventilation and prevent or reverse atelectasis. They may be useful for obese patients who are prone to atelectasis, patients recovering from chest injury or surgery, and weak or debilitated patients who are recovering from pneumonia. They are commonly prescribed in the hospital to improve ventilation after surgery or extubation. Some patients enjoy using these devices and would not otherwise practice deep-breathing exercises.

### Disadvantages and Side Effects

There are no contraindications to incentive spirometers; however, they should not replace pursed lip breathing exercises for patients with COPD. They are not necessary for patients who are motivated and able to take deep breaths on their own.

### Use and Care

The patient should be made aware of what he or she is trying to achieve with the incentive spirometer. Goals can be established for use of the device, such as periodically increasing the volume of inspired air by 200 ml. Patient instructions for proper use of incentive spirometers are the following:
1. Exhale normal tidal breath.
2. Place mouthpiece in mouth.
3. Inhale at a slow rate as long as possible, using lateral costal muscles to expand the chest.
4. Take mouthpiece out of mouth and exhale normally.
5. Pause for several seconds.
6. Repeat slow, deep breaths 5 to 10 times every 2 to 4 hours.
7. Cough after treatment period to clear any secretions that may be present.

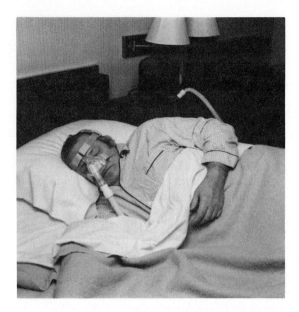

**Fig. 14-7**  Nasal continuous positive airway pressure device. (REMstar Choice, courtesy Respironics, Inc.)

## NASAL CONTINUOUS POSITIVE AIRWAY PRESSURE

Nasal continuous positive airway pressure (CPAP) is the application of positive pressure to the airways to hold them open and to prevent pharyngeal collapse. It is administered by a mask that is placed over the nose and held in place with a set of head straps (Fig. 14-7). The mask is connected by a large-bore tube to an airflow generator. A prescribed amount of resistance is incorporated into the circuit, resulting in continuous positive pressure against which the patient exhales. The devices are equipped with a dial to set the amount of resistance from 2 to 20 cm $H_2O$ pressure.

Nasal CPAP masks have one or more small openings to prevent rebreathing exhaled carbon dioxide. Some units use an adaptor between the mask and the tubing that serves this purpose (Whisper Valve, Respironics). Some units feature a 20- to 30-minute period over which the resistance gradually increases to a preset value. Nasal pillows and customized masks are available for difficult-to-fit faces. *Masks and pillows are available in pediatric sizes, as are nasal CPAP prongs, which may be appropriate for small infants.*

## Indications

Nasal CPAP is prescribed as a noninvasive therapy for obstructive sleep apnea (Riley, 1990) in lieu of maxillofacial surgery. The effectiveness of the therapy is determined by cessation of apneic episodes and maintenance of oxygen saturation within normal limits or above 85%. Nasal CPAP can dramatically improve sleep patterns and alleviate daytime somnolence. Long-term benefits include the prevention of complications of chronic hypoxemia and improved activity tolerance and quality of life. If nasal CPAP alone does not fully correct nocturnal oxygen desaturation, supplemental oxygen may be added to the circuit.

## Disadvantages and Side Effects

Side effects of therapy with nasal CPAP include the following:
- Claustrophobia
- Skin irritation under the mask; eye irritation if air leaks around the mask
- Dryness of the nasopharyngeal mucosa
- Pain and symptoms of sinus or inner ear infection

## Use and Care
### Use of the Device

Nasal CPAP should always be initiated in a monitored setting where continuous electrocardiography and oximetry can be performed. This also helps the patient understand how to use the therapy and reassures him or her that the proper prescription has been made. Many factors influence patients' compliance with and acceptance of nasal CPAP therapy (Nino-Murcia, 1989). Several actions may help promote patients' acceptance of the therapy and prevent problems:
- Educate the patient about sleep apnea and the potential benefits of therapy.
- Give the patient step-by-step instructions in

how to use and care for the device. It is important to leave written instructions with the patient. The patient should also have the telephone number of someone to call at any time if there are problems.
- Reassure the patient that he or she can still breathe through the mouth because it is not covered by the mask.
- Mark the straps with an indelible marking pen for the proper fitting.
- Patients may leave the mask in place and detach the tubing if they need to get up during the night.
- Refer patients to the local chapter of AWAKE, a sleep apnea support group (see Chapter 12).

### Care of the Device

The flow generator has an inlet dust filter that must be replaced or washed, depending on the brand. The mask is made of silicon to reduce the possibility of allergic contact dermatitis. Silicon cannot be cleaned with alcohol; therefore the mask should be washed every day with soap and water and dried thoroughly before wearing. The patient should also wash his or her face before putting on the mask. The tubing and valves also need to be washed regularly with soap and water. The nasal pillows, mask, and tubing should be washed with mild liquid detergent, rinsed, and disinfected for 20 minutes in a solution of 3 parts distilled water and 2 parts white vinegar once each week. All parts should be rinsed thoroughly after the vinegar soak and allowed to air dry.

## BILEVEL POSITIVE AIRWAY PRESSURE

Bilevel positive airway pressure (BIPAP) is a therapy similar to nasal CPAP with additional features that allow a higher pressure to be applied during inspiration than expiration, a backup respiratory rate, and a set inspiratory and expiratory ratio. There are dials to set the inspiratory positive airway pressure (IPAP) and expiratory positive airway pressure (EPAP), the respiratory rate, and the percentage of inspiratory time for each breath. When all these features are in place, the unit functions as a time-cycled, pressure-limited ventilator. A low-pressure alarm and external battery are available with some units.

## Indications

BIPAP is indicated for adult and pediatric patients who require high levels of CPAP (more than 10 cm $H_2O$) to eliminate sleep apneic episodes and associated hypoxemia, because they are more comfortable exhaling against a lower pressure. BIPAP is also indicated for patients who have extended periods of apnea and require additional respiratory support. It is reported to be safe and effective for patients with chronic respiratory failure from restrictive lung disease (Strumpf, 1990). In addition, it is shown to reduce $CO_2$ retention in patients who hypoventilate from obesity hypoventilation syndrome, restrictive problems of the chest wall, and neuromuscular disease (Waldhorn, 1992).

The BIPAP unit is portable, quiet, and less expensive and complicated than most of the portable volume ventilators used in the home, although more expensive than CPAP. The use of CPAP and BIPAP as alternatives to traditional volume ventilators is discussed in Chapter 16.

## Disadvantages and Side Effects

Nocturnal positive-pressure ventilation with a nasal mask using BIPAP does not appear to benefit patients with COPD and is poorly tolerated by them (Strumpf, 1991). Other side effects are the same as for nasal CPAP.

## Use and Care

The use and care of BIPAP devices are the same as for CPAP.

## POSITIVE EXPIRATORY PRESSURE

The positive expiratory pressure (PEP) unit consists of a cushioned seal mask or mouthpiece, a T-tube, an expiratory resistor, and one-way valves to direct the flow of air (Fig. 14-8). The patient breathes in and out through the mouthpiece (with or without a noseclip) or mask. The exhaled air is directed by a one-way valve through a resistor that has four settings. Each setting represents a different degree of resistance dictated by the size of the orifice through which the exhaled air flows. A manometer is used during training sessions to measure the amount of positive pressure applied to the airways during exhalation. The settings on the resistor are adjusted to enable the patient to maintain an expiratory pressure on the manometer between 10 and 20 cm $H_2O$.

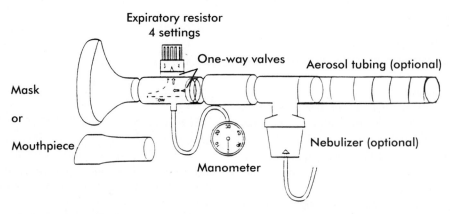

**Fig. 14-8** Positive expiratory pressure device. (Resistex, courtesy DC Lung Co, Inc, Sepastopol, Calif.)

The slight positive expiratory pressure keeps the airways from collapsing and facilitates airflow from obstructed airways, thereby enhancing the clearance of secretions. A nebulizer can be attached to the inspiratory side of the PEP unit so that bronchodilators can be delivered with inhalation.

## Indications

PEP therapy is used primarily as an alternative to traditional chest physical therapy. When combined with forced exhalation techniques in cystic fibrosis, it appears to be as effective as postural drainage with forced exhalation techniques for clearing secretions (Mortensen, 1991). It is more effective than diaphragmatic breathing techniques with forced expirations and cough in patients with chronic bronchitis (Christensen, 1990). It can be carried out anywhere, takes less time than conventional chest physiotherapy, and does not require the assistance of another person. Chest physical therapy is discussed in Chapter 7.

PEP therapy may also benefit patients who require lung expansion to prevent or treat atelectasis.

## Disadvantages and Side Effects

Increased air trapping may occur if expiratory time is too short. Some patients complain of fatigue because of resistance to exhalation, but this is usually resolved by keeping below 20 cm $H_2O$. PEP therapy should not be used during acute hemoptysis or if the patient has an acute pneumothorax. PEP therapy may aggravate sinusitis, ear infections, or epistaxis (Mahmeister, 1991).

## Use and Care

To take PEP treatments the patient is instructed to practice the following steps:
1. Place the mask on face or use mouthpiece (and noseclip if desired).
2. After a normal exhalation, take in a deep breath.
3. Hold the breath for 3 seconds.
4. Exhale actively but without excessive force, replicating the sensations experienced in the training session. Exhalation should take at least twice as long as inhalation. Do not induce coughing or wheezing.
5. Repeat the last three steps 10 to 15 times.
6. Huff four or five times to clear any secretions that have collected (see Chapter 7).
7. Repeat entire sequence 3 to 6 times.
8. The entire treatment should continue until the chest feels clear of secretions, usually about 20 minutes and should be taken bid or tid.

The mask or mouthpiece should be washed with soap and water and air dried daily. If a nebulizer is attached to the PEP unit for administration of bronchodilators during PEP therapy, the cleaning procedures recommended on p. 239 should be followed. PEP valves deteriorate after 1 to 2 months, depending on use, and the devices must be replaced.

## REFERENCES

Aitken ML et al: Recombinant human DNase inhalation in normal subjects and patients with cystic fibrosis: a phase I study, *JAMA* 8:1947, 1992.

American Association for Respiratory Care Consensus Conference: Aerosol consensus statement, *Chest* 100:1106, 1991.

Christensen EF, Nedergaard T, Dahl R: Long term treatment of chronic bronchitis with positive expiratory pressure mask and chest physiotherapy, *Chest* 97:645, 1990.

Dettenmeir P, Vogt-Yanta M, Shanahan E: Comparison of home nebulizer cleaning/disinfecting techniques reported to decrease bacterial growth, *Am Rev Respir Dis* 131:A166, 1985 (abstract).

Dolovich M: Clinical aspects of aerosol physics, *Respir Care* 36:931, 1991.

Hodson ME: Antibiotic treatment aerosol therapy, *Chest* 94(suppl 2):156S, 1988.

Kacmarek RM: Humidity and aerosol therapy. In Pierson DJ, Kacmarek RM: *Foundations of respiratory care*, New York, 1992, Churchill Livingstone.

Kacmarek RM, Hess D: The interface between patient and aerosol generator, *Respir Care* 36:952, 1991.

Li JTC: Inhalation of the cap of a metered-dose inhaler, *N Engl J Med* 325:431, 1991 (letter).

Mahlmeister MJ et al: Positive-expiratory-pressure mask therapy: theoretical and practical considerations and a review of the literature, *Respir Care* 36:1218, 1991.

Matthys H, Herceg R: Dosing strategies for aerosol delivery to the lung parenchyma with specific recommendations for pentamidine, *Respir Care* 36:989, 1991.

Mortensen J et al: The effects of postural drainage and positive expiratory pressure physiotherapy on tracheobronchial clearance in cystic fibrosis, *Chest* 100:1350, 1991.

Newman SP: Aerosol generators and delivery systems, *Respir Care* 36:939, 1991.

Nino-Murcia G et al: Compliance and side effects in sleep apnea patients treated with nasal continuous positive airway pressure, *West J Med* 2:165, 1989.

Riley RW, Nelson BP, Guilleminault C: Maxillofacial surgery and nasal CPAP: a comparison of treatment for obstructive sleep apnea syndrome, *Chest* 98:1421, 1990.

Schultz CH, Hargarten SW, Babbit J: Inhalation of a coin and a capsule from metered-dose inhalers, *N Engl J Med* 325:431, 1991 (letter).

Strumpf D et al: An evaluation of the Respironics BIPAP bi-level CPAP device for delivery of assisted ventilation, *Respir Care* 35:415, 1990.

Strumpf DA et al: Nocturnal positive-pressure ventilation via nasal mask in patients with severe chronic obstructive pulmonary disease, *Am Rev Respir Dis* 144:1234, 1991.

Waldhorn RE: Nocturnal nasal intermittent positive pressure ventilation with bi-level positive airway pressure (BiPAP) in respiratory failure, *Chest* 101:516, 1992.

Wilson AF, Mukai DS, Jahangir JA: Effect of canister temperature on performance of metered-dose inhalers, *Am Rev Respir Dis* 143:1034, 1991.

## SUGGESTED READINGS

Kacmarek R, Mack CW, Dimas S: *The essentials of respiratory care*, ed 3, St Louis, 1990, Mosby.

McPherson SP, Spearman CB: *Respiratory therapy equipment*, St Louis, 1990, Mosby.

Pierson DJ, Kacmarek RM: *Foundations of repiratory care*, New York, 1992, Churchill Livingstone.

Proceedings of American Association for Respiratory Care Consensus Conference on Aerosol Delivery, *Respir Care* 36, 1991.

# CHAPTER 15

# HOME OXYGEN THERAPY

GWENDOLYN J. McDONALD

Two major studies conclusively established the benefits of long-term oxygen therapy (LTOT) and specific criteria for its use in patients with chronic obstructive pulmonary disease (COPD) (Nocturnal Oxygen Therapy Trial Group, 1980; Medical Research Council Working Party, 1981). Long-term oxygen is highly beneficial for patients with chronic hypoxemia and is prescribed for significant numbers of home care patients. The indications for LTOT, the use and care of oxygen delivery systems in the home, and the problems associated with oxygen therapy are discussed in this chapter. Medicare reimbursement guidelines are not addressed in detail because they change so often. The home care nurse must be familiar with these regulations, however, because they are a key factor in the selection of an oxygen delivery system.

## BENEFITS OF HOME OXYGEN USE

The benefits of home oxygen are many and include the following:
- Marked improvement in long-term survival in COPD (Nocturnal Oxygen Therapy Trial Group, 1980; Medical Research Council Working Party, 1981)
- Reversal or reduction in severity of cor pulmonale and right ventricular failure
- Reduced red blood cell mass and hematocrit
- Marked improvement in cognitive function, memory, concentration, and judgment (which enhances learning and the retention of new skills)

- Marked improvement in motor coordination and reaction time
- Reduced severity and frequency of nocturnal desaturations and arrhythmias
- Improved sleep quality because of reduced frequency of arousals and increased rapid eye movement (REM) and total sleep time
- Possible improvement in school and work attendance in patients with cystic fibrosis (Zinman, 1989)
- *Faster weight gain in infants with bronchopulmonary dysplasia (Groothuis, 1987)*
- Reduced meal-related dyspnea in some adults (Castaldo, 1983); possible improvement in appetite and digestive function
- Improvement in exercise capacity and endurance, mostly in patients who desaturate with exercise (Marcus, 1992)
- Reduced dyspnea in some patients
- Reduced number of hospital days for some patients
- Some improvement in emotional functioning (Heaton, 1983; Grant, 1982)
- Improved quality of life for many

## INDICATIONS FOR LONG-TERM OXYGEN THERAPY
### Arterial Hypoxemia

The fundamental indication for LTOT is arterial hypoxemia. Arterial hypoxemia is defined as an abnormally low oxygen tension ($PaO_2$) in the arterial blood. This is distinct from hypoxia, which

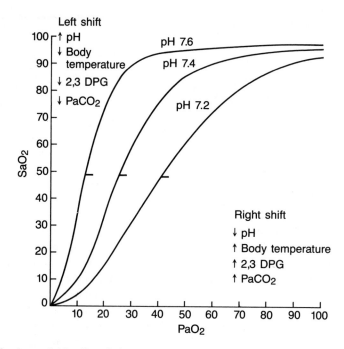

**Fig. 15-1** Oxyhemoglobin dissociation curve. (From Weilitz PB: *Pocket guide to respiratory care,* St Louis, 1991, Mosby.)

is inadequate tissue oxygenation. Small amounts of oxygen are dissolved in the blood, but most oxygen is attached to hemoglobin molecules as oxyhemoglobin. Dissolved oxygen exerts a pressure in arterial blood, which is expressed as $PaO_2$. $SaO_2$ refers to the relative degree to which the hemoglobin molecules are saturated with oxygen and is expressed as a percentage. For example, an $SaO_2$ of 90% means that the hemoglobin molecules contain 90% of the maximum amount of oxygen they are capable of containing. A normal $SaO_2$ exceeds 90% and in most healthy individuals is above 96%.

$PaO_2$ and $SaO_2$ are closely related, as is demonstrated by the oxyhemoglobin dissociation curve (Fig. 15-1). $PaO_2$ is the driving pressure that helps oxygen attach to the hemoglobin molecule. At a high $PaO_2$, hemoglobin is well saturated, and assuming a normal amount of hemoglobin is present, the oxygen content of the blood is high. However, as the $PaO_2$ drops below about 60 mm Hg, oxygen

saturation, and therefore oxygen content, drops precipitously.

$PaO_2$ and $SaO_2$ are affected by age and altitude. Children or young adults living at sea level have a normal $PaO_2$ of close to 100 mm Hg. However, the normal $PaO_2$ of older adults (70 to 80 years of age) is about 80 mm Hg and that of a young adult living at a 5000-foot elevation (as in Denver) is about 75 mm Hg.

Arterial hypoxemia exists when $PaO_2$ is below the normal, age-adjusted range of 80 to 100 mm Hg at sea level. In adults, mild hypoxemia ($PaO_2$ of 65 to 80 mm Hg, or $SaO_2$ of 93% to 95%) suggests pulmonary dysfunction but is not harmful and does not require long-term oxygen therapy because tissue oxygen levels are not compromised. In this range the patient is still well on the flat part of the $O_2$ dissociation curve, at which $PaO_2$ is high enough to saturate hemoglobin adequately. As $PaO_2$ drops below 55 to 60 mm Hg, $O_2$ saturation drops precipitously, the oxygen-carrying ability of the blood is dramatically reduced, and acute and chronic pathophysiologic changes resulting from tissue hypoxia begin to occur. Oxygen therapy is indicated when patients reach this steep part of the curve and are in danger of tissue hypoxia.

### Effects of Hypoxemia

The goal of long-term oxygen therapy is the reversal of severe hypoxemia. In turn, this prevents or reverses the many pathophysiologic changes that occur as a result of hypoxemia and that affect neuropsychologic functioning, exercise capacity, cardiopulmonary hemodynamics, and the function of other major organ systems.

Signs and symptoms of hypoxemia and problems associated with it vary depending on the severity and duration and on current metabolic demand. Metabolic demand increases with exercise, infection, fever, or basic activities such as eating or straining at bowel movements. Short-term effects include difficulty concentrating, generalized fatigue, muscle weakness, and digestive disturbance. *Infants demonstrate poor feeding*. Myocardial hypoxia increases the incidence of cardiac arrhythmias, particularly premature atrial and ventricular contractions.

The patient's exercise capacity is often markedly impaired, especially in those whose hypoxemia worsens with exercise. Patients may complain of fatigue, dyspnea, and muscle weakness with exercise and are at increased risk for arrhythmias. Dyspnea alone is an unreliable indicator of severe hypoxemia because it is often present in people without hypoxemia and may or may not be present in those who are hypoxemic. Similarly, cyanosis is a late and therefore unreliable indicator (see Chapter 2).

Nocturnal hypoxemia triggers arousals that disturb sleep quality and increase the incidence of cardiac arrhythmias. Hypoxia-related sleep disturbances are discussed in Chapter 12. Profound although often subtle changes in cognitive function, motor coordination, and mood are seen in chronically hypoxemic patients. Symptoms of depres-

sion, anxiety, and hypochondriasis are also prevalent and may be partly related to hypoxemia (Grant, 1982; Heaton, 1983).

Chronic hypoxemia profoundly changes the individual's cardiopulmonary hemodynamics, resulting in pulmonary hypertension, erythrocytosis, and ultimately cor pulmonale and right ventricular failure. Heart failure typically develops earlier in the patient who fits the chronic bronchitic "blue bloater" subtype of COPD. Cardiopulmonary effects are discussed in Chapter 10.

### Laboratory Criteria for Home Oxygen Use

LTOT is indicated for anyone who has documented hypoxemia or evidence of hypoxic organ dysfunction (such as cor pulmonale or erythrocytosis) after optimization of medical therapy and the resolution of an exacerbation (Fulmer, 1984). Oxygen may be prescribed for continuous use, with exercise, nocturnally, or with infant feedings, depending on the severity of the hypoxemia and the circumstances under which it occurs.

Specific criteria for home oxygen therapy are presented in Table 15-1. Arterial blood gas (ABG) measurements or oxygen saturation levels obtained by oximetry can be used to document oxygen need. ABG measurements are preferable (Second Conference, 1988) because they are more accurate and provide information on $PaCO_2$ and pH. Oximetry is less invasive; however, several factors affect the accuracy of oximetry, including the following:

- Smoking (increases carboxyhemoglobin levels and gives a falsely high $SaO_2$)
- Jaundice (gives an artificially low value)
- Impaired peripheral circulation
- Saturations below 70%
- Colored nail polish or acrylic nails

### Safety of Home Oxygen Use in the Patient with Hypercapnia

Patients with severe chronic hypercapnia are occasionally, although inappropriately, denied LTOT because a physician fears oxygen therapy may "turn off" the patient's ventilatory drive. Chronic

**Table 15-1**   Medical criteria for home oxygen use for adults

| Arterial oxygenation* | Conditions of use |
|---|---|
| $Pao_2$ less than 55 mm Hg or $Sao_2$ less than 88% | Continuous |
| $Pao_2$ 56-59 mm Hg or $Sao_2$ 89%-90% with evidence of cor pulmonale: Erythrocytosis with hematocrit of more than 56% Dependent edema caused by right ventricular failure "P" pulmonale on electrocardiograph Right ventricular hypertrophy on x-ray examination | Preferably continuous, but at least with sleep and exercise |
| $Pao_2$ less than 55 mm Hg or $Sao_2$ less than 88% with exercise, providing oxygenation or exercise capacity improves with oxygen use | With exercise |
| $Pao_2$ less than 55 mm Hg or $Sao_2$ less than 88% during sleep, or a drop of 10 mm Hg from waking levels, associated with symptoms of hypoxemia, provided oxygenation improves with oxygen use | Nocturnally and with sleep |

*All values obtained with the patient on room air and in a period of respiratory stability following optimization of therapy.

hypercapnia further blunts the responsiveness of $CO_2$ receptors in the medulla. This causes patients to rely primarily on $O_2$ receptors for stimulation of breathing. If $Pao_2$ is subsequently increased excessively as a result of oxygen therapy, the $O_2$ receptors sense that oxygenation is adequate and reduce the respiratory drive. Respiratory effort becomes less, hypercapnia and respiratory acidosis may worsen, and the patient may become difficult to rouse. However, low-flow oxygen can be safely administered as long as blood gases are carefully evaluated when oxygen therapy is initiated and the patient is well instructed in its use. Thus the presence of chronic hypercapnia, even when severe ($Paco_2$ 80 mm Hg or more), is *not* a contraindication to the use of home oxygen (Fulmer, 1984).

## Diagnostic Indications for Home Oxygen Use

Continuous oxygen therapy is often prescribed for hypoxemic patients with COPD or pulmonary fibrosis. Those with sleep-disordered breathing may or may not benefit from nocturnal oxygen (see Chapter 12). Medicare will not pay for oxygen prescribed for dyspnea, angina, peripheral vascular disease, or terminal illness, without evidence of hypoxemia.

*Children with bronchopulmonary dysplasia often are discharged with orders for home oxygen therapy, but most eventually develop sufficient healthy new alveoli to maintain their $Pao_2$ without supplemental oxygen. In contrast, once hypoxemia has developed in the child (or adult) with cystic fibrosis, oxygen therapy is usually required for the remainder of the patient's life. Less commonly occurring pediatric conditions for which oxygen therapy may be required include interstitial lung diseases, arteriovenous malformations in the lungs, and hypoplastic lung diseases (e.g., those resulting from a diaphragmatic hernia or oligohydramnios). Ventilator-dependent children with a variety of congenital abnormalities or lung diseases may also require oxygen therapy.*

The presence of cor pulmonale suggests the need for continuous oxygen therapy even when the daytime $Pao_2$ exceeds 55 mm Hg or 88% $Sao_2$. *Children whose daytime saturation level drops below 90% are typically started on oxygen therapy, at* least nocturnally, even in the absence of cor pulmonale. This early initiation of oxygen therapy is believed to delay the symptoms of cor pulmonale or attenuate their severity.

## Reevaluation of the Need for Home Oxygen Use

Many patients who meet blood gas criteria for home oxygen use following treatment for a respiratory exacerbation no longer require it after a 3- to 4-week convalescence. Indeed, gradual improvement in blood gases may continue for up to 3 months (Levi-Valensi, 1986). Thus it is reasonable to wait several weeks before deciding about the need for home oxygen use. However, if the $PaO_2$ is less than 50 mm Hg or if symptoms of cor pulmonale are present, the patient is usually discharged from the hospital with orders for home oxygen therapy.

All adults started on LTOT should be reevaluated in a month, again at 6 and 12 months, and annually thereafter to confirm the continuing need for oxygen therapy and the adequacy of the oxygen dose (Fulmer, 1984). There is no need to tell patients they will need oxygen therapy "permanently," unless hypoxemia has persisted for at least 3 months.

*The oxygen therapy needs of children are reevaluated as needed because their oxygen requirements change with both lung growth and the disease process. For example, the child with bronchopulmonary dysplasia is usually reassessed every 2 months while receiving LTOT, and the child with moderate to severe cystic fibrosis has his or her $SaO_2$ checked at each clinic visit depending on severity and course of the disease.*

## OXYGEN PRESCRIPTION

Oxygen is considered to be a medication and therefore requires a prescription. The dosage must be specified in liters per minute, and specific conditions of use (e.g., "continuously" or "with exercise") must be defined. Thus a typical prescription might read, "Oxygen continuously at 1 L/min, increasing to 2 L/min with sleep and exercise." For Medicare patients the prescription must also state the date the patient was last seen, the respiratory diagnosis, $PaO_2$ or $SaO_2$, and the conditions under which these values were obtained (e.g., "on room air at rest").

The goal of oxygen therapy is to maintain the $PaO_2$ between 65 and 80 mm Hg (American Thoracic Society, 1987). The prescribed flow rate should be the lowest that will achieve this goal without significantly increasing the $PaCO_2$ or reducing the pH. No additional benefit is realized by increasing $PaO_2$ above 70 to 80 mm Hg.

For most adults with COPD, flow rates between 1 and 3 L/min are sufficient. The flow rate is usually increased by 1 L/min with exercise and sleep to compensate for further desaturation that occurs under these conditions (American Thoracic Society, 1987).

Patients with restrictive lung diseases or lung cancer often require much higher flow rates (i.e., more than 5 L/min). *In contrast, small children may reach their target oxygen saturation level with only 0.25 or 0.5 L/min because their tidal volume is so much smaller. Flow rates may need to be increased during infant feedings or sleep. During weaning from oxygen, the infant will often still need to use oxygen with sleep, naps, or feedings.*

## CLARIFYING THE RELATIONSHIP BETWEEN FLOW RATE AND FRACTION OF INSPIRED OXYGEN

Ambient air is 21% oxygen. This is expressed as a fraction of inspired oxygen ($FIO_2$) of 0.21. The $FIO_2$ of inhaled air increases with increasing flow rates of supplemental oxygen (e.g., ranging from 24% to 50% with flow rates up to 6 L/min). However, the actual $FIO_2$ a patient receives depends on additional factors such as inspiratory flow rate and minute ventilation* (i.e., it cannot be predicted by flow rate alone). For example, when the inspiratory flow rate is fast or minute ventilation large, a greater volume of room air is inhaled along with the supplemental oxygen. This dilutes the oxygen, causing the $FIO_2$ of inspired air to be lower. Con-

---

*Minute ventilation = respiratory rate × tidal volume.

versely, when the inspiratory flow rate or minute ventilation is low (such as with *tiny infants* or those who take slow, shallow breaths), supplemental oxygen comprises a larger proportion of the inhaled volume and the inspired $FIO_2$ is higher (Fan, 1983). A higher $FIO_2$ usually increases the $PaO_2$, and vice versa. Thus $PaO_2$, $SaO_2$, or both need to be sampled when the breathing pattern or minute ventilation changes significantly.

## DESCRIPTION OF OXYGEN SYSTEMS
### Compressed Oxygen

Steel or aluminum cylinders containing 100% oxygen were the first devices available for delivery of LTOT. By compressing oxygen under very high pressures (1800 to 2400 psi at 70° F), a large volume can be stored in a small space. There are three types of tanks: a K tank holds 7070 liters, an H tank 6900 liters, and an E cylinder 655 liters (Fig. 15-2).

A regulator is required to convert high tank pressures to a level that can be safely and comfortably tolerated by the patient. Regulators operate in two stages, reducing tank pressure first to 400 psi, then to 50 psi. The E cylinder regulator is not interchangeable with those fitting the larger tanks.

### Liquid Oxygen Systems

Liquid oxygen is the system of choice for most ambulatory patients. Each system has two components: a reservoir and a smaller portable container that transfills from the reservoir (Fig. 15-3). Reservoir capacities range from 13,000 to 33,000 gaseous liters, while portable containers hold from 500 to 1000 L. A reservoir typically lasts 3 to 5 days, depending on the size, flow rate, environmental temperature, and frequency with which the portable unit is transfilled.

Liquid oxygen is prepared by supercooling 100% oxygen to $-297°$ F, thus changing the large volume of gaseous oxygen to a much smaller volume of liquid. The reservoir itself is simply a large "thermos bottle" designed to keep the liquid oxygen cold as long as possible. When the outlet valve is opened, the liquid oxygen moves through a series

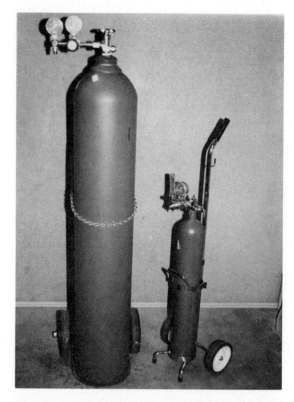

**Fig. 15-2** Compressed oxygen. H tank on left is secured by a chain to the stand; E cylinder on right is secured in wheeled cart.

of coils that absorb heat from the ambient air, gradually rewarming and vaporizing the oxygen. Flow rate capabilities typically range from 0.5 to 6 L/min. Some systems use a Thorpe tube to regulate the flow rate, whereas others use flow control knobs. The flow rate on the portable unit is regulated by a dial or buttons.

### Oxygen Concentrators and Enrichers

Oxygen concentrators are electrically powered devices that use filters or molecular sieves to separate oxygen from carbon dioxide, nitrogen, and water molecules in the ambient air (Fig. 15-4). Enrichers are similar devices with some important differences. Instead of a molecular sieve, enrichers

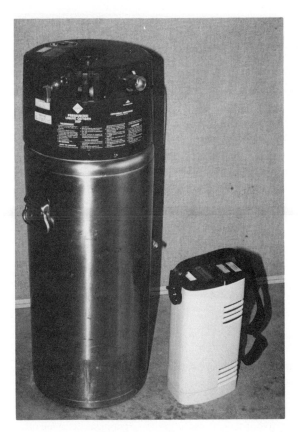

**Fig. 15-3** Liquid oxygen. Consists of reservoir containing enough oxygen for several days, depending on flow rate, and portable unit that transfills from reservoir.

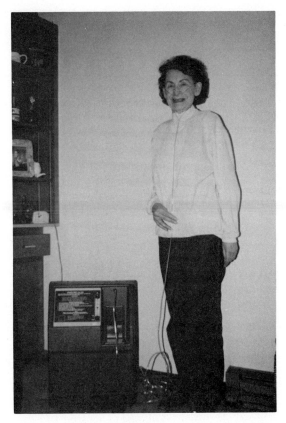

**Fig. 15-4** Oxygen concentrator. Newer models are smaller, quieter, and more efficient.

use a plastic membrane that filters out nitrogen and carbon dioxide but leaves water vapor. The newer models incorporate a heater and humidifier unit, which further humidifies the oxygen and may prevent mucosal drying. Because concentrators and enrichers make their own oxygen, the patient and vendor are freed from routine oxygen deliveries.

## CRITERIA FOR SELECTION OF THE OXYGEN SYSTEM

The choice of system is based on the oxygen dosage, mobility, safety, cost, reimbursement constraints, and preference of the patient or caregiver. Ease of use, noise, comfort, weight, and appearance of the system also are considered. Primary indications, advantages, and disadvantages of the various oxygen delivery systems are summarized in Table 15-2.

## Indications for Tank Oxygen

Tanks can be stored indefinitely without losing oxygen; thus they are an ideal backup system for the oxygen concentrator because they are needed only during a power outage. They may be the most economic system when patients require very low flow rates or use oxygen only intermittently. They are useful in outlying areas where frequent deliveries are impractical or in communities where liquid oxygen is unavailable or electric power unreliable.

**Table 15-2**   Considerations in selecting an oxygen delivery system

| | Compressed gas system (tanks) | Liquid oxygen system | Concentrator |
|---|---|---|---|
| Primary indication | Intermittent, infrequent use; homebound patients using 0.75 L/min or less continuously | Ambulatory patient; homebound patient using >5 L/min (used in combination with a concentrator) | Homebound patient using 0.75-5 L/min continuously<br>Enricher only: the "recalcitrant" smoker |
| Advantages | Can be stored indefinitely, without leakage; small aluminum tanks are light enough for portability | Portability; ideal for travel because vendors available for refills in most cities | Generally less expensive than liquid oxygen; requires no routine delivery, therefore ideal in isolated areas of country; attractive appearance<br>Enricher only: minimal fire hazard because of low $FIO_2$; high humidity output, which may help keep secretions loose |
| Disadvantages | Heavy, unattractive; arm strength needed to change regulator; expensive for continuous use; awkward to transport E tanks even with wheeled cart; small capacity of portable aluminum tanks | Considerable oxygen wastage due to venting; manual dexterity required for filling; expensive if patient uses >2 L/min continuously | Not portable; drop in $FIO_2$ at higher flow rates, therefore flow must be increased to compensate; generally not appropriate for rates above 4-5 L/min; noisy; electrically powered, therefore add to electric bill and are vulnerable to power outages; generates heat (advantage in winter, disadvantage in summer); requires start-up time of approximately ½ hr |
| Special features | Several tanks can be connected to increase time between deliveries | Portables transfilled from reservoir | Some small and light enough to lift into a car; some operate off automobile cigarette lighter or, with adaptor, off auto generator; newer models have built-in alarms to warn of drops in $O_2$ output |

**Table 15-2** Considerations in selecting an oxygen delivery system—cont'd

| | Compressed gas system (tanks) | Liquid oxygen system | Concentrator |
|---|---|---|---|
| Precautions | Must be stored in stand or secured to wall | Cannot be stored on side; increased venting in hot environment; potential for skin injury from "freezer burn" | Requires backup H tank in case of power outage; regular cleaning of filters needed; require servicing after every 2000 hr of use |

E tanks are used for portability in conjunction with a large tank or oxygen concentrator. They must be secured in a wheeled cart or in a frame attached to the back of a wheelchair. Despite the wheeled cart, they are heavy (more than 15 lb, empty) and awkward to move around. They are unsuitable for the ambulatory oxygen-dependent person *or for a parent who must manage other young children in addition to an oxygen-dependent baby.*

Small aluminum cylinders such as the D cylinder or the Mada (Mada Medical Products, Inc., Carlstadt, N.J.) are lighter (7½ to 11 lb) and therefore more portable than the unwieldy E tank. Most can be carried fairly comfortably in a shoulder bag. However, their capacities are relatively small. For example, the Mada holds just 190 L, enough for 1½ hours at a flow rate of 2 L/min. Some can be transfilled directly from an H or K tank, but this practice is generally discouraged because of the risks associated with transfilling from a high-pressure system.

## Indications for Liquid Oxygen Systems

Liquid oxygen is expensive. However, the portability of a liquid system is so superior that it remains the system of choice for any patient who is ambulatory and not homebound. Liquid oxygen offers no advantage for the patient who is homebound or reluctant use the portable component of the system. An additional monthly rental fee is charged for the portable unit, so if the unit is not being used, it is prudent to determine whether another system would be more appropriate.

## Indications for Concentrators or Enrichers

Many concentrators and enrichers are small enough to be transported by car, and some can be operated in a car, thus facilitating travel. However, they are not designed for portability, and an E cylinder or some other portable system (often not covered by insurance) must be provided for use outside the home. This basic lack of portability discourages activities outside the home and may prevent some patients from reaching rehabilitation goals. Thus concentrators are best suited for the homebound patient who needs portable oxygen infrequently and only for short periods.

Because routine oxygen deliveries are not needed, concentrators and enrichers are ideal for patients living in remote areas or in buildings for which access is difficult. However, the residential power supply must be reliable.

Concentrators are most efficient at low flow rates, when output is 93% to 97% pure oxygen. However, as the flow rate increases, efficiency drops; at liter flows above 4 L/min, output is only 75% to 90% oxygen. Because of the reduced efficiency at higher flow rates, concentrators are not recommended for patients requiring flow rates above 5 L/min.

The enricher's output is only 40% oxygen, but this remains constant regardless of flow rate. To compensate for the lower oxygen output, the actual flow rate is increased by a factor of three. Thus, if the flow rate is set at 2 L/min, the device actually delivers 6 L/min. This is well tolerated at low flow rates (1 to 2 L/min); in fact, some patients prefer the feel of the higher airflow and complain of "air hunger" if they are transferred to a lower flow system. However, at higher prescribed flow rates, the compensatory increase in the enricher flow rate is poorly tolerated.

*Because enrichers deliver humidified oxygen, they are used most often for infants or children needing high humidity.* Another advantage of the enricher is its relative safety in situations in which a fire hazard exists (e.g., an oxygen-dependent patient who is unable or unwilling to give up smoking). A cannula with an $F_{IO_2}$ of only 40% will not ignite even if exposed directly to a flame (West, 1983).

## Cost Considerations Influencing Choice of System

In an ideal world, patients are provided the oxygen system that best meets their needs for improved oxygenation and mobility. However, in the real world of health care reimbursement, the issue of cost versus benefit is inevitably raised and compromises are often made. The home care nurse is in a unique position to evaluate the relative merits of each type of oxygen system and to select the system (or combination of systems) that most effectively and economically meets a particular patient's needs.

Oxygen costs vary with geographic area and individual vendors and may include hidden expenses (e.g., for increased use of electricity). Reimbursement for oxygen is even more variable, ranging from none to 100% of "allowable" costs. It is important to differentiate between oxygen costs and oxygen reimbursement because the patient must often make up the difference between the two.

A low monthly cost is the major advantage of the concentrator. With other systems, cost increases according to the volume of oxygen used. However, because concentrators concentrate ambient oxygen, the only costs are the flat monthly rental fee and the cost of electricity to power the unit.

A formula to calculate the predicted monthly cost of tank or liquid reservoir systems when billing is based on actual monthly oxygen use rather than a flat fee is presented in Fig. 15-5. The economic "break-even" point of a liquid system versus a concentrator occurs at a continuous flow rate of approximately 2 L/min. Below this a concentrator is usually more expensive, especially if an E cylinder is also needed for portability.

Home oxygen therapy for Medicare patients is now reimbursed at a flat monthly rate based on liter flow. This has resulted in strong vendor reliance on oxygen concentrators, especially for the homebound patient. Most vendors are willing to provide liquid oxygen, alone or in combination with a concentrator, for ambulatory patients and for patients who have trouble maintaining an adequate oxygen saturation on a concentrator alone.

At flow rates above 5 L/min, cost can often be reduced and comfort increased by using a combination of a concentrator and a liquid system. A Y connector delivers oxygen to the patient from both systems simultaneously. Cost may also be reduced if a patient uses the more economical concentrator while at home and a portable liquid system while away from home.

A formula to calculate the projected monthly utility cost for electrically powered oxygen equipment is presented in Fig. 15-6 and must be con-

$$\text{\# L/min} \times 60 \text{ min/hr} \times \text{\# hr/day} \times 30 \text{ days/mo} = \text{\# L/mo}$$

$$\frac{\text{\# L/mo}}{\text{Reservoir capacity}} = \text{\# Reservoirs/mo}$$

$$(\text{\# Reservoirs/mo} \times \text{Cost/reservoir}) + \text{Basic monthly equipment rental fee} = \text{Predicted cost/mo}$$

**Fig. 15-5**   Calculating predicted monthly oxygen costs.

$$\frac{\text{Power consumption} \times \text{Hours/day}}{\text{of equipment (watts)}^* \qquad \text{use}} = \text{Kwts/day} \times \begin{array}{c}\text{local cost}^\dagger \\ \text{per Kwt Hr}\end{array} \times 30 \text{ days/mo} = \begin{array}{c}\text{Monthly cost to operate} \\ \text{equipment}\end{array}$$

Example: Given that Linde $O_2$ concentrator uses 400 watts, and current electric rate in Seattle is 4 cents/Kwt Hr, approximate cost to operate the concentrator is:

$$\frac{400 \times 24}{1000} = 9.6 \text{ Kwts/day} \times 0.04 \times 30 = \$11.52/\text{mo}$$

*Refer to manufacturer's brochure.
†Check with local power company.

**Fig. 15-6**   Calculating projected monthly increase in electric bill resulting from medical equipment operation.

sidered when calculating cost savings. In regions where electric power is expensive, this medical expense can be substantial and is not reimbursed by Medicare or other third-party payors. Many power companies offer discounts to people who require electricity for life support systems. The home care nurse should know whether this service is available and may need to help the patient apply.

## USE AND CARE OF OXYGEN EQUIPMENT
### Use and Care of Tank Oxygen
#### Changing Tanks

The procedure for changing oxygen tanks is as follows (Fig. 15-7):

- Remove the regulator from the empty tank using a large wrench (which should always be kept with the cylinder currently in use).
- Fit the regulator carefully on the full tank and tighten securely.
- Crack the main valve by turning it counterclockwise. This releases the oxygen into the regulator assembly. Do not stand directly in front of the tank when opening the valve (a sudden release of pressure from a defective regulator could blow the glass face off a gauge).
- Set the flow rate.

When patients lack the strength, manual dexterity, or cognitive ability to change regulators, several tanks can be connected together in sequence. Multiple tanks will last much longer, and tank changes can be performed by delivery personnel during regularly scheduled deliveries. The tank at the end of the sequence should always be used first so new tanks can be added easily. Once the tank in use is empty, the control valve is always turned off *before* the next tank in the sequence is turned on. Otherwise pressure equalizes between the two connected tanks and the patient is left with two half-filled tanks.

It is preferable to close the main valve when oxygen is not in use and "bleed" the regulator until the flow rate indicator drops to "0." This reduces wear on the regulator. However, it adds another potentially complicated step in the operation of the system. Thus, it is an optional practice and is often omitted for frail, elderly patients.

#### Reading the Flow Rate

A flow meter regulates the flow of oxygen from the tank (Fig. 15-8). For home use, flow meters calibrated from 1 to 5 or 1 to 7 L/min are preferable to those calibrated from 1 to 15 L/min. Settings

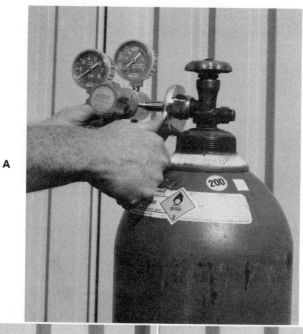

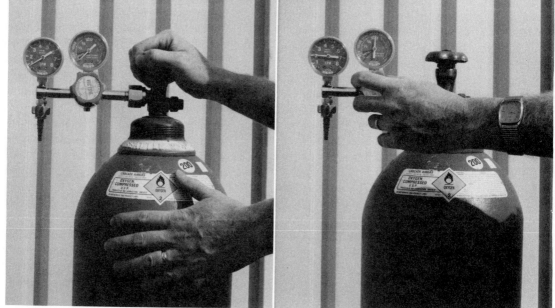

**Fig. 15-7**    Procedure for changing compressed oxygen cylinders. **A,** Regulator assembly is removed from empty tank. **B,** After regulator is tightened securely onto new tank, main valve is opened or "cracked" by turning regulator knob counterclockwise. **C,** Flow rate is set.

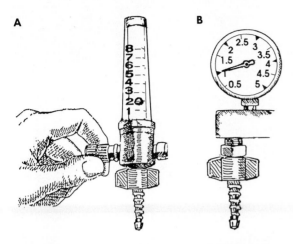

**Fig. 15-8**   Two types of flowmeters. **A,** Thorpe flowmeter. **B,** Bourdin gauge. When Thorpe flowmeter is used, flow rate is read at middle of float. (Courtesy Homedco, Seattle, Wash.)

are easier to see and the low flow rates used by most patients can be set more accurately. *In children, flow meters calibrated from 1 to 5 or 0.25 to 5 L/min are used.* Round Bourdin gauges measure pressure within the regulator rather than actual flow rate and register an artificially high flow rate whenever there is an added resistance to flow (e.g., with extra tubing or a humidifier) or tubing becomes kinked or obstructed. Because Thorpe tubes are "back-pressure compensated," they adjust for added resistance and measure flow rate accurately. If tubing becomes kinked or obstructed, the Thorpe flow rate indicator will drop to "0."

With the Thorpe tube, the flow rate is read at the middle of the ball, not the bottom, and must be set with the tank in the upright position. Once set, the flow rate will not change if the tank is placed on its side, although it will appear artificially high on the regulator.

### Reordering Oxygen

Patients must be taught to recognize when it is time to reorder oxygen. The pressure gauge on the regulator indicates the approximate pressure (in psi) remaining in the tank. The number of liters

remaining in an H tank can be roughly estimated by multiplying the psi by three (the precise conversion factor is 3.14). Remaining hours of oxygen use are then easily calculated by dividing liters remaining by liters used in an hour (e.g., 1 L/min = 60 L/hr). The conversion factor for an E cylinder is 0.28 L/psi. Below 500 psi, regulator calibrations are considerably less accurate, so psi cannot be used to predict remaining oxygen.

### Hazards of Tank Oxygen

Because of exceedingly high pressures, damage to a tank or regulator can result in sudden venting, sufficient to propel it like a missile. Serious injury and property damage can result. Because tank pressure increases by approximately 5 psi for every degree of cylinder temperature increase, tanks must be stored away from heat sources. They must also be well secured to a wall, stand, or other stabilizing device to prevent them from falling over.

## Use and Care of Liquid Oxygen Systems
### Vaporization of Liquid Oxygen

Some vaporization occurs even when the reservoir is not in use and is vented from the receptacle. Under normal conditions, liquid oxygen evaporates at a rate of approximately 1.1 lb a day; thus a full reservoir empties in approximately 20 to 30 days. Portable units vent more quickly because their insulation is less efficient. Each brand has some system by which the volume of oxygen remaining in the reservoir can be estimated.

### Operating the System

At flow rates above 5 L/min, the outlet valves on liquid systems tend to "freeze." If patients require higher flow rates, it is preferable to use two reservoirs, each delivering half the prescribed flow rate, blending the two flows with a Y connector, which is then attached to the nasal cannula.

Oxygen can be used directly from the reservoir or from the portable unit. The technique for transfilling the smaller portable container is relatively simple but does require training, intact cognitive functioning, and some manual dexterity. Some portable units pivot onto the side of their reservoir,

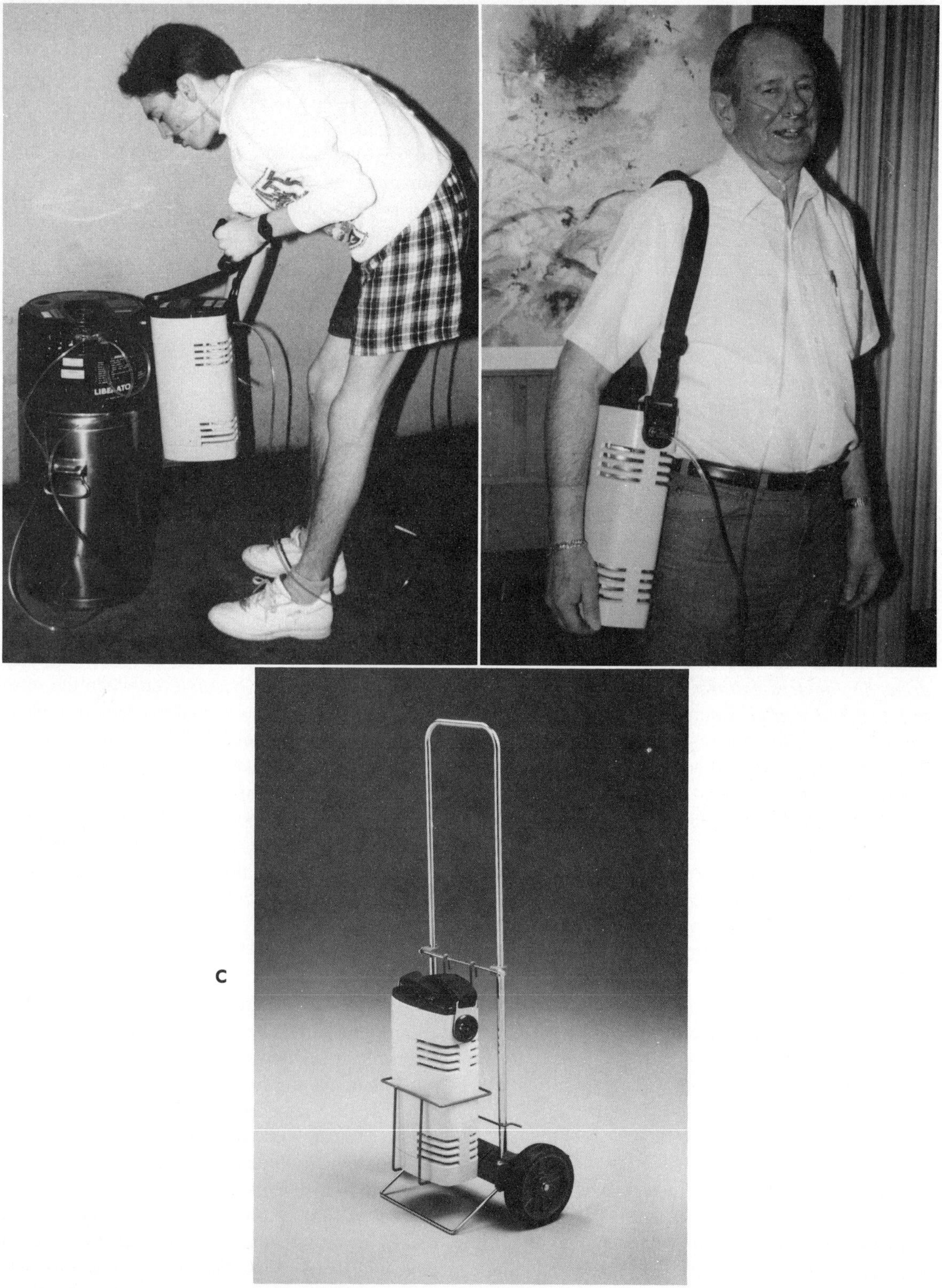

A B C

**Fig. 15-9** **A,** Filling liquid portable tank. Portable liquid containers can be carried, **B,** over the shoulder or, **C,** in vented backpack or wheeled cart.

whereas others latch onto the top (Fig. 15-9). Once in position, filling occurs automatically and with a soft hissing sound. Some systems allow filling to be terminated partway through the fill. This is a useful feature if the patient needs only 1 or 2 hours of portable oxygen. Some portable units come in more than one size. Smaller models are lighter and may be useful for patients who use very low flow rates or who rarely need more than 2 or 3 hours of portability at a time. To minimize oxygen wastage caused by venting, patients should use up the oxygen in the portable unit before switching back to the reservoir.

Most patients find that portable units are too heavy to be carried over their shoulder. Inexpensive grocery or luggage carts are good substitutes for the more costly wheeled carts sold by oxygen manufacturers. Vented backpacks are available and have the advantage of leaving both hands free (Airlift Unlimited, Evergreen, Colo.).

### Maintenance of Liquid Oxygen Systems

Inaccurate flow rates and problems with excessive venting can occur if equipment is poorly maintained by vendors (Massey, 1988). However, patient maintenance responsibilities are minimal. Most liquid systems are equipped with a small plastic drainage tube to direct any liquid oxygen condensate into a jar. This should be emptied regularly. Leakage in excess of a few milliliters a day should be reported promptly to the vendor.

### Minimizing Risks

Most precautions concerning the use of liquid oxygen relate to venting. Excess venting, especially in an enclosed area, increases ambient oxygen concentration and therefore the risk of fire. Movement and high environmental temperatures increase venting. Thus liquid oxygen should be stored in a cool, well-ventilated area of the house and at least 6 feet from electrical outlets or open flames.

As venting occurs, frost similar to dry ice may collect around the vent nipple and can cause skin damage. Direct skin contact with this frost should be avoided.

Occasionally, small particles of dust or debris get into the oxygen release valve or excess ice collects around the valve, causing it to stick open and vent profusely. A cloud of oxygen spewing into the air is an alarming sight, but the situation poses no particular danger if properly handled. The patient should eliminate any source of nearby sparks or flame, then leave the room and simply let the reservoir vent until it is empty. The vendor should then be notified.

### Transportation of Liquid Oxygen

Special precautions are needed if liquid oxygen is to be transported in a car, especially during hot weather when internal car temperatures can exceed 200° F. Windows must be left open for ventilation, the car's electrical system should be in good working order to reduce the risk of sparks, and smoking is prohibited.

## Use and Care of Oxygen Concentrators and Enrichers
### Operation of the System

Once the concentrator is plugged into a wall outlet, a warm-up period of about half an hour is required before the maximum oxygen concentration is achieved. Motor noise can be minimized by placing the machine on carpeting or by adding an extra length of tubing and placing the concentrator in a separate room. Most concentrators come with wheels so they can be moved easily from one room to another.

A backup K tank is usually provided with concentrators and enrichers for use in case of a power failure. Although 1 or 2 hours without supplemental oxygen is rarely harmful, a backup system permits continuation of usual activities and may minimize patient anxiety concerning power outages.

### Maintenance of the System

An external filter is located in an accessible spot on the outside of the machine. About once a week (more often if the environment is dusty), it must be rinsed thoroughly under running water, squeezed dry, and replaced. Aerosol sprays should not be used in the vicinity of the equipment because particles will be pulled into the system and may clog internal filters. Equipment must be checked and serviced by the supplier after every 2000 hours of use and requires a "major tune-up" in the shop at least annually.

### Determining the Accuracy of Oxygen Delivery

Similar to any other mechanical device, home oxygen equipment can malfunction. On the other hand, patients may believe that equipment is malfunctioning when breathlessness has increased for some other reason. For these reasons, home care staff must be able to differentiate equipment problems from changes in a patient's physiologic state.

The accuracy of the flow rate can be checked with a liter meter. $FiO_2$ is easily measured with an oxygen analyzer. Both devices are inexpensive and will improve the assessment capabilities of home care staff. They should be purchased by the home care agency if possible.

The ultimate test of the efficacy of home oxygen is the achievement of a $PaO_2$ or an oxygen saturation level that remains within the therapeutic range. Oxygen saturation is monitored with a pulse oximeter. Although more expensive than a liter meter or oxygen analyzer, it is an excellent investment for any home care agency with a high volume of respiratory referrals. $SaO_2$ is checked at rest and with exercise, in different positions (i.e., sitting, supine, or perhaps in Trendelenburg's position if used for postural drainage), and at different flow rates.

### ADJUNCT EQUIPMENT FOR THE DELIVERY OF HOME OXYGEN
### Oxygen Tubing and Cannula

A standard nasal cannula comes with approximately 7 feet of tubing, which is adequate for a portable system or a bedfast patient. An extra 50 feet of extension tubing is needed for ambulation within the house. This additional length adds some resistance to flow, but the use of a back-pressure-compensated flow meter will maintain an accurate oxygen output. Thus flow rate does *not* need to be increased when extra lengths of tubing are added.

The cannula is positioned with the prongs curving back into the nares. The tubing loops up and over the ears and is secured by snugging it up under the chin. Prongs of the nasal cannula should be observed for mucous secretions that occlude the openings and inhibit the flow of oxygen. Secretions can often be removed by washing the cannula in warm soapy water, rinsing in clear water, and blowing the excess water out with a compressor. Generally, however, the cannula will need to be replaced periodically as secretions accumulate.

Tubing is checked regularly for kinks, obstructions, leaks, or disconnections. Increased environmental humidity, humidifier use, or use of the enricher increases the likelihood of water condensation in the tubing. Water that fully obstructs tubing also obstructs oxygen flow and may cause a significant drop in $PaO_2$. It is easily removed by briefly turning up the flow rate or by connecting the tubing to an air compressor (if available) and blowing the water out. If the problem continues, an in-line water trap will prevent droplets from collecting.

The risk of tripping over oxygen tubing is minimized by keeping it out of major traffic pathways. Also a tape tab, attached to the oxygen tubing at shoulder level, can be pinned to clothing so that the tubing falls behind the patient rather than in front. Some patients devise elaborate systems for suspending tubing over doorways and heavily used areas.

High oxygen costs and self-consciousness about wearing cannulae have led to the development of more efficient and less noticeable oxygen delivery systems. One innovative device (Oxy-Frames, Engineered Specialty Products, Inc., Tallevast, Fla.) incorporates the oxygen tubing into fake eyeglass frames (Fig. 15-10). Another, the Nocturnal Cannula (Engineered Specialty Products, Inc., Tallevast, Fla.), consists of tubing secured by a headband and extending down along the nose rather than looped over the ears. It is useful for patients whose tubing tends to slip off at night, and for those with skin and ear irritation from a nasal cannula.

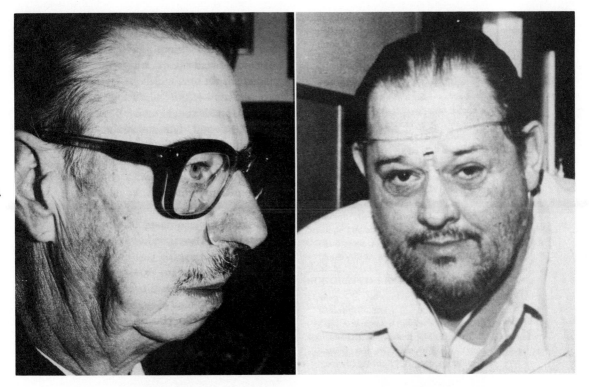

A

B

**Fig. 15-10** **A,** Oxy-Frames. Oxygen tubing is concealed alongside eyeglass frames. **B,** Nocturnal cannula. Headband helps to secure cannula, reducing likelihood of displacement during night. (Courtesy Saul Weiss, VA Medical Center, Pittsburgh, Pa.)

## Oxygen-Conserving Devices

Traditional nasal cannulae deliver oxygen throughout both inspiration and expiration. Yet only the first half of inspired air actually participates in alveolar gas exchange. The last half fills airway dead space where the supplemental oxygen it contains is essentially wasted and oxygen delivered during exhalation is lost to the ambient air. In response to this problem of wastage, three types of oxygen-conserving devices have been developed:

- Reservoir cannulae
- Demand (or pulse) oxygen-delivery systems
- Transtracheal catheters

Reservoir cannulae and demand systems are designed to deliver a bolus of oxygen during the first half of inspiration. This markedly reduces flow rate requirements, reducing oxygen cost proportionately (Tiep, 1987; O'Donohue, 1988; Hoffman, 1988; Herrick, 1989). Lower flow rates permit the use of lighter, smaller cylinders that are less obvious and easier to carry. Liquid portable units last two to four times as long with oxygen-conserving devices, permitting patients far more mobility than is possible with standard nasal prongs.

## Reservoir Cannulae

Two reservoir cannulae—the Oxymizer and the Oxymizer Pendant (Chad Therapeutics, Chatsworth, Calif.)—are available (Fig. 15-11). The Oxymizer incorporates an oxygen-filled reservoir, which sits on the upper lip like a little pillow,

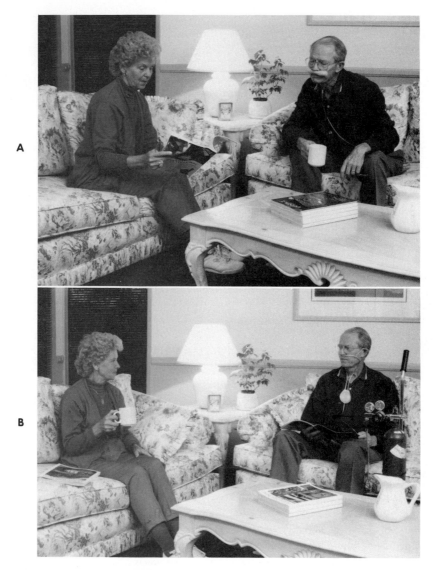

**Fig. 15-11** **A,** Oxymizer. **B,** Oxymizer Pendant. Oxygen-conserving devices can markedly increase hours of oxygen use available from small portable cylinders. (Courtesy Chad Therapeutics, Chatsworth, Calif.)

whereas the Oxymizer Pendant hangs down on the chest. A 20 ml bolus of oxygen is pulled from the reservoir bag at the beginning of each breath. Oxygen savings have been demonstrated to be about 3:1 over traditional nasal cannulae, but cosmetic concerns and problems with bulk and excessive pull on the ears have resulted in poor patient ac-

ceptance (Claiborne, 1987). The Oxymizers cost significantly more than the traditional nasal cannula and must be replaced weekly.

## Demand Devices

Demand devices incorporate a battery-operated electronic or fluidic sensor at the nasal cannula that activates a brief burst of oxygen flow at the start of inspiration. They can be built into the oxygen reservoir or portable unit or contained separately in a special belt pack (O'Donohue, 1988). Examples include the following:

- Pulsair and PdO$_2$ (Cryo/2 Corp., Fort Pierce, Fla.): These devices deliver 16.5 ml for each L/min flow setting. The Pulsair I weighs 7 lb and lasts about 11 hours at 2 L/min of pulsed flow. The Pulsair II, weighing approximately 10 lb, lasts about 25 hours. Both can be converted back to continuous delivery by flicking a switch. The Pulsair systems are built into the Cryo/2 portable liquid system, whereas the PdO$_2$ is designed for use with compressed gas cylinders.
- Oxymatic (Chad Therapeutics, Inc., Chatsworth, Calif.): This device delivers 35 ml of oxygen with one of four breaths, two of four breaths, three of four breaths, or four of four breaths, depending on the setting.
- PortoMate and Omni (John Bunn Co., Tonawanda, N.Y.): These devices deliver a set flow rate during the first half of each respiratory cycle.
- Companion 5 and 6 (Puritan-Bennett Corp., Lenexa, Kan.) and DO$_2$ (Minnesota Valley Engineering, New Prague, Minn.): These devices deliver a variable pulse volume adjusted for both flow rate and respiratory rate.

As with the reservoir cannula system, nasal breathing is needed to trigger these devices. Thus they may be unreliable at times when mouth breathing often predominates (e.g., at night and with exercise). SaO$_2$ should be carefully assessed at rest, with exercise, and with sleep following the initiation of one of these delivery devices.

Oxygen use with demand systems may be as low as one seventh that required with nasal prongs (Tiep, 1987; O'Donohue, 1988; Herrick, 1989). Substantial oxygen savings with demand systems have also been demonstrated for patients with restrictive lung disease, especially with exercise (Carter, 1989). Some patients are bothered by the clicking noise that accompanies activation.

## Transtracheal Oxygen

A technique for the administration of oxygen via a transtracheal catheter was developed by Heimlich and offers distinct advantages over traditional delivery systems (Heimlich, 1982). Approximately 8000 patients in the United States currently use tracheal oxygen (O'Donohue, 1989). By introducing oxygen directly, the trachea becomes its own reservoir. Less oxygen is lost to ambient air and an acceptable PaO$_2$ can be achieved with a flow rate that is one quarter to one half that required with a standard nasal cannula. Thus each tank of oxygen lasts much longer and the overall cost is markedly reduced. Because the tracheal insertion site is inconspicuous, cosmetic appearance is also improved.

Heimlich's "microtrach" (Ballard Medical Products, Midvale, Utah) and the SCOOP (Transtracheal Systems, Denver, Colo.) are percutaneous devices (Fig. 15-12). A subcutaneous technique has also been developed using a silicone rubber catheter, the Johnson Intratracheal oxygen catheter (ITO$_2$C, Cook, Inc., Bloomington, Ind.). The catheter is inserted on the anterior chest and tunnelled up to the trachea where it is sutured in place through a tiny incision (Johnson, 1987). Once the tracheal incision has healed, there is no visible evidence that oxygen is being used.

Because these are invasive procedures, there is concern about the potential for complications. Those complications most often encountered include the following:

- Obstruction of the catheter from mucous balls
- Increased cough
- Loss of the catheter tract following catheter displacement

Other reported complications include bronchospasm, hoarseness, hemoptysis, cutaneous inflammation and infection, keloid formation around the scar, retroflexion of the tube upward in the trachea, endotracheal mass (Fletcher, 1988), subcutaneous emphysema from accidental tube displacement or air leakage around a new stoma (Hoffman, 1987; Christopher, 1987; Heimlich, 1989). Design improvements have reduced or eliminated some of

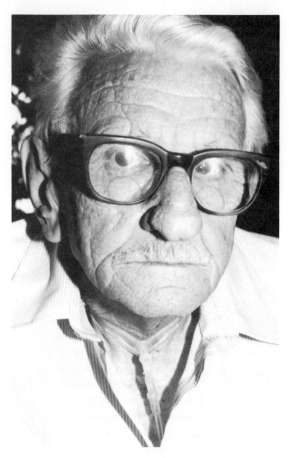

**Fig. 15-12** SCOOP transtracheal oxygen system. Transtracheal systems deliver oxygen directly into trachea and often allow patient to use lower liter flows. External catheter can be hidden under clothing.

these problems. Patient acceptance tends to be good, however, even when complications have developed. Improved acceptance is likely to result in better patient compliance and may improve the long-term outcome.

Potential advantages of transtracheal devices include the following (Hoffman, 1987; Heimlich, 1988; Johnson, 1987; Christopher, 1986):

- Less dyspnea
- Elimination of nasal and ear irritation
- Improved taste, smell, and appetite
- Improved sleep
- Improved mobility
- Improved self-esteem
- Marked reduction in hematocrit in patients with polycythemia
- Reduced hospital days
- Adequate $PaO_2$ in patients with refractory hypoxemia on nasal cannula

Careful selection of candidates and rigorous patient education and follow-up are essential for all transtracheal delivery systems. Success depends on a well-motivated, emotionally stable patient who is capable of following self-care instructions. Poor candidates for transtracheal oxygen delivery are patients with severe bronchospasm, copious sputum production, a compromised immune system (including those receiving steroid doses in excess of 30 mg/day), serious cardiac arrhythmias, uncompensated respiratory acidosis (pH less than 7.33), prolonged bleeding times, or excessive anxiety (Hoffman, 1988; Christopher, 1987).

Specific care for each type of transtracheal device is described in the product literature. Percutaneous catheters can be inserted in an outpatient setting, but they require scrupulous care and patient education in the first few weeks. Careful skin cleansing around the insertion site is important. The subcutaneous catheter must be placed or removed in an operating room or outpatient surgery, but the follow-up self-care protocol is simpler and displacement less likely. Routine saline irrigations are performed two to three times daily with all devices and seem to help some patients clear secretions. Percutaneous catheters must be replaced regularly every 1 to 3 months. Subcutaneous catheters are replaced only if they are displaced. The costs of the initial insertion, follow-up care, and routine tube replacement may outweigh the savings realized from the subsequent reduction in oxygen flow rate. Thus studies evaluating the long-term cost savings of these devices are being conducted.

## Face Masks

Face masks, especially Venturi masks, are rarely used at home because they may cause claustrophobia, are esthetically unappealing, interfere with eating and talking, and often require high flow rates to achieve an acceptable level of oxygenation. A face mask is sometimes used for terminally ill cancer patients. Such a mask may be a temporary alternative while sores from a nasal cannula heal. A tracheostomy collar is used with a tracheostomy.

## Humidifiers

Humidifiers add negligible humidity to supplemental oxygen (Darin, 1982), and subjective complaints (dry or sore throat, headache, or sputum production) are no different with unhumidified than humidified oxygen (Campbell, 1988). Therefore humidification of oxygen delivered by nasal cannula is generally unnecessary, at least for flow rates of 5 L/min or less. An empiric trial of humidification is reasonable for a patient with symptomatic complaints at higher flow rates or with extremely low environmental humidity. Humidifiers are necessary when using transtracheal oxygen because these devices preclude nasopharyngeal humidification of the gas; however, for convenience, they are usually not used when outside the home. Liquid oxygen reservoirs do not incorporate any type of humidifier.

### Humidifier Care and Cleaning

The humidifier jar is washed two to three times a week in warm, soapy water, then rinsed and dried thoroughly. Vinegar or quaternary ammonium soaks are often recommended for bacterial decontamination but are probably unnecessary. The clean humidifier is refilled with either distilled water or boiled and cooled tap water. Tap water can be used in disposable humidifiers but will corrode nondisposable equipment. Prepackaged sterile humidifiers are more expensive but can be used for 1 to 2 weeks. They may be a better alternative for patients who lack the motivation, strength, or coordination to clean their humidifiers. The humidifier must be replaced carefully because a damaged or improperly tightened seal will cause an oxygen leak.

## ADAPTATIONS FOR CHILDREN USING OXYGEN
### Nasal Cannula

*School-age children use the same equipment as adults except that the nasal cannula is smaller. Special neonatal and pediatric cannulae are available for young children. Alternatively, a makeshift cannula can be fashioned by cutting off the nasal prongs, making a slit between the two holes, and positioning the slit below the nares.*

### Flow Meters

*Flow meters with small calibrations are needed for young children because their flow rates are usually so much lower. The Timeter (Allied Health Care, St. Louis, Mo.) (0.1 to 1 L/min; ⅛ to 3 L/min; 25 to 200 cc/min) or the Veriflow (Richmond, Calif.) (⅛ to 3½ L/min; 1/32 to ½ L/min) is available for the regulation of extremely low flow rates. When a child returns home from the hospital using oxygen therapy, the saturation should be rechecked with the child using the home system. Oxygen saturation achieved from a hospital wall outlet may not be exactly the same as that achieved with the same flow rate from home equipment, and the home flow rate may need to be adjusted accordingly.*

### Crib Oxygen Tents

*Active infants may dislodge oxygen tubing or become tangled in it as they move around the crib. If an infant or small child is unable to keep a cannula in place, humidified oxygen can be bled into a crib tent. Tents permit greater freedom of movement for a child but are often frightening unless the child has grown up with one. They are difficult to clean and use significantly more oxygen. It is also more difficult to maintain a steady state oxygen concentration because oxygen is lost each time the tent is opened. An oxygen analyzer is used for the routine monitoring of tent oxygen concentration, and a high- and low-oxygen alarm may be indicated.*

*The Oxyhood (Olympic Medical, Seattle, Wash.) is a Plexiglas box that covers only the child's*

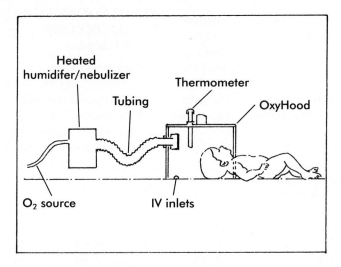

**Fig. 15-13**   Oxyhood permits oxygenation while leaving infant's torso exposed for treatment and monitoring. Open neck prevents accumulation of carbon dioxide. Lid opens for quick access to baby. Comes in three infant sizes. (Courtesy Olympic Medical, Seattle, Wash.)

*head (Fig. 15-13). It requires a flow rate of 10 to 12 L/min of air into which oxygen can be bled. The Oxyhood is sometimes useful for children with bronchopulmonary dysplasia who are being weaned from oxygen and may need it only at night.*

## Parental Mobility

*Parental mobility is a prime concern in selecting a portable system for young children. The parent may need to juggle infant, oxygen, groceries, stroller, and possibly other children. An E cylinder is awkward; thus a system that can be carried over the parent's shoulder or in a backpack is preferable.*

## ADVERSE EFFECTS ASSOCIATED WITH OXYGEN USE

Home oxygen is a safe and effective intervention with potential benefits that far outweigh the risks. Although minor discomforts and more serious sequelae do occur, most can be prevented with good patient and caregiver education. Adverse effects may include the following:

- Unresolved hypoxemia: This is often caused by an inadequate flow rate, poor patient compliance, or both.
- Unjustifiably high oxygen costs: This can result from a flow rate that exceeds oxygen need, poor patient compliance, or improper selection of the system.
- $CO_2$ narcosis from reduced hypoxic ventilatory drive in response to an excessive flow rate: Symptoms of $CO_2$ narcosis include lethargy, drowsiness, morning headache, confusion, nightmares, and combativeness. Use of sedatives and alcohol increases the risk. Any oxygen-dependent patient who retains $CO_2$ needs instruction in the risks of exceeding the prescribed flow rate of oxygen and in the signs and symptoms of $CO_2$ narcosis. Patients with a normal $Pa_{CO_2}$ are not at risk for oxygen-induced $CO_2$ narcosis.

- Injuries resulting from fire or explosion: Oxygen will not ignite or explode spontaneously but does support combustion. When injuries occur, it is usually because a spark or flame was introduced into an oxygen-enriched atmosphere. Therefore oxygen should be kept at least 6 feet from electrical outlets, open flames, and sparks. Smoking is, of course, prohibited. Singed eyebrows and facial burns can easily occur when patients smoke while using oxygen, and deaths have been reported.
- Nasal irritation: Complaints of nasal dryness, a sore or stuffy nose, occasional nose bleeds, sore throat, hoarseness, and symptoms of rhinitis or sinusitis are common. These symptoms may be worse in the winter when household heating systems reduce ambient humidity to unusually low levels.
- Painful sores in the nares: Sores in the nares are a fairly common problem.
- Ear lesions: Deep, painful lacerations may develop over the ears if the nasal cannula is pulled too tightly or if it is too heavy.
- Skin sensitivity: Skin sensitivity to the polyvinyl chloride composition of the cannula can occur.
- *Skin breakdown: Skin breakdown can occur on the cheeks of infants because of cannula changes, which require the daily removal of tape from face.*
- Oxygen toxicity: Prolonged use of a high concentration of oxygen ($FIO_2$ of more than 50%), or just 24 hours of 100% oxygen are known to cause significant damage to the lung parenchyma and play a major role in the development of infant and adult respiratory distress syndrome. *Low-flow oxygen administered over long periods of time contributes to the development of bronchopulmonary dysplasia in infants who survive infant respiratory distress syndrome* (Fulmer, 1984). Low-flow oxygen does not cause clinically significant damage in adults.

## Prevention of Adverse Effects
### Injuries from Fire or Explosion

Professional opinions differ as to how one should approach the problem of the oxygen-dependent patient who is unable or unwilling to stop smoking. Options include the following:

- Establish a contract with the patient in which he or she agrees, at a minimum, to remove the cannula while smoking and never to smoke in bed.
- Switch to an oxygen enricher, which is less a fire hazard because the concentration of oxygen it produces is only 40%.
- The physician may refuse to prescribe home oxygen. This is common practice in England and Australia.
- Post signs warning that oxygen is in use to discourage others from smoking.

Other strategies to prevent fire or explosion include the following:

- Remove frayed electrical wiring and ground all electrical equipment to reduce the risk of sparks.
- Never use petroleum products (e.g., oil, grease) on oxygen equipment because of the risk for combustion. A water-soluble lubricant is preferable to Vaseline for dry lips or nostrils.
- Store liquid systems in a cool, well-ventilated place so that high oxygen concentrations do not accumulate in ambient air and saturate nearby curtains or bedclothes. Portable units should not be exposed to conditions that create static electricity. A mesh carrying bag is safer than a solid fabric bag because vented oxygen is more readily dispersed.

### Nasal Irritation

Symptoms of nasal irritation may be relieved with a commercial bedside vaporizer (see Chapter 14 for precautions regarding equipment care). Painful sores in the nares may be relieved by occluding one of the nasal prongs and alternating flow between nostrils or by switching to a single-prong cannula or the biflow nasal mask (Intec Medical,

Inc., Blue Springs, Mich.), a small soft "cup" that is placed under the nares. A thin layer of healing ointment may also reduce discomfort from irritation, but thick layers increase the risk for aspiration.

### Ear Lesions

If ear lesions occur, loosen the cannula, cleanse the lesion, and gently pad it with a cotton ball or moleskin to prevent any further contact with the tubing. Zinc oxide or A&D ointment may further protect the area and promote healing. Oxy-ears (American Medical Products, Phoenix, Ariz.), which are small foam cylinders that fit over the cannula, and the Nocturnal Cannula headband (p. 263) are other options for temporary relief of ear lesions.

### Skin Sensitivity

Skin hypersensitivity can be managed with hypoallergenic tape such as Tegaderm (3M Corp, St. Paul, Minn.), pink HY tape (HY Tape Co., Yonkers, N.Y.), Dermaclear transparent tape (Johnson and Johnson, New Brunswick, N.J.), or a layer of Opsite (Smith and Nephew, Massillon, Ohio), which is used as a base to which regular tape is applied. Coloplast (Coloplast Inc., Tampa, Fla.) or corya gum may also be applied to the cheek, and the cannula taped to the gum. Alternately the cannula can be wrapped with the hypoallergenic tape or a different brand of cannula may be used. Hydrocortisone cream may also relieve the discomfort of skin sensitivity.

## PATIENT EDUCATION

Rigorous education of patients and caregivers is essential to ensure safe, effective, and appropriate use of home oxygen. Lack of skill in the use of equipment is greatest in patients using oxygen less than 7 months, whereas knowledge deficits are greatest after 7 to 12 months of use (O'Toole, 1983). These findings reinforce the importance of follow-up teaching, especially during the first year of oxygen therapy.

Patients must know the following information:
- Rationale and expected benefits of use, especially if these are not obvious to the patient: Because the beneficial effects of oxygen in reversing pulmonary heart disease develop subtly over several weeks, it is often difficult to convince patients that they should use oxygen continuously, especially during periods of sleep or rest—the very times when they are likely to feel the least subjective need for it.
- Oxygen is a drug and must be used as prescribed: While removing oxygen for short periods of time is not harmful, significant changes in pulmonary vascular resistance and cardiac function can be seen when oxygen therapy has been discontinued for only 3 hours (Selinger, 1987).
- Oxygen should not be discontinued with activity or during meals or sleep: Oxygen should be continued during these times because the oxygen demand increases during activity and meals and oxygen saturation normally falls during sleep.
- Signs and symptoms of hypoxemia and hypercapnia: Patients should also know what to do if these occur.
- When and how to reorder oxygen: Patients should understand how to calculate the amount of oxygen remaining in a reservoir and how to reorder oxygen.
- How to troubleshoot common equipment problems: Patients should be able to anticipate, identify, and fix common equipment problems.
- Sources and limits of reimbursement: Patients should be aware of the costs of oxygen therapy and the amounts that they will have to pay out of pocket.

Patients must be able to perform the following:
- Set the flow rate correctly. Pediatric flow meters are easier to read and can be set more precisely. With liquid systems, flow can often be set by feel (i.e., counting clicks on the dial), permitting safe use by the visually impaired; also, a flow lock can be added that will au-

tomatically deliver a preset flow rate as soon as the reservoir is turned on. Use of a flow lock can also prevent the confused or noncompliant patient from increasing the flow rate excessively.

- Fill and transport the portable liquid system. Most patients will need a wheeled cart.
- Determine whether oxygen is flowing through the cannula (e.g., by observing bubbles when prongs are held under water or by feeling the flow when prongs are placed against the cheek); recognize leaks in the system; and remove water from tubing.
- Effectively clean cannulae, humidifiers (if used), and concentrator filters.

## EMOTIONAL IMPACT OF HOME OXYGEN USE

It is generally assumed that long-term oxygen therapy improves the patient's quality of life. However, for some patients, initiation of home oxygen therapy has a profoundly negative emotional impact. In a survey of oxygen-dependent male veterans, 83% reported a diminished quality of life with home oxygen therapy (O'Toole, 1983). Other patients report a significant reduction in body image and the performance of social activities with home oxygen therapy (Marchionno, 1985). Thus any evaluation of the benefits of oxygen use for a patient must include the overall impact on his or her quality of life.

For some, especially young people with cystic fibrosis, being told they need home oxygen therapy marks the "beginning of the end," a signal that they are entering a terminal phase of their illness. Anxiety over a poor prognosis may be ameliorated by emphasizing the role of oxygen in prolonging life (by preventing or alleviating cor pulmonale), improving sleep quality, and enhancing ability to exercise and manage activities of daily living.

Some patients feel self-conscious or increasingly vulnerable using oxygen in public. Patients can overcome embarrassment by beginning with outings to safe, supportive destinations (e.g., the clinic or COPD support group meetings) where there are others using oxygen therapy. Visits to supportive family and friends also help to bridge the gap.

Fear based on the myth that oxygen is combustible or explosive can be dispelled by clarifying misconceptions and teaching safe use. Fear of becoming addicted to or dependent on oxygen is also countered by a clarification of misconceptions. It sometimes helps to remind patients that *everyone* is dependent on oxygen and that oxygen delivery systems merely compensate for the normal work their damaged lungs can no longer do. A discussion of the physiologic role of oxygen, with specific reference to the patient's own blood gas values while on and off oxygen, is often convincing.

## TRAVELING WITH OXYGEN

Home oxygen therapy need not be a constraint against traveling. Indeed, it may be precisely the intervention that makes travel once again possible. Travel with oxygen does require careful planning, however.

The realistic potential for travel can be a major motivating factor for many homebound oxygen-dependent patients and should be included by the home care nurse in discussions of long-term rehabilitation goals. COPD support groups and local offices of the American Lung Association are often good sources of travel information and advice. Several excellent resources on travel have been included in the suggested readings at the end of this chapter.

## REFERENCES

American Thoracic Society: Standards for the diagnosis and care of patients with COPD and asthma, *Am Rev Respir Dis* 136:225, 1987.

Campbell EJ, Baker D, Crites-Silver P: Subjective effects of humidification of oxygen for delivery by nasal cannula, *Chest* 93:289, 1988.

Carter R et al: Demand oxygen delivery for patients with restrictive lung disease, *Chest* 96:1307, 1989.

Castaldo W, DeGregorio B, Brandstetter RD: Meal induced hypoxemia in COPD patients, *Am Rev Respir Dis* 124:94, 1983 (abstract).

Christopher KL et al: Transtracheal oxygen therapy for refractory hypoxemia, *JAMA* 256:494, 1986.

Christopher KL et al: A program for transtracheal oxygen delivery, *Ann Intern Med* 107:802, 1987.

Claiborne RA et al: Evaluation of the use of an oxygen conservation device in long-term oxygen therapy, *Am Rev Respir Dis* 136:1095, 1987.

Darin J, Broadwell J, MacDowell R: An evaluation of water-vapor output from four brands of unheated prefilled bubble humidifiers, *Respir Care* 27:41, 1982.

Fan LL, Voyles JB: Determination of inspired oxygen delivered by nasal cannula in infants with chronic lung disease, *J Pediatr* 103:923, 1983.

Fletcher EC, Nickeson D, Costarangos-Galarza C: Endotracheal mass resulting from a transtracheal oxygen catheter, *Chest* 93:439, 1988.

Fulmer JD, Snider GL: ACCP/NHLBI national conference on oxygen therapy, *Heart Lung* 13:550, 1984.

Grant F, Heaton RK, McSweeny J: Neuropsychiatric findings in hypoxemic chronic obstructive pulmonary disease, *Arch Intern Med* 142:1470, 1982.

Groothuis JR, Rosenberg AA: Home oxygen promotes weight gain in infants with bronchopulmonary dysplasia, *Am J Dis Child* 141:992, 1987.

Heaton RK et al: Psychological effects of continuous oxygen therapy in hypoxemia chronic obstructive pulmonary disease, *Arch Intern Med* 143:1941, 1983.

Heimlich HJ: Respiratory rehabilitation with transtracheal oxygen system, *Ann Otol Rhinol Laryngol* 91:643, 1982.

Heimlich HJ: Oxygen delivery for ambulatory patients, *Postgrad Med* 84:68, 1988.

Heimlich HJ, Carr GC: The microtrach: a seven year experience with transtracheal oxygen therapy, *Chest* 95:1008, 1989.

Herrick TW, Yeager H: Home oxygen therapy, *Am Fam Physician* 39:157, 1989.

Hoffman LA, Wesmiller SW: Home oxygen: transtracheal and other options, *Am J Nurs* 88:464, 1988.

Hoffman LA et al: Patient response to transtracheal oxygen delivery, *Am Rev Respir Dis* 135:153, 1987.

Johnson LP, Cary JM: The implanted intratracheal oxygen catheter, *Surg Gynecol Obstet* 165:74, 1987.

Levi-Valensi P et al: Three-month follow-up of arterial blood gas determinations in candidates for long-term oxygen therapy, *Am Rev Respir Dis* 133:547, 1986.

Marchionno PM et al: Effects of continuous oxygen therapy on body image and life-style in patients with COPD, *Am Rev Respir Dis* 131:A163, 1985 (abstract).

Marcus CL et al: Supplemental oxygen and exercise performance in patients with cystic fibrosis with severe pulmonary disease, *Chest* 101:52, 1992.

Massey LW, Hussey JD, Albert RK: Inaccurate oxygen delivery in some portable liquid oxygen devices, *Am Rev Respir Dis* 137:204, 1988.

Medical Research Council Working Party: Long-term domiciliary oxygen therapy in chronic hypoxic cor pulmonale complicating chronic bronchitis and emphysema, *Lancet* 1:681, 1981.

Nocturnal Oxygen Therapy Trial Group: Continuous or nocturnal oxygen therapy in hypoxemic chronic obstructive disease, *Ann Intern Med* 93:391, 1980.

O'Donohue WJ: The future of home oxygen therapy, *Respir Care* 33:1125, 1988.

O'Donohue WJ: New problems in home oxygen therapy, *Am Rev Respir Dis* 140:1813, 1989.

O'Toole VA et al: Self-care practices of COPD patients receiving continuous oxygen therapy via a liquid oxygen system, *Am Rev Respir Dis* 127(4, part 2):149, 1983 (abstract).

Second Conference on Long-Term Oxygen Therapy: Further recommendations for prescribing and supplying long-term oxygen therapy, *Am Rev Respir Dis* 138:745, 1988.

Selinger SR et al: Effects of removing oxygen from patients with COPD, *Am Rev Respir Dis* 136:85, 1987.

Tiep BL, Lewis MI: Oxygen conservation and oxygen-conserving devices in chronic lung disease: a review, *Chest* 92:263, 1987.

West GA, Primeau P: Nonmedical hazards of long-term oxygen therapy, *Respir Care* 27:906, 1983.

Zinman R et al: Nocturnal home oxygen in the treatment of hypoxemic cystic fibrosis patients, *J Pediatr* 114:368, 1989.

**SUGGESTED READINGS**

Petty TL: Home oxygen: a revolution in the care of advanced COPD, *Med Clin North Am* 74:715, 1990.

*Respir Care* 28(7):1, 1983. Entire issue devoted to papers from the 1982 ACCP International Symposium on Long-Term Oxygen Therapy.

Spofford B et al: Transtracheal oxygen therapy: a guide for the respiratory therapist, *Respir Care* 32:345, 1987.

Tiep BL: Long-term home oxygen therapy, *Clin Chest Med* 11:505, 1990.

**Travel for the Patient with Chronic Lung Disease**

Gong H: Air travel and oxygen therapy in cardiopulmonary patients, *Chest* 101:1104, 1992.

Livingstone G: *Airline travel with oxygen: lung disease care and education briefing paper,* New York, 1991, The American Lung Association.

Santoro K: A vacation cruise for COPD patients, *Respir Ther* 15:31, 1985.

# CHAPTER 16

# MECHANICAL VENTILATION IN THE HOME

NANCY A. MIZUMORI • ELLAN J.P. NELSON •
WILLIAM S. PRENTICE • LYNN M. WITHEY

Home health care is a realistic and preferable option to the hospital for many ventilator-dependent patients. The goal of home health care is to provide safe, effective, and psychosocially rewarding care in the home setting. The success of home mechanical ventilation depends on many variables, including a medically stable patient, coordinated discharge planning, a smooth transition from hospital to home, a funding source, family support, and access to community health care resources.

Benefits of home ventilator care include the following:

- Marked reduction in the cost of care, compared with hospital care (Plummer, 1989)
- Freedom from exposure to microorganisms endemic to hospitals
- Enhanced quality of life, because patients:
    Live in a more normal environment
    Regain a sense of control over their environment
    Can participate in daily activities with their families and begin to establish new roles for themselves within the limitations of their disability

Problems inherent in the home care of a ventilator-dependent patient are primarily those of ensuring safety and adequacy of the environment, ensuring caregiver expertise, and preventing caregiver burnout.

## INDICATIONS FOR HOME VENTILATORY SUPPORT

A variety of disorders can realistically be treated with home ventilatory support. These include the following:

- Neuromuscular disorders
    Poliomyelitis
    Muscular dystrophy
    Amyotrophic lateral sclerosis
    Myasthenia gravis
    Spinal cord lesions
    Phrenic nerve lesions
    Undifferentiated neuromuscular disease
- Obstructive pulmonary disorders
    End-stage chronic bronchitis and emphysema
    Bronchopulmonary dysplasia
- Restrictive pulmonary disorders
    Interstitial pulmonary fibrosis
    Kyphoscoliosis
    Chest wall deformities
- Sleep apnea syndromes
    Central sleep apnea
    Mixed central and obstructive sleep apnea

### Clinical Stability

Patients who depend entirely on ventilatory support should not be considered for home care unless they are clinically stable. Criteria for clinical stability are shown in the box on p. 274.

In addition, the patient and family must be mo-

---

### Criteria of Clinical Stability for Ventilator-Dependent Patients

Absence of significant sustained dyspnea or severe dyspneic episodes and/or tachypnea

Acceptable arterial blood gases with $FIO_2$ $\leq 0.40$

Psychologic stability

Absence of life-threatening cardiac dysfunction or arrhythmias

No major changes in management expected for 1 month

Ability to clear secretions

Evidence of gag and cough reflex or protected airway

Absence of significant aspiration

*Progression on growth curve and developmental progress (infants and children)*

---

Modified from O'Donohue WJ et al: *Chest* 90:1S, 1986.

tivated and able to participate in the home care program. A safe home environment; adequate community resources such as home nursing care, respite care, or both; and a reliable equipment vendor must be available. Financial support must be available to meet nursing, equipment, and supply costs.

## DISCHARGE PLANNING FOR THE VENTILATOR-DEPENDENT PATIENT

Responsibility for all aspects of discharge planning rests with a multidisciplinary team. The discharge planning team includes the patient, at least one responsible family member, the physician, the patient's primary hospital nurse, the respiratory therapist, the social worker, the discharge planning coordinator, the equipment vendor representative, and the home care nurse. The active involvement of home care staff is essential to the success of the transition.

Regardless of the level of care needed, it is extremely important to have a patient care coordinator with expertise in both pulmonary care and the management of ventilator-dependent patients to partic-

ipate in the discharge planning process and to organize the activities of the multidisciplinary home care team (Plummer, 1989). Organization of care psychologically comforts both the patient and caregivers and makes everyday situations easier to handle. Without careful discharge planning the transition from hospital to home is usually unsuccessful.

Each member of the team brings different skills and carries different responsibilities for the discharge planning process. Regular communication through team conferences helps all members formulate plans and prevents duplication of time-consuming discharge activities. The team leader assigns specific activities to various team members. These activities include the following:

- Setting a tentative discharge date
- Investigating and confirming funding sources
- Contacting the home care agency and equipment vendor to arrange for nursing care and equipment and for their participation in subsequent discharge planning activities
- Interviewing the patient and family
- Inspecting the home to evaluate the safety and adequacy of the home environment (This is often done jointly by clinicians from the home care agency and the equipment vendor. Important elements of the home assessment are listed in the box on p. 275.)
- Organizing and supervising the training of family and professional caregivers
- Teaching the family and patient signs and symptoms of potential respiratory or other medical problems and appropriate interventions if problems occur
- Arranging with community agencies for services that may be needed to enhance growth and development and help the patient adjust to the new life situation
- Contacting the fire department, paramedics, and power company, as indicated, to establish emergency plans
- Supporting and counseling the patient and family as indicated

It is important to know the patient's concerns,

### Requirements for a Safe and Functional Home Environment

Ramps for wheelchair access

Doorways and hallways wide enough to accommodate a wheelchair

Adequate electrical system, including:

Enough power to run the equipment without blowing circuit breakers or fuses

If fuses used, extras kept by fuse box

Three-prong outlets for all respiratory equipment

If extension cords required, must be heavy duty, with connections taped and secured along walls to prevent tripping

A backup battery in case of power failure

A patient-operated audible alarm system

All equipment "childproofed" so children cannot alter settings

No smoking in the patient's immediate environment

feelings about discharge, and motivation to remain at home. It is also necessary to know whether the patient can ambulate, eat and dress independently, manage bowel and bladder control, suction self, and connect or disconnect the ventilator. The patient should achieve as much independence in personal care activities as possible before discharge.

Individual interviews are usually needed to determine how the patient and family perceive their needs and the type of home care support they feel will be most appropriate. The family member who will be primarily responsible for the ventilator-dependent patient should be interviewed to determine the following:

- Overall commitment to the patient going home
- A plan for educating as many family members as possible regarding ventilator use and maintenance, tracheostomy care, suctioning, and other patient needs
- Any potential problems within the environ-

ment or family support system that could affect patient safety

- Persons available to provide backup support for the primary caregiver
- Financial situation of the family and insurance coverage; whether they can meet out of pocket expenses for items not covered for insurance, including higher electric bills
- Anticipated impact of having necessary care providers in the home

The presence of a supportive family is one of the most critical variables affecting the success or failure of home ventilator care. Home care is more likely to succeed if the patient and family are motivated and can work together. Discharge planning must be family oriented with members involved in all aspects of care and decision making. It is important for family members to participate in conferences and be oriented to the equipment and procedures. Careful assessment of the needs and reactions of each family member is also important.

Because the attitudes and abilities of a family are such critical determinants of the success of caring for a ventilator-dependent patient, the family must be supported if they decide against home care. Not all families are able to accept such responsibility.

### Equipment Vendor

Early in the discharge planning process a determination is made about the type of home care equipment that is needed. Patient needs may also change after discharge, and the home care nurse must be able to work with the vendor to secure the appropriate equipment. It is extremely important that the vendor has access to a specialist, usually a nurse or respiratory therapist, who understands the patient's medical problem and how to manage the equipment and make the transition from hospital to home.

As part of the discharge planning team, the equipment vendor's primary responsibility is to arrange for the appropriate ventilator and equipment. Vendors that provide the following services are preferable:

- Make predischarge assessment visits to see the patient in the hospital and to visit the home
- Arrange for the patient to use the specific ventilator that will be used at home in the hospital for at least 72 hours, but preferably for a week before discharge (O'Donohue, 1986)
- Teach the family, patient, and home care nurses ventilator operation and maintenance: cleaning, circuit changes, ventilator monitoring, and troubleshooting
- Determine home stock of disposable items such as suction catheters, sterile water, and ventilator circuit parts, and teach the family how and when to order additional supplies
- Deliver other respiratory equipment, a backup ventilator, and supplies to the home
- Troubleshoot ventilator malfunctions; assume 24-hour on-call responsibility for ventilator problems
- Make regular assessment visits to ensure that equipment is functioning properly; perform routine maintenance and safety checks on equipment
- Participate with other caregivers in assessing patient response to home care
- Obtain oximetry readings periodically, if necessary, to evaluate oxygen saturation or obtain blood for arterial blood gas analysis
- Provide liaison between the physician, patient, and family as indicated

## MECHANICAL VENTILATORS

There are a variety of options for home mechanical ventilation, including negative- and positive-pressure devices. Selection is based on severity of the underlying problem, anticipated duration of need, whether ventilation is needed continuously or intermittently, cost, complexity of care required, and acceptance by the patient.

### Negative-Pressure Ventilation

Negative-pressure ventilation is applied with a tank ventilator, shell, or body wrap that surrounds the chest and upper abdomen with negative pressure. The negative pressure pulls against the chest wall, causing the thorax to expand. This in turn causes intrathoracic pressure to fall and air to flow into the lungs through the mouth and nose until the pressure difference is equalized. The principle is similar to that of normal respiration, in which contraction of respiratory muscles causes intrathoracic pressure to drop and air to enter the lungs.

### Types of Devices

■ *Tank Ventilator.* The tank ventilator, or "iron lung," is the most powerful negative-pressure ventilator available (Fig. 16-1). Patients who cannot be ventilated on other negative-pressure units can often be ventilated by the iron lung. The patient's entire body, except for the head and neck, is placed inside the sealed tank. The disadvantages of the tank are its size and the fact that the entire body is enclosed. Because it restricts body movement, the tank is primarily used as a nighttime ventilator. Currently manufacturers make units that can sit on top of a bed.

■ *Cuirass (or Shell) Ventilator.* The cuirass negative-pressure ventilator offsets some of the problems associated with the tank. It consists of a rigid shell that fits over the patient's chest and upper abdomen. The shell attaches to a negative-pressure ventilator, such as the Puritan Bennett Multi-Vent, the Life Care NEV-100, or the Monaghan 170-C (Fig. 16-2). Advantages of the cuirass include its smaller size and the increased freedom of movement for the patient. Shell ventilators are less powerful than tanks and require careful fitting of the cuirass to ensure a good seal.

■ *Body Wrap (or "Poncho").* The body wrap, or "poncho," applies negative pressure to the chest (Fig. 16-3). A poncho or bag is put on, with a plastic grid placed over the chest under the wrap. The wrap is then sealed tightly at the arms, neck, and pelvic area, and a negative-pressure ventilator is connected to the bag. The body wrap is more powerful than the cuirass and does not require custom fitting. However, it requires that the patient be in a flat position, which often results in musculoskeletal discomfort severe enough to require the use of nonsteroidal antiinflammatory drugs (NSAIDs).

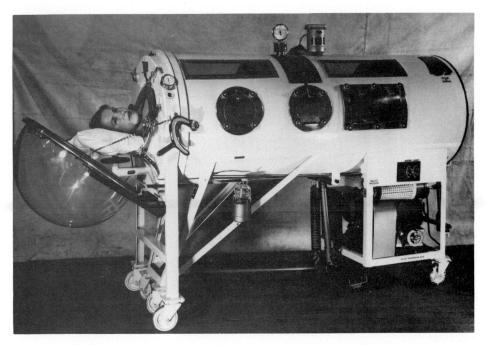

**Fig. 16-1**    Iron lung. (Courtesy J.H. Emerson Company, Cambridge, Mass.)

### Indications for Use

Negative-pressure ventilation is most often used for patients with neuromuscular diseases, kyphoscoliosis, or central hypoventilation (Hill, 1986). It may also benefit some patients with respiratory muscle fatigue resulting from chronic obstructive pulmonary disease (COPD) (Braun, 1984). For patients experiencing respiratory muscle fatigue, periodic mechanical ventilation provides an opportunity for respiratory muscles to rest. When used nocturnally, many patients are able to sustain their ventilatory effort during the day, and symptoms of hypoxemia and hypercapnia decrease or disappear. An advantage of negative-pressure ventilation is that a tracheostomy tube is not required.

### Complications Associated with the Use of Negative-Pressure Ventilation

The following are complications seen with the use of negative-pressure ventilation:

• Upper airway obstruction: This is the major

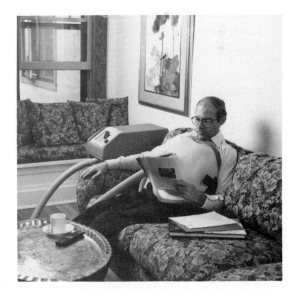

**Fig. 16-2**    Chest shell. (Courtesy Life Care, Lafayette, Colo.)

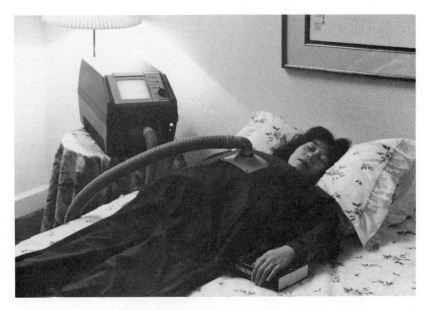

**Fig. 16-3**    Poncho. (Courtesy Life Care, Lafayette, Colo.)

adverse reaction of negative-pressure ventilation, *especially in children;* it is caused by collapse of the trachea during sleep (O'Donohue, 1986).

- Aspiration: Aspiration may occur if patients attempt to eat or drink during negative-pressure ventilation. If continuous negative-pressure ventilation is needed, older children and adults may be trained to coordinate eating and breathing; *however, young children usually require a gastrostomy tube for feedings.*
- Skin breakdown: The primary nursing concern with use of the cuirass is skin breakdown from chafing (Curigan, 1986). A thin undershirt or stockinette over the chest and abdomen helps prevent skin problems.
- Leaks: Leaks occur most often around the clavicle and the iliac crest with the cuirass and around the neck, arms, and legs with the body wrap. Leaks cause a loss of negative pressure, which results in a reduced tidal volume. When a leak occurs, the patient usually feels air being sucked into the cuirass during inspiration. Pa-

tients with spinal deformities may require a custom-fitted cuirass to prevent leaks. *Children require adjustments with growth.*
- Claustrophobia: Claustrophobia can be a problem with any of the negative-pressure devices. An anxious patient may experience overt panic.

### Maintenance

Negative-pressure ventilators require minimal maintenance. As with any device, they should undergo routine preventive maintenance. The cuirass and poncho wraps need to be inspected for wear and replaced as needed.

### Positive-Pressure Ventilation

Positive-pressure ventilation uses pressures greater than atmospheric to force air into the lungs. Portable positive-pressure units are smaller than negative-pressure ventilators and are able to operate from battery power. Continuous positive-pressure ventilation usually requires a tracheostomy to maintain effective ventilation. However,

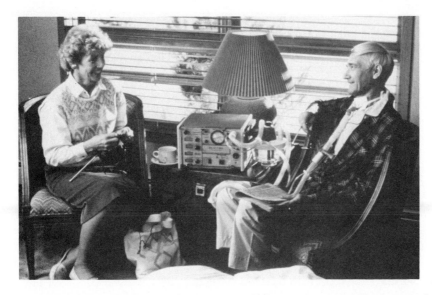

**Fig. 16-4**    PLV-100, a portable positive-pressure ventilator. (Courtesy Life Care, Lafayette, Colo.).

tracheostomies greatly increase complications by causing increased sputum production, tracheal stoma problems, tracheal erosion, and bacterial colonization. Because of these problems, there is increasing interest in periodic positive-pressure ventilation, delivered by a mouthpiece, face mask, or nasal mask.

### Periodic Positive-Pressure Ventilation

Clinical indications for this less invasive form of positive-pressure ventilation include neuromuscular disease, obstructive sleep apnea, central hypoventilation, and restrictive chest wall diseases (e.g., kyphoscoliosis). It does not appear to be useful in COPD (Strumpf, 1991). Criteria for its use include the need for nocturnal ventilation only and minimal pulmonary secretions (Ellis, 1987; Kerby, 1987).

Continuous positive airway pressure (CPAP) and bilevel positive airway pressure (BIPAP) are the devices used to deliver periodic positive airway pressure ventilation (see Fig. 14-7). Unlike negative-pressure devices, they do not cause obstructive sleep apnea. They also tend to be easier to apply and are usually more portable than negative-pressure devices. CPAP and BIPAP are discussed in Chapter 14.

### Continuous Positive-Pressure Ventilation

■ *Types of Devices.* Current portable ventilators can operate on either a volume-limited or pressure-limited basis. With volume-limited positive-pressure ventilation, a preset volume of air is delivered during the inspiratory cycle (Fig. 16-4). The ventilator is set to automatically adjust the pressure required to deliver the preset volume of air. Volume ventilation is especially useful for patients with excessive secretions or bronchospasm. Patients with "stiff lungs" caused by fibrosis or pneumonia require higher inspiratory pressures and are usually ventilated by a volume-limited unit. With pressure-limited ventilation, air flows into the lungs until a preset pressure is reached. Pressure-limited ventilation is most useful with an uncuffed tracheostomy tube. Inspired air leaks around an uncuffed tube, but the pressure-limited system

**Table 16-1**   Features and modes of operation of portable ventilators

| | Companion 2801 | Aequitron LP10 | Life Care PLV 100 | Bear 33 |
|---|---|---|---|---|
| Modes of ventilation | Control<br>Assist<br>SIMV<br>Pressure limit<br>Sigh | Control<br>Assist<br>SIMV<br>Pressure limit | Control<br>Assist<br>SIMV<br>Pressure limited with external control | Control<br>Assist<br>SIMV<br>Pressure limit<br>Sigh |
| Volumes | Tidal volume: 50-2800 ml<br>Sigh: 125-2800 ml | Tidal volume: 100-2200 ml<br>Sigh: Not provided | Tidal volume: 50-3000 ml<br>Sigh: Not provided | Tidal volume: 100-2200 ml<br>Sigh: 1.5 × tidal volume delivered 6 times/hr |
| Breaths per minute | Normal rate: 1-69<br>SIMV rate: 1-69 | Normal rate: 1-38<br>SIMV rate: 1-38 | Normal rate: 2-30<br>SIMV rate: 2-30 | Normal rate: 2-40<br>SIMV rate: 2-40 |
| Flow (liters per minute) | 40-125 | Flow regulated by adjusting inspiratory time | 20-120 | 20-120 |
| Pressure limit (cm $H_2O$) | 10-70 | 15-90 | 10-100 | 10-80 |
| Digital data display | Flow<br>1:E ratio<br>Volume | None—the control knobs are calibrated; parameters are verified with optional printer or handheld spirometer | Volume<br>Rate—machine and spontaneous<br>1:E ratio<br>Flow | Flow<br>1:E ratio<br>Volume<br>Rate<br>Peak flow<br>Assist sensitivity<br>High- and low-pressure alarm |
| Alarm volume | Adjustable | Fixed | Fixed | Fixed |
| Microprocessor | Yes | Yes | Yes | Yes |
| Volume limited | Yes | Yes | Yes | Yes |

compensates for the leak by delivering air until the preset pressure is reached.

■ *Features of Positive-Pressure Ventilators.* Ventilators have a variety of features that can be adjusted to meet the physiologic needs of the patient. The type of ventilator that will best meet the needs of the patient for use in the home environment should be determined well before the patient leaves the hospital. The features and modes of operation of several portable ventilators are summarized in Table 16-1.

1. *Respiratory rate control.* The respiratory rate can be controlled or assisted. With controlled ventilation the patient receives a preset number of breaths per minute. The control for respiration is typically used for patients with neuromuscular disease who cannot initiate inspiration.

In the assist control mode the ventilator senses negative inspiratory efforts made by the patient and cycles on to assist each breath. Should the patient fail to breathe, however, the ventilator will initiate the breath. For example, if the ventilator is set for a backup rate of 12 breaths per minute and the patient triggers the ventilator at least every 5 seconds, the control rate will not engage; but if more than 5 seconds elapses, the ventilator delivers a breath.

Synchronized intermittent mandatory ventilation (SIMV), a feature of most portable ventilators, is not recommended for home use because this mode of ventilation increases work of breathing.

2. *Flow rate control.* Flow refers to the rate (expressed in liters per minute) at which the inspiratory volume is delivered. The flow rate determines inspiratory time (i.e., the faster the flow rate, the shorter the inspiratory time). Patients with rapid breathing rates may require a flow rate above 60 L/min. If the flow rate is inadequate, the set tidal volume may not be delivered. Some machines permit adjustment of inspiratory time rather than flow rate. The shorter the inspiratory time, the faster the flow of air delivered by the ventilator.

3. *Inspiratory pressure limit.* The inspiratory pressure limit can be adjusted on volume-limited ventilators. It is usually set 10 to 20 cm $H_2O$ greater than the cycling pressure. If the inspiratory pressure required to inflate the patient's lungs exceeds the preset pressure limit, a valve opens and excess pressure is released, reducing the potential for barotrauma. Usually ventilators incorporate a high-pressure alarm that sounds when the pressure limit is reached. Most portable ventilators, other than the Puritan Bennett Companion Series, do not have a separate adjustment for the high-pressure alarm. When the pressure limit setting is adjusted, the high-pressure alarm is automatically set at the same level.

A low-pressure alarm activates when the pressure within the patient circuit fails to reach a preset level. The low-pressure limit is set 5 to 10 cm $H_2O$ below the inspiratory cycling pressure. Low-pressure alarms activate when the ventilator fails, there is a leak in the circuit, or the patient becomes disconnected. All of these events require immediate intervention. Because of its importance, the alarm must be tested periodically during the day. It can be tested by removing the patient from the ventilator. In 10 to 15 seconds the alarm will sound. Alarms must be audible throughout the house if the patient is left unattended.

4. *Sigh mode.* A sigh is a periodic deep breath. Although it is normal for persons breathing spontaneously to take sighs, it is not clear that all patients on ventilators need them. Currently, implementation of the sigh mode is based on physician preference. As a general rule, if adult patients are ventilated at 10 to 15 ml/kg ideal body weight and *children at 8 to 12 ml/kg,* sighing is not required. Some portable ventilators are capable of delivering sighs, whereas others are not.

5. *Power modes.* Ventilators operate from either conventional home electricity (AC) or 12-volt battery power (DC). Patients at home should always have an external battery connected to the ventilator that will operate the ventilator for 12 to 18 hours. This ensures that the ventilator will continue to operate should a power outage occur. Ventilators also have a built-in internal battery for emergency backup, which provides power for about 1 hour. Both the internal and external batteries recharge when the ventilator is connected to AC power. If the external battery is used for a long period, however, it should be recharged with a battery charger.

The ventilator automatically selects its own power source, using AC power first if it is available. If not available, it draws power from the external battery. If an external battery is unavailable or the power is low, the ventilator switches to the internal battery. Indicator lights identify the power source being used. Portable ventilators sound an alarm when the power mode changes.

6. *Ventilator circuit.* A ventilator circuit connects the patient to the machine (Fig. 16-5). The circuit has three components: a humidifier, which heats and moistens the delivered air; an exhalation valve, which controls the direction of the airflow; and tubing, which delivers the moistened air from the humidifier to the patient.

7. *Supplemental oxygen port.* Supplemental oxygen can be bled into the circuit of any portable ventilator or can be added to room air as it enters the system. If bled into the circuit, it increases the

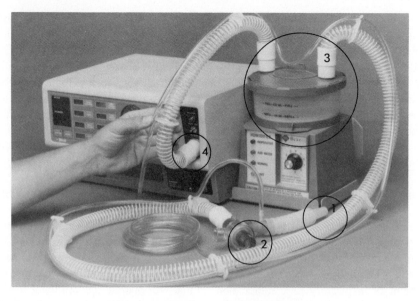

**Fig. 16-5**  Components of ventilator circuit. *1*, Patient-machine connection. *2*, Exhalation assembly, which contains mushroom valve. *3*, Humidifier with inlet and outlet tubing ports. *4*, Tubing-machine connection. Air leaks may occur at any of these areas.

delivered tidal volume. This addition is not clinically significant for adults but may be for small children. *Thus small children should have oxygen added as air enters the ventilator.*

### Potential Problems Associated with the Use of Positive-Pressure Ventilators

The following are potential problems associated with the use of positive-pressure ventilators:

- Barotrauma (lung injury resulting from pressure) is a major risk of positive-pressure ventilation. *Thus tidal volumes should be monitored frequently, especially with children.*
- Impaired cardiac return may result from high intrathoracic pressures, especially in patients with significant air trapping (e.g., patients with COPD) or who are dehydrated. This, in turn, results in impaired cardiac output and hypotension.

### Maintenance

■ *Changing the Ventilator Circuit.* The circuit is typically changed every 24 to 48 hours, although two to three times a week may be sufficient (O'Donohue, 1986). The procedure is as follows:

1. Place clean equipment on a towel and check each component to make sure it is correctly assembled.
2. Fill the humidifier with sterile distilled water.
3. Check the pressure gauge on the ventilator and note the reading.
4. Disconnect the patient from the ventilator circuit and, if possible, have someone ventilate the patient with a hand-operated resuscitator. This is necessary if the patient is completely ventilator dependent. If a second person is unavailable, have the clean circuit assembled and ready before the patient is disconnected so that the change over takes as little time as possible. Give the patient periodic breaths from the resuscitator bag as often as necessary.
5. If required, reset the disconnect alarm each time it sounds during the change of the circuits (reset only needed on LP6 and LP10).

6. Remove each component of the old circuit from the ventilator and immediately replace it with the same component from the clean circuit.

7. Slide the old humidifier off the heater and replace it with the clean humidifier.

8. Check the circuit for air leaks by occluding the tracheostomy connector and observing the maximum pressure setting.

9. If the maximum pressure limit is reached, indicating there are no air leaks, connect the ventilator circuit to the patient.

10. Check the pressure gauge again; the reading should be approximately the same as before the circuit change.

■ *Cleaning the Ventilator Circuit.* Double- or triple-quaternary ammonium disinfectant solutions can be used for cleaning home ventilatory equipment. These are inexpensive, nonirritating detergents that have good bactericidal properties against gram-positive and gram-negative organisms. The solutions are easy to prepare and are reusable for 2 weeks. However, they must be stored in a clean, airtight container.

1. Disassemble the circuit parts and wash vigorously in warm, soapy water using a liquid detergent. A bottle brush is helpful to remove secretions. Do not submerge the ends of small-bore tubes.

2. Rinse the parts well in hot water.

3. Soak in quaternary solution for 20 minutes only. Longer submersion can damage the circuit.

4. Rinse the parts well in hot water.

5. Clean the mushroom valve and assembly separately. Cover the valve stem, then wipe the valve with alcohol. Check the valve for leaks, holes, or tears that would cause the circuit to malfunction.

6. Briskly twirl the large-bore tubes to eliminate excess water, then hang to dry. The suction machine can be used to dry small-bore tubes.

7. Reassemble the circuit parts after they are thoroughly dried and store in a clean plastic bag. Circuit parts can also be stored between two clean towels.

The ventilator circuit can also be cleaned by dishwasher, using the following steps:

1. Disassemble the circuit, placing large parts in the main dishwasher racks and smaller parts in the small baskets.

2. Make sure that the small parts do not fall through the holes. Place these in a mesh bag if they cannot be contained within the dishwasher baskets.

3. Run the dishwasher at the hottest temperature setting using liquid dishwasher detergent.

4. After the dry cycle, open the dishwasher door slightly to reduce condensation.

5. Remove the circuit after about half an hour.

6. Hang large-bore tubes to air dry and use the suction machine to dry small-bore tubes.

7. Reassemble the parts after they are thoroughly dried and store in a clean plastic bag.

## Troubleshooting Equipment Problems

Most ventilator equipment manufacturers provide detailed instructions that describe potential equipment problems and corrective action. However, skill and confidence in correcting problems are best learned through supervised practice sessions at the hospital before discharge and at home in the first couple of weeks when anxiety is the highest. Commonly occurring equipment problems are demonstrated, and the caregiver is guided through the process of identifying and correcting each one.

■ *Air Leaks.* The most common problem encountered with a ventilator circuit is an air leak. Under normal circumstances air passes through a closed circuit to the patient. An air leak within the circuit causes a drop in pressure, triggering the low-pressure alarm. Most air leaks are corrected by checking the components of the circuit and retightening or reconnecting them when necessary. The most common sites for leaks (as depicted in Fig. 16-5) are the following:

- Unsecured patient-to-machine connection
- Thermometer or heat probe that is incorrectly inserted or accidentally left out
- Leak in mushroom valve or tear in diaphragm
- Humidifier jar that is not properly tightened

- Loose connections at any point in the circuit, including connection with machine
- Area around the tracheostomy tube

Leakage of air around a cuffless tube is common in adults and in children who have been ventilated for several months. To compensate for air leaks around the tracheostomy tube, the tidal volume on the ventilator is set higher than the usual tidal volume. Patients using cuffless tubes should have their exhaled tidal volume measured routinely to be certain that they are receiving adequate ventilator volumes. *The usual tidal volume for infants and children is 10 ml/kg (O'Donohue, 1986).*

■ *Increased System Pressure.* If pressure increases above the high-pressure setting, the high-pressure alarm sounds and the pressure does not go any higher. The causes can be a kink or an obstruction in the ventilator tubing, increased airway secretions, water in the circuit, or coughing during inspiration.

■ *Mechanical Failure.* As with any mechanical device, ventilators can malfunction, and they tend to do so once or twice a year. If the ventilator power light goes out and the ventilator fails while other household electrical equipment and lights continue to operate, the problem is clearly in the ventilator. Either a circuit breaker or a fuse has blown or an internal electric malfunction has occurred. Occasionally the internal battery fails to take over when it should. Anytime a mechanical failure occurs, use the hand-operated resuscitator or switch the patient to the backup ventilator (if available) and notify the equipment vendor immediately. If the problem is a power failure, ensure that the ventilator is connected to the external battery, and if indicated, notify the power company. A flashlight should be kept near the ventilator in case of power outages. Matches or candles should not be used.

■ *Indications for a Backup Ventilator.* A backup ventilator should be provided (1) for any patient who is not routinely off the ventilator for at least 4 continuous hours a day and (2) when a replacement ventilator cannot be provided within 2 hours (Plummer, 1989). A high degree of patient or parental anxiety concerning equipment failure may also be an indication for backup equipment.

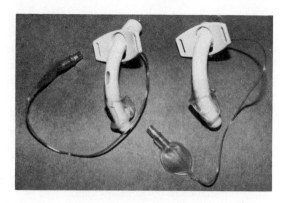

**Fig. 16-6**   Shiley tracheostomy tubes. Cuffed tube on left is fenestrated. (From Dettenmeier PA: *Pulmonary nursing care,* St. Louis, 1992, Mosby.)

## PATIENT WITH A TRACHEOSTOMY
### Types of Tracheostomy Tubes

Tracheostomy tubes can be plastic or metal, cuffed or cuffless, and fenestrated or nonfenestrated. Plastic tubes are made from polyvinyl chloride (PVC), nylon, or Silastic. Plastic tubes may have cuffs that prevent air from escaping through the upper airway (Fig. 16-6). Metal tubes are manufactured from stainless steel and do not have cuffs. A fenestrated tube (Fig. 16-6) is a tube with a window or opening in the posterior wall of the outer cannula. With the inner cannula removed and the outer cannula plugged, exhaled air is diverted through the opening and up through the vocal cords, allowing the patient to speak. Fenestrated tubes that are currently available are indicated only for patients who can breathe without the ventilator for brief periods of time.

### Tracheostomy Plugs and Buttons

If a patient is able to breathe without the ventilator for long periods, the tracheostomy tube can be plugged. When the tube is plugged, the patient can speak, the oropharyngeal airway warms and humidifies inhaled air, and lint and particles are prevented from entering the tracheostomy tube. If the tracheostomy is cuffed, the cuff must be deflated to allow airflow around the tube.

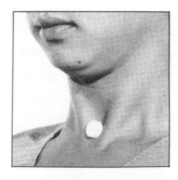

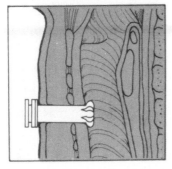

**Fig. 16-7**  Olympic Trach-Button. (Courtesy Olympic Medical, Seattle, Wash.)

In some instances it is desirable to preserve the tracheostomy stoma after the tube has been removed (e.g., if the physician anticipates a need to reinsert the tube at a later date). A tracheostomy button will keep the stoma patent. The Olympic Trach-Button (Olympic Medical, Seattle, Wash.) consists of a firm, hollow, Teflon outer cannula with a mushroom expansion lock that inserts just into the tracheal wall. A closure plug is inserted to occlude the cannula (Fig. 16-7). A Kistner button (Pilling Instruments, Fort Washington, Penn.) can also be used.

### Indications for Selection of Tube

The type of tracheostomy tube used depends on the patient's circumstances. The choice needs to be reevaluated at least once a year. *For children, the type or size of tube changes frequently because* *of growth in airway diameter, changes in ventilation needs, and development of granulation tissue.*

PVC or Silastic tubes are most frequently used in home care because they are soft, conform to the trachea more readily, and cause less tracheal trauma. Also, they do not require an inner cannula. However, metal tubes with inner cannulas are still used in various regions of the United States. They can be easily cleaned and are less expensive because they can be reused. They also tend to cause less local tissue reaction (O'Donohue, 1986).

Cuffless tracheostomy tubes are generally used for patients with neuromuscular problems and for children. *Cuffed tracheostomy tubes are rarely used in children under 8 years of age because the cricoid cartilage is the narrowest part of a child's trachea and serves as a "natural cuff." Pediatric tracheostomy tubes with diameters of less than 5 mm usually provide an adequate seal for positive-pressure ventilation, at least initially (Persky, 1985).* The advantages of cuffless tubes are that they need to be changed less frequently and they rarely result in tracheal irritation. A cuffless tube is preferred in the home setting.

A cuffed tube is necessary if ventilation cannot be maintained in the presence of an air leak. It also helps prevent aspiration in the dysphagic patient.

### Problems Associated with Use of Tracheostomy Tubes

The following are problems associated with the use of tracheostomy tubes:

- Drying of tracheal mucosa: Because the normal humidification mechanisms of the upper airway are bypassed when the patient has a tracheostomy, drying and crusting of the tracheal mucosa may occur and predispose the patient to obstruction, bleeding, and infection.
- Increased mucus: The tracheostomy itself promotes increased mucus production.
- Infection: The tracheostomy quickly becomes colonized with bacteria. Cellulitis and mediastinitis are more likely complications in the patient who has impaired defense mechanisms from corticosteroid therapy.

• Tracheal erosion: Overinflation of the cuff may result in tracheal irritation, ischemia, or necrosis. A low-pressure cuffed tube with a small occluding volume minimizes these complications.

## Speaking with a Tracheostomy

Air leaks around the tracheostomy tube permit the patient to speak during inhalation while using the ventilator. Speech occurs when enough of the ventilator-delivered tidal volume escapes around the tube and goes over the vocal cords. Voice quality depends on the amount of air going over the cords and the flow rate of the ventilator. Faster flow rates cause the speech cycle to be short. The placement of a Passy-Muir speaking valve (Passy-Muir Inc., Irvine, Calif.) in the circuit allows the patient to speak also during exhalation. (Fig 16-8). Another option is the Olympic Trach-Talk (Olympic Medical, Seattle, Wash.) (Fig. 16-9).

## Humidification

The humidifier that is part of the ventilator circuit warms and moisturizes inspired air during mechanical ventilation. When the patient is not being ventilated or if additional humidification is required during ventilation, other systems such as warm or cool mist are useful. Patients off ventilators usually have to use the humidifier when they sleep to ensure adequate humidification. Adequate humidification is particularly important with a new tracheostomy, when significant crusting and obstruction are most likely to occur.

### Artificial Nose

Artificial noses or in-line condensers (Fig. 16-10) may be used as an alternative method to humidify inspired air. They are corrugated filterlike devices that fit snugly over the end of the tracheostomy tube or are placed in-line between the exhalation valve and the patient. During exhalation, moisture from exhaled air condenses onto the filter surface. During inhalation, air passes back through the moisture-laden filter and is warmed and humidified, replicating the natural function of the upper airway.

An artificial nose is used in situations in which humidification is difficult to maintain, such as during transporting or weaning. *It is especially helpful for children with smaller tracheostomy tubes and those who tend to build up secretions on the inside of the tracheostomy tube*. It can also be used during waking hours by ventilated patients with uncuffed tracheostomy tubes, allowing the patient to move around without a bulky humidifier. The nose should be changed daily or more frequently if it becomes soiled with secretions. If the patient has copious secretions or is using a Passy-Muir valve, an artificial nose is not used.

## Tracheostomy Care

The specifics of tracheostomy care differ regionally and between agencies and institutions. However, basic principles remain the same. Careful handwashing before carrying out any aspect of tracheostomy care is essential. *Tracheostomy care for a young child is more easily accomplished by keeping the infant snugly wrapped in a blanket during the procedure*.

### Care of the Stoma

To prevent infection and skin excoriation, the area around the tracheostomy tube should be kept clean and dry. The stoma is cleansed at least daily with a cotton-tipped applicator and water or a 1:1 solution of hydrogen peroxide and water. The stoma should be inspected for redness and formation of granulomas. If skin breakdown is present, cleaning must be done more frequently and povidone-iodine ointment (Betadine) or polymyxin B-Bacitracin (Polysporin) cream applied. A lint-free dressing is often placed around the tube. Dressings are changed one or more times a day, depending on the amount of drainage.

### Changing Tracheostomy Ties

Twill and Velcro ties are available for tracheostomy tubes. Velcro ties can be washed and reused; however, it is important to be sure the Velcro is still functional before it is reused. A procedure for changing twill tracheostomy ties follows:

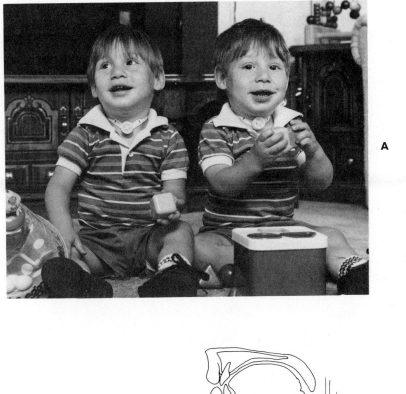

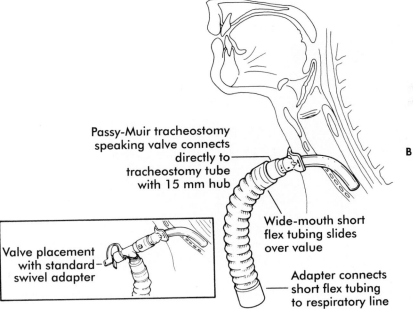

**Fig. 16-8** Passy-Muir tacheostomy speaking valve enables speech by redirection of exhaled air around tracheostomy tube and through nose and mouth. **A,** Used with tracheostomy tube alone. **B,** Used with fully ventilator-dependent patient. (Courtesy Passy-Muir, Inc., Irvine, Calif.)

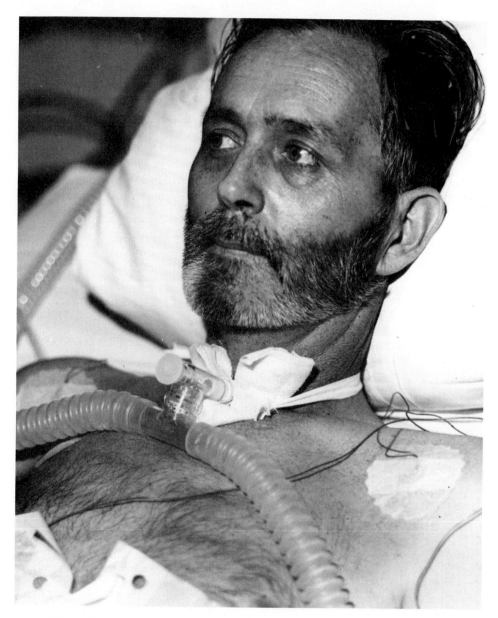

**Fig. 16-9**   Olympic Trach-Talk. (Courtesy Olympic Medical, Seattle, Wash.)

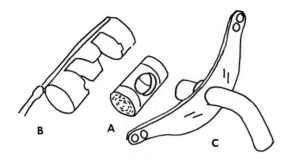

**Fig. 16-10** "Artificial nose." **A,** Thermal humidifying unit, or "artificial nose." **B,** Optional oxygen attachment. **C,** Tracheostomy tube, to which artificial nose attaches.

1. Cut twill ties according to the circumference of the patient's neck. Ties are cut at an unequal length. This allows the knot to be tied at the side of the patient's neck rather than in the back, making it more readily accessible.
2. Cut a slit approximately 1 inch from each end of the ties.
3. Working one side at a time, cut and remove the old tie while holding the tracheostomy tube in place.
4. Pull the slit end of the new tie through the hole on the tube's wing flap, then thread the other end of the tie through the slit and pull tight. Tweezers or a small hemostat may be helpful.
5. Repeat the procedure for the other wing flap.
6. Tie the new ties in a square knot, allowing one fingerbreadth of space between the patient's neck and the ties.

**Changing the Tracheostomy Tube**

The tracheostomy tube or the outer cannula is usually changed for the first time by the physician about 1 week after insertion. Sterile tracheostomy changes are unnecessary, at least for adults, because the trachea becomes colonized with normal flora within days of the initial tracheostomy. If the first tracheostomy change goes smoothly, subsequent changes can be made by the home care nurse or by the caregiver with the assistance of the home care nurse. The frequency with which the tube is changed depends on factors such as secretion volume, airway size, and the presence of a cough. For adults, cuffed tubes usually require replacement every 4 to 8 weeks. Uncuffed tubes can be kept in place up to 6 months. *Children typically require more frequent changes, ranging from three times a week to once a month. Tracheostomy changes for young children should always be performed with two people present.* The following procedure can be used for changing the outer cannula:

1. If the tube is cuffed, check for leaks by using a syringe to inflate the new cuff with air, then deflate.
2. Remove the inner cannula, insert the obturator into the outer cannula of the new tube, and attach the tracheostomy tube ties.
3. Apply a water-soluble lubricant sparingly to the external cannula and obturator of the new tube.
4. With the patient's neck extended slightly, give three full breaths with a hand-operated resuscitator.
5. Cut the old tracheostomy tube ties, deflate the cuff (if present), and gently slide the tube out.
6. Slide the new tube in by curving it back and downward, but *do not* force.
7. Immediately remove the obturator, insert the inner cannula, and lock it in place.
8. Fasten the tracheostomy ties and place the patient back on the ventilator.
9. Inflate the cuff (if present) with the prescribed amount of air.
10. Observe the patient for any respiratory difficulty. Auscultate breath sounds in both lungs to be sure that ventilation is adequate.

**Cleaning the Tracheostomy Tube**

As with other aspects of tracheostomy care, specific procedures vary, based on empiric experience. Few controlled studies of the efficacy of specific protocols or cleaning solutions have appeared in the literature. However, basic elements of any cleaning procedure must include removal of secretions, followed by thorough washing. Because bacteria thrive best in a warm moist atmosphere, air drying is a necessary final component to the procedure. Tracheostomy tubes can also be washed in the dishwasher, but it is important to be sure that any secretions are brushed and rinsed out beforehand. A procedure for manual cleaning is as follows:

1. Separate and soak the tracheostomy tube and obturator in hydrogen peroxide for approximately 1 hour.
2. Use a small brush as needed to remove secretions.
3. Rinse the tube and obturator in hot water.
4. Air dry.

Some health care providers feel that disposable tracheostomy tubes should not be reused, and manufacturers will not guarantee disposable equipment that has been reused.

### Cleaning the Inner Cannula

Begin by giving the patient three full breaths with a manual resuscitator. Remove the inner cannula and soak it in hydrogen peroxide. Suction the outer cannula. Clean the inner cannula with a pipe cleaner or small brush, then rinse under tap water. Shake dry and replace. A temporary inner cannula that can be used to maintain ventilation while the regular cannula is being cleansed is available for the Shiley tracheostomy tube.

### Suctioning the Tracheostomy

The tracheostomy is suctioned as needed to remove accumulated secretions. *Children usually need suctioning before naptime and bedtime and on awakening*. Brief suctioning within the tracheostomy tube is called "top suctioning" and is usually sufficient. However, deeper suctioning is occasionally necessary. The trachea may be instilled with sterile normal saline solution whenever secretions are thick and dry. However, if secretions are dry even with adequate oral hydration, increased humidification may be necessary. Clean, rather than sterile, suctioning technique is usually acceptable for the home care patient.

1. Gather all equipment for suctioning and place on a clean surface:
   Suction machine

   Clean catheter
   Clean glove
   Clean paper cup containing fresh tap water
   Sterile saline solution, if needed
2. Turn on the suction machine and check for the correct setting. Recommended vacuum settings are the following:
   7 to 15 inches Hg for adults
   *5 to 10 inches Hg for children*
   *3 to 5 inches Hg for infants*
3. Put on clean glove (optional) and connect suction catheter to the suction machine connecting tube.
4. If necessary, instill 1 to 2 ml of sterile saline solution into the tracheostomy tube.
5. Give three full breaths with the hand-operated resuscitator or ventilator.
6. Without applying suction, insert catheter gently to just beyond the end of the tracheostomy tube.
7. When the patient coughs or if obstruction is met, withdraw the catheter by rotating it while applying suction. The total time for suctioning should be no longer than 10 to 15 seconds at a time *(5 seconds for a child)* (O'Donohue, 1986).
8. Give the patient three full breaths.
9. Repeat above steps until the airway is clear.
10. Rinse suction catheter with water. Use the vacuum to draw air through the catheter until the inside is dry.
11. Wipe the outside of the catheter with a $4 \times 4$ or a lint-free tissue and place between the folds of a clean towel or in a clean, covered basin for storage.

Suction catheters are typically changed every 8 to 24 hours. Over time, however, even once daily changes become expensive. Therefore patients with mature tracheostomies may be able to reclean, disinfect, and reuse catheters. Catheters should be cleaned by thorough washing in soap and water. Rubber and plastic catheters can be boiled in water for 10 minutes. They can be stored in a plastic bag or container after they are thoroughly dry. Size 6 to 10 French suction catheters may be too small to clean properly for reuse.

# NURSING CARE OF THE VENTILATOR-DEPENDENT PATIENT AT HOME
## Role of the Nurse

To accept responsibility and liability for safely managing a home ventilator program, nurses must expand their clinical knowledge and skills regarding ventilator-dependent patients. A detailed orientation to the operation, troubleshooting, and maintenance of the ventilator and other equipment is essential. The nurse must have an understanding of the patient's physiologic and psychosocial needs and must be able to perform all care procedures, including emergency care. The necessary technical skills are acquired through specialized training and supervised clinical practice. Recent hospital experience caring for ventilator-dependent patients is extremely helpful but not essential. In some communities, where formal training programs have been developed, improved knowledge, skill, and confidence as a result of the specialized training have been documented (Dettenmeir, 1986).

## Avoiding Common Problems for Ventilator-Dependent Patients
### Planning for Emergencies

The family can improve their response to any type of emergency by following these recommendations:

- Install a telephone in the patient's room (or in the room where the patient spends the most time) with a list of emergency phone numbers nearby. If a second telephone cannot be installed, emergency numbers should be kept near the main household phone. In addition, keep a list of current ventilator settings readily accessible.
- Place all emergency equipment (e.g., a hand-operated resuscitator and spare tracheostomy tube) in the patient's room so they are easily located in an emergency. Check emergency equipment periodically for cleanliness and function.
- Develop written emergency procedures for physiologic problems and ventilator malfunction.

- If the patient is prone to life-threatening physiologic emergencies, train family and caregivers in cardiopulmonary resuscitation (CPR). Periodically review CPR techniques.

### Planning for Outings

Newly ventilator-dependent patients are understandably apprehensive about venturing out. They may fear the possibility of an emergency occurring while away from home. More likely, however, they are self-conscious and fearful about going out into the "real" world among "normal" people. The ventilator, tubes, and wheelchair make patients feel conspicuous and different. To ease these apprehensions about going out, caregivers can remove unnecessary equipment, such as the humidifier, and streamline the system by winding up and concealing electrical cords. Besides being safer, this makes the equipment somewhat less noticeable.

A checklist should be developed and consulted when the patient and family go out. An outing checklist should include, but not be limited to, the following items:

*Things to do*
- Evaluate the destination for wheelchair accessibility and possible internal power source.
- Secure ventilator on wheelchair or cart.
- Check "going-out" bag.
- Suction patient's airway if necessary.
- Streamline ventilator.

*Things to include in "going-out" bag*
- Hand-operated resuscitator
- Portable suction machine
- Adequate supply of catheters and gloves for suctioning
- Normal saline ampules (if tracheal instillation required)
- Spare tracheostomy tube with ties in case the patient's tube comes out
- Lubricant to insert tracheostomy tube
- Scissors to cut tracheostomy ties in case of emergency
- Collapsible plastic cup
- Three-prong electrical adapter
- Emergency phone numbers
- List of ventilator settings

The checklist decreases the likelihood of forgetting something and helps ensure that the destination is accessible. These considerations are especially important if the family is traveling a long distance. An outing checklist also provides psychologic reassurance that emergencies are adequately prepared for. Maintaining a "going-out bag" alleviates the task of gathering essential items every time an outing is planned.

When planning a trip, caregivers should always check the weather report for the possibility of rain or snow. Unless the ventilator has a splash-proof casing, it must be protected from getting wet. The ventilator itself can be protected with a plastic cover or rubber raincoat, but the air inlet filter must always remain uncovered. Ventilators are usually not affected by extreme cold unless they are exposed to low temperatures while not in operation for a prolonged period. If this occurs, allow the ventilator to warm up at room temperature for half an hour before using.

### Bathing

Bathing the patient creates a problem because of the potential dangers that arise when using electricity near water. Yet this problem is easily overcome if steps are taken to minimize dangers. Patients are either sponge or tub bathed. Because of the advantages and disadvantages of each, a bathing schedule combining both methods is ideal. The frequency of each method depends on the situation of the patient and the caregiver. A sponge bath is a straightforward procedure and is not discussed here. Although a tub bath can be quite a physical undertaking, it can be accomplished with minimal danger. A tub bath is carried out using a handheld shower nozzle with the patient sitting directly in the tub or on a bath seat. The tubing circuit may get wet, but the exhalation valve must not be immersed. The following precautions should be taken for a safe tub bath:

- Use the ventilator's internal battery as the power source, and do not use the humidifier. This eliminates the possibility of electrical cords getting wet.

- Keep the ventilator as far away from the bathtub as possible. Add an extra length of large-bore tubing to allow the ventilator to be placed further away.
- Keep the ventilator off the floor so that contact with puddles is avoided.
- Cover the ventilator (but not the air inlet filter) with plastic.
- Use a portable, battery-operated suction machine if the patient's airway needs to be suctioned during the bath.

### Hiring Assistants

If the patient's care is not complex and professional caregivers are not employed, the patient and family may want to hire someone without formal medical training. Assistants may be found by advertising on college campuses and through resource centers for the disabled, church organizations, employment agencies, and help wanted columns. Health care agencies and nursing or physical therapy schools may also be of assistance. Unfortunately, the turnover rate for assistants is generally high.

If the patient is old enough, he or she should be involved in interviewing potential employees. Compatibility with the patient is extremely important so that the patient feels comfortable with the individual. Unless the assistant is hired through an agency, the patient, family, or both must determine that the person is honest, reliable, punctual, and a quick and capable learner. The last is important because of the amount of information the caregiver must learn. Although personality characteristics are difficult to determine in one or two interviews, much can be learned about a person if the right questions are asked. In addition, references should be checked thoroughly.

### Spinal Cord–Injured Patients

Spinal cord lesions above the C4 level are normally associated with lifelong ventilator dependency and quadriplegia. The patient's inability to survive for more than a few minutes without using the ventilator increases the risks and stress associated with care. Discharge planning is complex. Often there are problems in finding suitable caregivers and helping the patient and family make necessary psychologic adjustments. Caregivers must be skilled in patient positioning, assisting with bowel and bladder programs, nutrition, contracture prevention, and the psychologic implications of spinal cord injuries.

Unless the patient's body position is changed every 1 to 2 hours, pressure sores will develop. Pressure sores form easily and heal slowly. Special mattresses can minimize problems but are not a substitute for frequent position changes. Loss of bowel and bladder control results in incontinence and fecal impaction. Bowel and bladder programs initiated in the hospital need to be continued at home. Foods high in protein promote skin integrity and decrease the likelihood of pressure sores. High fluid intake prevents urinary tract infections and formation of calculi and may help keep secretions thin. Full range of motion exercises are necessary two to three times daily to preserve joint mobility. Padded footboards are used to prevent footdrop.

High spinal cord–injured patients' inability to bathe, toilet, dress, and feed themselves results in feelings of helplessness and often great frustration. They may be intensely afraid of becoming disconnected from the ventilator when left alone. Profound alterations in body image and feelings of worthlessness, guilt, or depression are common. Spinal cord–injured adults must adjust to major losses in their roles as spouse, parent, breadwinner, and friend. They may respond to these losses with anger, manipulation, and regressive behavior. Loss of sexual function can be particularly devastating. Psychosocial issues and sexuality are discussed in Chapters 17 to 19.

## Care of Ventilator-Dependent Children

*The care of the ventilator-dependent child is a particularly challenging responsibility. Children may have more difficulties with respiratory infections and dysfunction than adults because their pulmonary systems are less well developed. Greater instability in a ventilator-dependent child often re-*

*sults in more frequent hospitalizations. Ventilator-dependent children often have associated gastro-esophageal reflux, which may require treatment (O'Donohue, 1986). Because the margins for error are smaller with children, skill in technical procedures is extremely important. Also, because infants and young children cannot describe what is wrong, skill in physical assessment and recognition of equipment problems is essential. Issues of growth and development unique to children must also be considered in implementing the plan of care.*

*As the ventilator-dependent child grows and the lungs develop, larger tracheostomy tubes are needed and adjustments must be made in ventilator settings and oxygen concentration. The F$IO_2$ and tidal volume settings may also need to be adjusted if the child develops an infection. Thus the pediatrician or pulmonologist must be actively involved in the home care plan.*

### Growth and Development

*Infants with chronic lung disease are often delayed in their growth and development and require home physical therapy to assist in achieving normal developmental skills. Pediatric physical and occupational therapists can teach caregivers to stimulate and train infants in nippling techniques, rolling, crawling, and other developmental exercises.*

### Weaning from the Ventilator

*As the ventilator-dependent child grows, weaning from the ventilator is often possible. Sometimes this weaning occurs naturally as a result of the child's growth; ventilator or oxygen settings may remain unchanged but because new alveoli are developing, lung function improves and the relative contribution of the ventilator volume to total ventilation is reduced. For others, a weaning protocol may be needed. Children are best weaned during periods of growth stability. Increased ventilation may be needed during growth spurts or if the child regresses, fails to maintain normal height and weight, or develops an infection.*

*The child's response to weaning efforts is closely monitored to ensure adequate ventilatory function. Serum bicarbonate levels are used for indirect evaluation of a steady state. Capillary blood gases are followed to determine carbon dioxide and acid-base trends, and oximetry is used to follow oxygen saturation levels.*

### Weaning from the Tracheostomy

*Once the physician determines the child is ready, weaning from a tracheostomy can often be accomplished at home by replacing the tube with progressively smaller tubes on a regular schedule. For example, a smaller tube may be substituted every week at the time of the routine tracheostomy change. Once the child has been weaned to the smallest tube, the tracheostomy tube is plugged for increasing periods each day. When it can be plugged for many hours at a time or all night without causing any increase in the work of breathing, the tube can be removed. The child should be able to tolerate having the tube plugged for a full 24 to 48 hours before the tube is removed.*

### Humidification

*To prevent drying of mucous membranes, inspired ventilator air must be saturated with warmed water vapor. The small airways of children become obstructed more readily than adult airways. Water accumulates rapidly in the smaller-bore tubing circuits used for children and must be emptied more frequently.*

### Safety

*Small objects, medications, and cleaning solutions must be kept out of reach of the child. Powders or aerosols should not be allowed because they may cause airway irritation. Fuzzy blankets or clothing should be avoided because lint can be inhaled. A child with a tracheostomy should be kept away from sandboxes or the beach, especially on windy days. Ventilator controls need to be secured so that the child or siblings cannot tamper with the settings. To reduce the risk of infection and prevent accidental extubation, other children*

*must be prevented from touching the tracheostomy tube.*

*The child may be bathed in a tub with continuous observation. If the ventilator is not required for short periods, a 4 × 4 placed over the tracheostomy tube or an artificial nose helps protect it from splashing water. Boating, rafting, and swimming are not advised because of the risk of water splashing into the tracheostomy tube or of drowning caused by accidental submersion.*

### Recognition of Infection

*Children who develop respiratory infections can quickly develop high fevers. The parent or care-giver should contact the physician if the child exhibits signs and symptoms of infection. These include fever over 101° F, increased cough, change in sputum color or odor, rash, drainage, and un-usual odor around the tracheostomy stoma. Rapid breathing that persists after suctioning may also indicate infection, although tachypnea often occurs with fever as the result of other causes. If persistent irritability or lethargy occurs, the physician should be called.*

### Recognition of Respiratory Distress

*If signs and symptoms of respiratory distress occur, the caregiver immediately suctions the tracheostomy tube. If the catheter meets resistance, the tube should be changed because it may be obstructed. Signs and symptoms of respiratory distress in children are presented in Table 3-4 (p. 61).*

### Mobility

*It is important for the child to be as mobile as possible. Wheelchairs and carts especially adapted for portable home ventilators are available and can be obtained through a rehabilitation center or equipment vendor. Families may need encouragment at first to try excursions outside the home.*

*Whenever possible, ventilator-dependent children should attend regular schools. This requires preparation and close cooperation of school staff, but it can often be arranged.*

## Respite Care

Because home care of a ventilator-dependent patient can be demanding, family caregivers need time for themselves on a regular basis. Some feel compelled to provide constant care for the patient. To assume full responsibility for 24-hour care over an extended period of time is unrealistic and inevitably results in exhaustion and "burnout," particularly in single-parent families or families with other young children. Respite care is often needed to restore the family's energy so that members can continue to meet the patient's emotional and physical needs.

Occasionally private insurance companies and health maintenance organizations (HMOs) pay for respite care, although this coverage is difficult to obtain. Third-party payors may cover respite care if they can be convinced that the alternative is rehospitalization. If funding is unavailable, families should be encouraged to rely on trusted relatives or friends who can be trained to care for the patient on a regular basis. Whenever possible, the patient should participate in the selection of the alternative care provider.

### REFERENCES

Braun NM, Marino WD: Effects of daily intermittent rest of the respiratory muscles in patients with severe chronic airflow limitation, *Chest* 85:595, 1984.

Curigan L, Sparapani M: The chest cuirass and related nursing management, *Rehabil Nursing* II:17, 1986.

Dettenmeier PA, Feldman-Malen J, Vogt-Yanta M: Management of patients on mechanical ventilation from hospital to home: courses 1 and 2, *Am Rev Respir Dis* 138:A353, 1986.

Ellis ER et al: Treatment of respiratory failure during sleep in patients with neuromuscular disease: positive pressure through a nosemask, *Am Rev Respir Dis* 135:148, 1987.

Hill NG: Clinical applications of body ventilators, *Chest* 90:897, 1986.

Kerby GR, Mayer LS, Pingleton SK: Nocturnal and pressure ventilation via nasal mask, *Am Rev Respir Dis* 135:738, 1987.

O'Donohue WJ et al: Long-term mechanical ventilation: guidelines for management in the home and at alternative community sites, *Chest* 90:1S, 1986.

Persky M: Airway management and post inhalation sequelae. In Zimmerman S, Gilden J, editors: *Critical care pediatrics,* Philadelphia, 1985, WB Saunders.

Plummer AL, O'Donohue WJ, Petty TL: Conference report: consensus conference on problems in home mechanical ventilation, *Am Rev Respir Dis* 140:555, 1989.

Strumpf DA et al: Nocturnal positive pressure ventilation via nasal mask in patients with severe chronic obstructive pulmonary disease, *Am Rev Respir Dis* 144:1234, 1991.

### SUGGESTED READINGS

Donner CF, Howard P, Robert D: Consensus conference on recommendations for home mechanical ventilation, *European Respiratory Review* 2, No 10, Dec 1992.

Johnson D, Giovannoni RM, Driscoll SA: *Ventilator assisted patient care: planning for hospital discharge and home care,* Rockville, Md, 1986, Aspen Publications.

Make BJ, Gilmartin ME: Rehabilitation and homecare for ventilator-assisted individuals, *Clin Chest Med* 7:679, 1986.

McCoy P, Feenan L: Alterations in respiratory function. In McCoy P, Votroubek W, editors: *Pediatric home care,* Rockville, Md, 1990, Aspen Publications.

Thomas VM et al: Caring for the person receiving ventilatory support at home: care givers' needs and involvement, *Heart Lung* 21:180, 1992.

# Quality of Life Issues

# CHAPTER 17

# PSYCHOSOCIAL CONSIDERATIONS IN THE CARE OF THE ADULT WITH CHRONIC PULMONARY DISEASE

LINDA K. FAHR

People with chronic lung disease struggle daily to cope with the disheartening and frustrating effects of their illness. Nurses and other caregivers face the challenge of facilitating this process of coping and adaptation. The purpose of this chapter is to provide insight into the behavioral responses, coping patterns, and psychosocial problems frequently experienced by adults with pulmonary disease and to discuss the recognition and management of anxiety and depression, common coexisting problems in people with chronic lung disease that markedly impair functional capacity and quality of life.

## PSYCHOSOCIAL MANIFESTATIONS OF CHRONIC LUNG DISEASE

Patients with chronic lung disease are likely to respond in a variety of ways—some adaptive, some maladaptive—to the multiple problems with which they must grapple. Response patterns vary greatly between patients. Patterns also evolve over time as a manifestation of the grieving process or as a reflection of worsening disease severity.

### Loss of Self-Esteem

Chronic pulmonary disease is characterized by symptoms and changes in physical appearance that may alter body image and threaten self-esteem.

Examples include chronic productive cough, barrel chest configuration, clubbing of extremities, fluid retention, cushingoid changes, and the need to use oxygen therapy equipment in public.

Pulmonary disability also poses a major threat to self-esteem. Initially, dyspnea may only limit physical stamina and threaten athletic prowess, but eventually it threatens job security and the ability to manage even simple activities of daily living. These disabilities are particularly difficult for people who place great importance on their role as breadwinner.

### Overdependence

For some the added attention, freedom from responsibility, and comfort of being taken care of may outweigh the need for independence and diminish more healthy, independent behaviors. Some comforting aspects of illness may be hard for a patient to give up. As limitations forced by the illness increase dependence, the patient is likely to become more childlike, demanding, and difficult to please.

### Anger and Frustration

Anger is part of the grieving process, and its expression is often a necessary step toward coping with the losses associated with chronic pulmonary disease. Fear of alienating spouses by expressing anger may cause patients to lash out instead at home care staff. Conversely, patients may feel safe in expressing anger toward spouses who cannot easily abandon them, but may be careful to control outbursts directed at the health care providers on whom they depend for ongoing care. Some patients learn to repress emotion in an effort to avoid uncomfortable symptoms (termed the emotional straitjacket effect) (Dudley, 1980), but this can be counterproductive because anger and frustration mount and feelings finally are expressed at inappropriate times.

### Guilt

Individuals who have contributed to their pulmonary disease by smoking may feel guilt or remorse about their habit. This guilt may be reinforced by family or friends who may view the patient as a malingerer. The adage that "sick lungs don't show" may lead patients to adopt illness behaviors to convince others that their disability is real, a response that only adds to the feelings of guilt.

### Somatization

A preoccupation with somatic complaints is a common feature in patients with chronic lung disease and is exaggerated in hypoxemic patients (McSweeny, 1982). It is a predominant feature of depression (Katon, 1984). Anxious patients with many somatic complaints and poor overall quality of life are likely to overuse emergency care services (Traver, 1988). Somatic complaints may be a way of masking a more painful affective state, such as depression, or it may be that an increased awareness of symptoms relating to one body system produces an increased awareness of symptoms relating to other body systems. Caregivers often feed into this preoccupation by routinely asking about symptoms, creating a symptom-focused mindset for both patient and caregiver.

### Noncompliance with the Treatment Regimen

Noncompliant behavior takes various forms in patients with pulmonary disorders, ranging from refusal to see the physician to the manipulation of medications in attempts at self-treatment. For some, noncompliance represents denial of the seriousness of the problem. For others it is an expression of independence and control. Noncompliance may also be a cry for help or a means of expressing anger, or it may represent a last attempt to withdraw from a painful and seemingly hopeless situation. In end-stage chronic obstructive pulmonary disease (COPD) it may signal the patient's resignation to death. Noncompliance is discussed in Chapter 21.

### Manipulative Behavior

Some individuals with advanced disease become manipulative, presumably in an attempt to control the few aspects of their lives that seem within their control. Unfortunately, this behavior is usually counterproductive, giving rise to feelings of intense frustration in those who are being manipulated. Some caregivers eventually tire of the game playing and withdraw from the patient; others remain caught in the "manipulation trap" and succumb to burnout.

## ROLE OF NEUROPSYCHOLOGIC DEFICITS

Many patients with COPD who have moderate or severe hypoxemia have neuropsychologic deficits suggestive of cerebral dysfunction (Prigitano, 1983; Grant, 1982). These deficits are presumably caused, at least in part, by insufficient cerebral oxygenation.

Cognitive functions most affected in COPD are the ability to acquire and retain new information, to form new concepts and think flexibly, and to perform complex perceptual-motor maneuvers and engage in simple perceptual discriminations—all skills that are important in learning to adapt to a complex chronic illness. Decrements in motor speed, strength, and coordination also are often present. Patients tend to perform best on tests of verbal ability and intermediate verbal memory, suggesting that the deficits may be easy to overlook if caregivers are rushed or not alert to subtle indicators of cognitive difficulty.

The tendency of some patients with advanced COPD to be obstreperous, inflexible, or seemingly lacking in insight about the effects of their behavior on their condition may be related to a mild organic brain disorder. Major personality changes such as paranoia or apathy may also reflect increased cerebral dysfunction.

## DEFENSE MECHANISMS AGAINST PSYCHOLOGIC DISTRESS

When anxiety or psychologic discomfort reaches a certain degree of intensity, the individual begins to use defense mechanisms (Table 17-1). These defense mechanisms are unconscious and involuntarily employed by the patient. Clinically apparent anxiety may be seen in terms of failure of defenses.

### Role of Psychosocial Coping Assets

People with chronic lung disease vary widely in their ability to cope effectively with their disease. Some manage productive and fulfilling lives despite severe physiologic impairment, whereas others with relatively mild physical impairment are profoundly impaired functionally. Clearly, disease severity is not the most important determinant of how well a patient copes. More important factors include age, socioeconomic status, educational level, neuropsychologic functioning, and the presence of psychosocial assets.

Psychosocial assets include external social supports and internal, personality-based characteristics that enhance an individual's ability to cope with adversity. Financial security, comfortable and adequate housing, educational achievement, and social support (i.e., being loved, feeling esteemed, being part of a mutual "defense system" that one can use if needed) are examples of external supports. Flexibility, good judgment, congeniality, freedom from oversensitivity, the ability to adapt to things that cannot be changed, and a willingness to accept reasonable responsibility are examples of personality-oriented assets. Patients who possess many psychosocial assets are able to deal more effectively with their illness and are more responsive to rehabilitative efforts than are patients with few such assets.

Attitudes and beliefs are an outgrowth of psychosocial assets and can affect functional ability. Indeed, attitudes and beliefs were found to greatly outweigh measures of mood or ventilatory capacity as predictors of 12-minute walk distance in a group of patients with chronic bronchitis (Morgan, 1983). The patients who walked farthest were those with positive attitudes, confidence in the value of treatment, and a belief in the value of exercise. Those who had a negative attitude toward treatment or a fear of exercise walked shorter distances.

## PSYCHOSOCIAL PROBLEMS COMMON TO OLDER ADULTS
### Loss

Patients of all ages with lung disease experience sudden and gradual losses. Unique to the older patient, however, are the more frequent loss of friends and family through death, loss of income and self-esteem resulting from premature retirement, and loss of status in a culture that focuses on youth, vigor, and productivity.

### Financial Concerns

The older adult with respiratory disease often faces early disability and retirement and may have to live prematurely on a fixed income. Additionally, older adults spend a disproportionate share of income on health care. Some patients are forced to sell their homes or other treasured assets to pay medical bills. Financial concerns are major contributors to anxiety and depression.

### Normal Effects of Aging

Increased frailty, diminished taste, sight, and hearing, and other "normal" effects of aging add to the disability associated with chronic lung disease and further impair the patient's quality of life. With aging there is also an increased likelihood of neurologic deficits and the inevitable progression of COPD.

### Coexisting Medical Diagnoses

Multiple diagnoses add greatly to the overall burden of illness. Because so many patients with chronic lung disease are older and have smoked,

**Table 17-1**   Common psychologic defense mechanisms

| Mechanism and description | Adaptive functions | Maladaptive effects |
|---|---|---|
| **Denial** Avoidance of potential threat by subconsciously refusing to recognize, intellectually or emotionally, that it exists | Protects against overwhelming anxiety | Often compromises compliance with therapy; tends to disintegrate when inconsistency with reality eventually becomes more apparent, resulting in depression, personality disorganization, and even suicidal ideation |
| **Repression** Exclusion from consciousness of unacceptable feelings or impulses (e.g., anger) | Eliminates need to deal with intense emotions and may reduce associated dyspnea | Prevents resolution of underlying problems; adds to psychic turmoil |
| **Intellectualization** Use of overly intellectual approach to one's illness | Reduces anxiety by distancing and depersonalizing problems; diminishes personal threat of illness | Isolates patient emotionally; interferes with ability to deal with affective response to illness |
| **Regression** Adoption of earlier modes of behavior that the patient found comforting or useful (e.g., overdependence, infantile behavior) | May be helpful during acute phase of illness | Prevents progress towards optimal independence in activities of daily living; when used chronically, alienates caregivers |
| **Displacement** Patient focuses on less threatening symptom (e.g., excessive concern about bowel function) | Reduces anxiety by deflecting attention away from more frightening symptoms (e.g., dyspnea) | Can result in unnecessary diagnostic workups; can compromise compliance as patients focus on measures to relieve their symptom of concern and ignore measures related to more physiologically threatening symptoms |
| **Introjection** Patient turns feelings onto self in punitive fashion; may blame self for illness and believe punishment is deserved; may be symptom of depression | | Adds to guilt and psychic distress |
| **Projection** Patient blames others or environment for illness; refuses to accept responsibility for events occurring in the course of the illness | "Absolves" patient of responsibility for illness or for illness-enhancing behaviors | Alienates others, resulting in social isolation; may facilitate continuation of self-destructive behaviors (e.g., smoking) |

coexisting diagnoses such as lung cancer, hypertension, and cardiovascular disease are common. Problems resulting from the treatment of coexisting illnesses can further complicate the situation. Nutritional deficiencies are common in an older frail population and can affect both physical and emotional well-being.

## Loneliness and Social Isolation

With the development of exertional dyspnea, older patients who may already be limited in their physical activities begin to cut back even more. Social activities are often the first to go. Unwillingness to risk the increase in dyspnea that may result from animated social interaction causes many to avoid even those social situations that do not require physical activity. Thus patients with COPD are often viewed as socially withdrawn and difficult to get along with. Although relatives tend to expect less of breathless patients, they may still be unhappy with a patient's social functioning. A circular process is set in motion whereby patients' tendency to withdraw encourages others to leave them alone, reinforcing their loneliness and social isolation.

## PSYCHOSOCIAL PROBLEMS COMMON TO THE YOUNGER ADULT

The two chronic lung diseases that have the greatest psychosocial impact on young adults are cystic fibrosis and chronic, severe steroid-dependent asthma. Major issues of concern are body image, meaningful work, courtship, marriage, and parenthood. Young men may feel especially sensitive about their lack of strength, muscular development, and athletic prowess. Both men and women are often embarrassed by expectoration of sputum and sensitive about taking medication or treatments in public. Opportunities for socialization with healthy peers may be limited because of the constraints imposed by the illness, thereby interfering with normal adult social development. Attending school and obtaining academic degrees can become major hurdles for those with significant pulmonary dysfunction. Such patients may also be

limited in the occupational roles for which they can prepare, and once they are employed, excessive use of sick time may threaten job security.

## Lack of Medical Insurance

Once teenagers reach 18 years of age or are no longer full-time students (and therefore dependents), most insurance companies will no longer include them on their parents' policy. Yet medical insurers typically exclude coverage for a preexisting illness, making it difficult to obtain health insurance. Faced with this dilemma, some accept or remain on a job they may not want, simply because it provides medical benefits. Others opt to go on disability benefits as a means of securing medical coverage, although they may still be physically capable of part-time work. Still others struggle to continue working despite severe disability, fearful of losing what coverage they have. Patients without coverage often defer needed medical care.

## Dating, Marriage, and Family Issues

Young adults with cystic fibrosis must grapple with major philosophic issues surrounding courtship, marriage, and family. Although their life expectancy is increasing, few live into their fourth decade. With increasing age comes an increasing severity of illness and the knowledge that time is running out. This knowledge often results in reluctance to initiate or maintain relationships for fear of rejection when the illness is revealed to the partner, or an unwillingness to enter a relationship that may end in loss and heartache. Some individuals cope by denying the seriousness of the problem both to themselves and to their prospective partners. Others confront the realities head on. Maturity and a great deal of love are required by couples entering into a committed relationship.

Most men with cystic fibrosis are infertile, and thickened cervical mucus may reduce fertility in women. Also, women with markedly compromised lung function usually cannot tolerate the physiologic stress of pregnancy and may suffer life-threatening complications. Thus marriage for someone with cystic fibrosis brings with it the possibility that the couple will remain childless. However, women with well-preserved lung function (e.g., forced vital capacity [FVC] of at least 70% predicted) appear to tolerate pregnancy quite well and increasingly are choosing to become pregnant. Therefore genetic counseling is needed for patients with cystic fibrosis. Several issues emerge in the decision concerning pregnancy. For example, is the couple willing to do the following:

- Bear a child who is a carrier for the gene?
- Risk having a child who may also have cystic fibrosis?
- Risk an accelerated decline in lung function during the pregnancy?
- Begin a family knowing that one parent may not live long enough to finish raising the child?

Genetic issues in cystic fibrosis are discussed in Chapter 19.

## ASSESSING PSYCHOSOCIAL ADJUSTMENT

Careful observation of patients in their home setting often yields clues to psychosocial problems and the adequacy of patients' adjustment to these problems. The nurse must create opportunities to talk with the patient and spouse or family members separately because each may feel more free to talk about feelings and concerns when alone. A simple, direct explanation of the purpose for private discussions usually makes this process easier. It is important to determine what the patient views as the problem of greatest concern and to explore this issue in some depth. Does the patient believe the problem can be dealt with? What has already been tried? Did it help? What could be tried now? Similar questions must be asked of the spouse.

It is also important to talk with the patient and family together, observing their patterns of interaction. Who responds first to questions? Does the patient have an opportunity to talk or appear to have a useful role within the family? Do family members talk much to each other? From these observations the nurse can make inferences regarding independence, interdependence, and dependence

conflicts; can obtain a sense of unresolved tensions; and can assess the level of overall patient and family adjustment to the illness.

### Assessing for the Presence of Nonpersonhood

Careful observation of family interaction with the patient also uncovers clues to "nonpersonhood." A nonperson is described as an object without normal human privileges, a family member who has a physical or mental deficit that limits participation in family interactions (Dolphin, 1984). Family members often discount the nonperson to the point that participation in family activities and decision making is no longer allowed. Family members may answer for patients as though they were not present or refer to them by pronouns ("he" or "she") rather than by name or family title. Conversation about patients flows over and around them, and critical remarks are made in their presence. Nonverbal clues to nonpersonhood include the following:

- Physical isolation of the patient to areas of the home where there is little contact with family members; no effort by family members to establish contact in the course of their daily activities
- Unkempt, depersonalized physical appearance of the patient
- Lack of warmth and caring in family interactions with the patient, for example:

  Few smiles, minimal eye contact

  Patient's behavior (either positive or negative) may elicit no reaction

  Patient's requests are ignored or actions to fulfill them postponed

  Decisions are made for, rather than with, the individual (e.g., moving an elderly disabled patient to a son's or daughter's home without asking how the patient feels about such a move)

Patients with chronic lung disease, with their tendency toward social isolation, seem particularly at risk for nonpersonhood.

# ANXIETY

Anxiety and panic disorder are often present in patients with chronic lung disease (Karajgi, 1990) and may become so pervasive as to dominate the individual's entire life. High anxiety complicates home care because anxious patients are much less receptive to teaching, have more somatic complaints, and are more likely to place frequent calls to care providers or use emergency care services for minor changes in symptoms.

## Etiology
### Dyspnea, Anxiety, and Deconditioning Feedback Loops

Anxiety in patients with chronic lung disease is related primarily to dyspnea and the associated fear of suffocation and death, although disease-related psychosocial and family issues often add to its severity. Respiratory complaints such as air hunger and suffocation (common symptoms of anxiety in the non–medically ill) are heightened in the patient with respiratory disease (Sheehan, 1983). Patients with COPD often feel they have little control over either dyspnea or anxiety. As a consequence, dyspnea increases anxiety and the fear of breathlessness; these in turn make the perception of dyspnea even more acute. A vicious cycle is created, often culminating in an episode of hyperventilation, which may worsen bronchospasm or otherwise alter alveolar ventilation (Fig. 9-1). If the underlying airway obstruction is not too severe, a true hyperventilation syndrome associated with a low $PaCO_2$ may result. Such negative feedback responses lead to the avoidance of activity and ultimately result in deconditioning. This so-called phobia of physical activity greatly complicates the management of patients with respiratory disease.

### Role of Emotional Arousal

Intense emotions such as anger, fear, frustration, and excitement can increase dyspnea by increasing sympathetic stimulation. To minimize respiratory symptoms arising from states of increased emotional arousal, patients may use any of a set of mechanisms designed to control the arousal itself. These include avoiding interpersonal contact or situations likely to result in intense emotions, reducing physical activity to avoid dyspnea, and several protective defense mechanisms such as denial or repression that operate outside of awareness (Table 17-1). Each of these operates to lessen the impact of emotionally loaded events. Although use of these mechanisms is adaptive to a degree, overuse interferes with normal social interaction and is maladaptive. Maladaptive use of these mechanisms is a major source of dysfunctional illness behavior.

## Assessment of Anxiety
### General Characteristics

The anxious patient usually looks intensely uncomfortable and exhibits a number of physiologic manifestations. "Pushed speech" (accelerated rate and volume) or pinched-sounding or shaky speech (caused by muscular tension around the larynx) may be present. Anxious patients with chronic lung disease often have a fear of death or a sense of impending doom. They may develop obsessive compulsive traits, phobias, and ritualistic behaviors or may become excessively worried about their disease state and functional abilities.

### Symptoms of Generalized Anxiety Syndrome

Some anxious patients with chronic lung disease develop true generalized anxiety disorder. This psychiatric disorder is characterized by pervasive and excessive anxiety that occurs in response to normal life circumstances, lasts for many months, and is accompanied by symptoms of motor tension, autonomic hyperactivity, or increased vigilance. The specific diagnostic criteria of the American Psychiatric Association are listed in the box on p. 306.

### Characteristics of Panic Disorder

Patients with chronic lung disease may also experience panic attacks that are typically accom-

## Diagnostic Criteria for Generalized Anxiety Syndrome

A. Unrealistic or excessive anxiety concerning more than two normal life circumstances on most days for 6 or more months (i.e., diffuse, durable symptoms)

B. At least six of the following 18 symptoms often present when the patient is anxious:

**MOTOR TENSION**

1. Trembling, twitching, or feeling shaky
2. Muscle tension, headaches, achiness, or soreness
3. Restlessness
4. Easy fatigability

**AUTONOMIC HYPERACTIVITY**

5. Shortness of breath or smothering sensations
6. Palpitations or accelerated heart rate
7. Sweating or cold clammy hands
8. Dry mouth
9. Dizziness or light-headedness
10. Nausea, diarrhea, or other abdominal distress
11. Flushing (hot flashes) or chills
12. Frequent urination
13. Trouble swallowing or sensation of lump in throat; pressure in the chest

**VIGILANCE AND SCANNING**

14. Feeling keyed up or on edge
15. Exaggerated startle response
16. Difficulty concentrating or "mind going blank" because of anxiety
17. Trouble falling or staying asleep
18. Irritability

C. No organic factors to explain symptoms (e.g., hyperthyroidism, caffeine intoxication)

Modified from American Psychiatric Association: *Diagnostic and statistical manual,* ed 3 revised, Washington, DC, 1987, The Association.

panied by respiratory symptoms such as dyspnea, chest heaviness, or a smothering feeling. These attacks may occur spontaneously but are more often precipitated by specific triggers such as strong odors, crowds, tobacco smoke, or being left alone and feeling that help may be unavailable if needed. Another common trigger is being in too small a space (e.g., an elevator, a shower enclosure, or a bathroom when the door is closed).

### Screening Tool for Anxiety

The Patient Rated Anxiety Scale (PRAS) is a simple 35-item screening tool that may help to identify patients experiencing syndromal anxiety (Sheehan, 1983). It includes many distressing somatic symptoms that are often present in chronic lung disease but that also occur in both anxiety and depression. Patients with high scores on the PRAS (maximum is 72) are likely to benefit from a more thorough diagnostic evaluation and treatment.

## Nursing Interventions
### Supportive Interventions

A number of supportive interventions can be used to help patients overcome anxiety and prevent it from incapacitating them or markedly reducing their quality of life. Several of the following are described in detail in Chapter 8.

■ *Breathing Techniques and Panic Control.* Any technique that decreases dyspnea can decrease anxiety. Patients with COPD may benefit from coaching in pursed lip breathing combined with conscious relaxation of tense neck and shoulder muscles. These techniques slow respiratory rate and provide a sense of relaxation and control over the sensation of dyspnea. Gentle massage of the neck and shoulder muscles, coupled with reminders to relax, often enhances relaxation. Patients with COPD should be taught to use pursed lip breathing at the first awareness of either dyspnea or increasing anxiety. Family members should also learn the techniques so they can coach the patient during times of increased anxiety or panic.

■ *Pacing and Energy Conservation.* Patients often become highly anxious during simple activities.

Pacing of activities combined with pursed lip breathing conserves energy and helps reduce anxiety. Breathing instruction should be reinforced at every opportunity.

■ *Relaxation Training.* Relaxation techniques are often helpful for anxiety reduction. Jacobsen's classic "tense-relax" technique incorporates sequential contraction and relaxation of specific muscle groups (Jacobsen, 1938; Sexton, 1987). It is a well-founded method that appears to be used most effectively by patients who do not have severe, ongoing dyspnea. It may also help those whose shoulder and neck muscles are unusually tense and those with a higher degree of anxiety or panic (Freedberg, 1987).

Patients with COPD who cannot exert the effort required by the Jacobsen method can use other relaxation techniques to reduce anxiety. Progressive muscle relaxation has been shown to reduce dyspnea, respiratory rate, heart rate, and symptoms of anxiety in patients with COPD (Renfroe, 1988). Techniques that evoke mental images of peaceful or calm surroundings and mental states—such as "I feel calm and relaxed," "My legs are heavy and warm," and "My breathing is easy and regular"—can be very effective. Relaxation should be practiced in an uncluttered environment. Patients should be positioned comfortably and wear loose clothing. Soft background music may enhance a relaxed atmosphere. Patients may relax more effectively if they use a bronchodilator and empty their bladder before practicing relaxation.

Relaxation is best learned through one-on-one instruction by an experienced clinician. Relaxation tapes can then be used to reinforce the exercise and guide daily practice sessions. Commercial tapes are readily available; however, a tape recording made by the patient's relaxation coach is often more effective because the technique is reinforced by a familiar voice.

■ *Meditation.* In patients with asthma, meditation techniques have been shown to improve measures of pulmonary function and decrease heart rate, blood pressure, oxygen consumption, and respiratory rate. People who regularly practice transcendental meditation (TM) tend to use medical services much less frequently than others, perhaps because of a reduction in anxiety associated with an improved sense of control over one's body (Orme-Johnson, 1987).

TM typically employs the use of a mantra, a word or phrase with a positive connotation that is repeated silently for a 20-minute period twice daily. It is used to block interfering thoughts from the mind. *The Relaxation Response* (Benson, 1975) is a classic that can be used by the patient and the practitioner to learn the art of meditation. Many bookstores and New Age vendors offer other meditation and relaxation tapes and books.

■ *Biofeedback Training.* Biofeedback uses medical technology to communicate information about some aspect of physiologic functioning (e.g., heart rate, muscle tension, or skin temperature) in such a way that the individual can begin to alter that function. Biofeedback training may help some respiratory patients reduce muscle tension and anxiety (Knapp, 1985). People with asthma have been able to reduce airway resistance with biofeedback training (Janson-Bjerklie, 1982).

Biofeedback is best taught at a well-qualified laboratory, but it can be practiced at home once the technique has been mastered. It is probably most effective when combined with other relaxation approaches.

### Counseling and Psychotherapy

When patients remain highly anxious despite the implementation of supportive interventions described previously, counseling with a mental health professional may be indicated. Social workers, psychiatric nurse practitioners, clinical nurse specialists, psychologists, and psychiatrists who are especially interested or experienced in dealing with the problems of chronic illness will be able to help the patient and family deal with unrelenting anxiety. Interested professionals in the community can work together with the local Lung Association to formulate a list of mental health professionals who are skilled at counseling highly anxious pulmonary patients.

### Pharmacologic Treatment

■ *Anxiolytics.* In most instances anxiolytics are *not* recommended for patients with chronic lung disease. Benzodiazepines such as diazepam (Valium), hydroxyzine (Atarax, Vistaril), chlordiazepoxide (Librium), clorazepate dipotassium (Tranxene), and alprazolam (Xanax) tend to be overused and prescribed primarily because physicians feel helpless to control the symptoms in any other way. If anxiolytics are used (e.g., to overcome an acute situational crisis), they should be prescribed for a short period only and the patient's response must be closely monitored.

Side effects of benzodiazepines include drowsiness, fatigue, weakness, dizziness, ataxia, confusion, slurred speech, headache, insomnia, and nausea. They can exacerbate respiratory depression by reducing respiratory drive. They can also worsen anxiety, potentiate depression, and produce behavioral disorganization or even a paradoxic rage. In an unstable patient, anxiolytics can readily confuse and complicate the clinical picture. Long-term use results in drug dependence, and habituated patients must have the drug tapered off very slowly.

■ *Antidepressants.* Anxiety frequently coexists with depression in patients with chronic lung dis-

ease (Borson, 1992). When this occurs, the home care nurse is immediately alerted to the anxiety but may fail to note the underlying depression. If anxiety alone is treated, especially if that treatment includes anxiolytic agents, depressive disability is likely to persist or even worsen. A tricyclic antidepressant is preferred (see following discussion) because this class of drug is effective in treating both depression and anxiety.

## DEPRESSION

Patients with chronic lung disease experience fatigue, dyspnea, diminished exercise tolerance, and losses in almost every aspect of their lives. The knowledge that their illness is irreversible enhances these losses and may create feelings of hopelessness and the fear of losing control. The most adaptive response to pervasive loss is a process of grief and mourning. Depression is an adaptive step in this process, but it can be maladaptive if delayed, absent, or prolonged.

The prevalence of major depressive illness in the general population is estimated to be between 1% and 4%. Not surprisingly, prevalence rates are much higher in people with chronic illnesses, and in COPD they are estimated to be between 10%

**Table 17-2**  Depressive disorders common to patients with chronic lung disease

| Type of depression | Description |
|---|---|
| Situational depression | Depression occurring in response to specific circumstance such as divorce or loss of loved one; tends to be viewed as normal, although intense response to major stressor; responds well to support and various behavioral interventions; antidepressants usually not needed |
| Dysthymia | Chronic mild depression with symptoms enduring for at least 2 yr; also called "depressive neurosis"; responds well to antidepressants |
| Major or endogenous depression | More severe type of depression, associated with more symptoms and usually accompanied by sleep disturbance; may evolve insidiously from a situation, reflect an escalation of dysthymia, or occur in the absence of any apparent precipitant or precursor symptoms; symptoms must have persisted for at least 2 wk to meet diagnostic criteria, but have often been present much longer; responds well to antidepressants |
| Major depression with melancholia | Symptom complex, as defined above, in which there is slowing down of activity or psychomotor retardation |

and 15% (Borson, 1986). The prevalence of depressive symptoms, however, may be as high as 42% (Light, 1985).

Types of depression most commonly seen in patients with chronic lung disease are summarized in Table 17-2.

## Etiology

Patients with a family history of depression or a history of alcohol abuse are at greatly increased risk for major depression. Depression in the young is most prevalent in women, especially those who are separated or divorced or in an unhappy marriage (Weissman, 1987). In the elderly, risk factors include poor health, physical disability affecting employment, marital separation and divorce, bereavement, loneliness, and poverty (Kennedy, 1989). The probability of an individual developing depression in association with lung disease is likely to be greatly increased in the presence of other risk factors.

## Depression and Smoking

Some interesting associations between smoking and depression have recently been noted—namely, that people with a history of major depression are more likely to be heavy smokers and are less likely to respond to smoking cessation interventions, such as pharmacologic treatment with clonidine (Glassman, 1988; Hughes, 1986).

## Depression and Ventilatory Drive

Depression has been associated with measurable abnormalities of ventilatory regulation, including blunting of ventilatory drive (Jellineck, 1985). In a patient with chronic hypercapnia, this could be sufficient to destabilize blood gases and precipitate respiratory failure.

## Depression and Dyspnea

Depression in medically healthy patients is often associated with complaints of dyspnea and sensations closely akin to dyspnea, such as an oppressive sense of heaviness in the chest (Borson, 1992). Thus patients with chronic lung disease who are depressed are likely to experience more severe dyspnea than nondepressed pulmonary patients. The presence of disproportionate dyspnea (i.e., dyspnea greatly in excess of what would be expected on the basis of measurable pulmonary function impairment) has been found to correlate highly with depression in patients with chronic bronchitis (Burns and Howell, 1969). In one group studied, it was often accompanied by hysteric features and excessive somatic complaints.

## Depression and Efficacy of Pulmonary Rehabilitation

Mood and general outlook on life improve with pulmonary rehabilitation. Depressed individuals, however, may be unable to mobilize themselves enough to benefit from rehabilitation efforts and often fail to complete rehabilitation programs in which they have enrolled (Shenkman, 1985).

## Depression as a Contributor to Excess Mortality

Depression in adults with severe asthma may result in a delay in seeking emergency care, increasing the risk of death in an acute exacerbation (Janson-Bjerklie, 1992).

## Assessment of Depressive Illness
### Characteristic Behaviors of the Depressed Patient

Feelings of helplessness and hopelessness characterize the emotional state of the depressed patient but are often not evident during a casual interview. Patients may have frequent crying spells or withdraw into themselves and become preoccupied with their own concerns, causing relationships to deteriorate and social interactions to diminish. Sexual activity may be limited both from loss of libido and from dyspnea. The cognitive state of the depressed patient may be marked by difficulty in concentrating, memory impairment, indecisiveness, and low self-esteem. Passivity and dependence may appear in previously active, independent people. Suicidal ideation may be present, and occasionally patients kill themselves.

### Neuropsychologic Deficits Associated with Depression

Neuropsychologic impairment resulting from depression must be distinguished from neuropsychologic deficits caused by hypoxemia, fatigue, or sleep disturbance. Depression tends to result in problems with arousal, attention, and mental concentration, whereas hypoxemia is more likely to impair higher cognitive functions such as abstract reasoning, complex perceptual-motor integration, motor speed, coordination, strength, and memory (Grant, 1982; Prigitano, 1983).

### Factors Complicating the Diagnosis of Depression in Chronic Obstructive Pulmonary Disease

A number of factors tend to confound the diagnosis of depression in the patient with COPD, resulting in significant missed diagnoses:

- Mood disorders tend to be chronic and relatively mild, with symptoms such as chest heaviness, fatigue, insomnia, or difficulty with breathing that are as easily attributable to COPD as to depression.
- Somatic complaints often predominate and lead to a misdirection of diagnostic efforts; this is particularly apparent with coexisting anxiety.
- Health provider contacts with the patient are often brief and tend to focus on physical symptoms.
- Older patients, especially men, are often reluctant to admit to feelings of depression.

Important clues to the presence of depression in patients with chronic lung disease are summarized in the box. A high incidence of somatic complaints is particularly suggestive (Katon, 1984). Home care staff must be alert to these subtle indicators of mood problems.

### Screening Tools

Questionnaires designed to screen patients for symptoms of depression can be helpful. Several are available; most can be administered in just a few minutes and are easy to score. The home care nurse

---

> ### Clues to Depression in Chronic Lung Disease
>
> 1. Disproportionate dyspnea
> 2. A "heavy feeling" in the chest
> 3. Increased frequency of phone calls, physician visits, and "emergencies"
> 4. An increase in nonspecific complaints (e.g., vague aches)
> 5. Diurnal variation in mood (usually feel more blue in the mornings)
> 6. Frequent and early morning awakenings
> 7. More neuropsychologic impairment
> 8. Poorer response to pulmonary rehabilitation efforts
> 9. A high score on a depression screening tool

---

is encouraged to become familiar with screening tools, to select one or two, and to use them routinely whenever symptoms suggest the possibility of depression or anxiety.

However, it is important to remember that a screening tool cannot diagnose a mood disorder; it can merely suggest its presence. Referral for a more thorough evaluation of mood should be considered for any patient whose score on a screening test suggests significant mood dysfunction.

■ *Geriatric Depression Scale.* The Geriatric Depression Scale (GDS) was developed specifically for use with elderly people (Yesavage, 1983) (Fig. 17-1). It excludes questions about somatic symptoms, which may confound the interpretation of depression scale scores in medically ill patients. Because items must be answered yes or no, it does not allow for the expression of relatively modest attitudinal changes. A score of 11 or more is suggestive of depression.

■ *Beck Depression Inventory.* The Beck Depression Inventory (BDI) (Beck, 1961) includes somatic symptoms common to chronic lung disease; thus it may result in falsely high scores. A score of 17 or more, however, is suggestive of depression.

| | Norms | |
|---|---|---|
| Normal | 5.75 | 4.34 |
| Mildly depressed | 15.05 | 6.50 |
| Very depressed | 22.85 | 5.07 |

Choose the best answer for how you felt the past week

| | | | |
|---|---|---|---|
| 1 | Are you basically satisfied with your life? | YES | NO |
| 2 | Have you dropped many of your activities and interests? | YES | NO |
| 3 | Do you feel that your life is empty? | YES | NO |
| 4 | Do you often get bored? | YES | NO |
| 5 | Are you hopeful about the future? | YES | NO |
| 6 | Are you bothered by thoughts you can't get out of your head? | YES | NO |
| 7 | Are you in good spirits most of the time? | YES | NO |
| 8 | Are you afraid that something bad is going to happen to you? | YES | NO |
| 9 | Do you feel happy most of the time? | YES | NO |
| 10 | Do you often feel helpless? | YES | NO |
| 11 | Do you often get restless and fidgety? | YES | NO |
| 12 | Do you prefer to stay at home, rather than going out and doing new things? | YES | NO |
| 13 | Do you frequently worry about the future? | YES | NO |
| 14 | Do you feel you have more problems with memory than most? | YES | NO |
| 15 | Do you think it is wonderful to be alive now? | YES | NO |
| 16 | Do you often feel downhearted and blue? | YES | NO |
| 17 | Do you feel pretty worthless the way you are now? | YES | NO |
| 18 | Do you worry a lot about the past? | YES | NO |
| 19 | Do you find life very exciting? | YES | NO |
| 20 | Is it hard for you to get started on new projects? | YES | NO |
| 21 | Do you feel full of energy? | YES | NO |
| 22 | Do you feel that your situation is hopeless? | YES | NO |
| 23 | Do you think that most people are better off than you are? | YES | NO |
| 24 | Do you frequently get upset over little things? | YES | NO |
| 25 | Do you frequently feel like crying? | YES | NO |
| 26 | Do you have trouble concentrating? | YES | NO |
| 27 | Do you enjoy getting up in the morning? | YES | NO |
| 28 | Do you prefer to avoid social gatherings? | YES | NO |
| 29 | Is is easy for you to make decisions? | YES | NO |
| 30 | Is your mind as clear as it used to be? | YES | NO |

**Fig. 17-1**   Geriatric Depression Scale. (From Yesavage J et al: *J Psychiatr Res* 17:37, 1983.)

■ *Zung Self-Rating Depression Scale.* The Zung Self-Rating Depression Scale (SDS) (Zung, 1965) may not be especially reliable in patients over 70 years of age. A score of 60 or more in an older medically ill population suggests clinical depression.

■ *Center for Epidemiological Studies Depression Scale.* The Center for Epidemiological Studies Depression Scale (CES-D) is useful for older patients. It allows for a range of severity with each item. A score of 16 or more suggests depression (Radloff, 1986).

### Diagnostic Criteria for Major Depression

The diagnosis of a major depression is usually based on psychiatric interview, using the diagnostic criteria described in the box.

## Nursing Interventions

Treatment of major depression usually begins with medication, specialized psychotherapy, or both and incorporates other therapies as needed.

### Counseling and Psychotherapy

Counseling and individual or group psychotherapy can be helpful in activating a depressed patient. Selection of a therapist whose clinical approach and personality are compatible with the patient is a key factor in success. Family counseling may be indicated to deal with the impact of nonproductive, deeply entrenched patterns of family interaction.

Support groups, such as Better Breathers, can reduce social isolation and help restore a sense of hope and community. Similarly, pulmonary rehabilitation programs can diminish feelings of helplessness and hopelessness by helping patients set realistic goals and increase self-care skills and functional ability. Referral to such community resources should be a routine part of home care discharge planning as patients regain their ability to pursue activities outside the home.

### Pharmacologic Treatment

Clinicians often view depression in people with chronic lung disease as a normal response to the stress of severe chronic illness (i.e., a situational

---

**Diagnostic Criteria for Depressive Disorders**

**MAJOR DEPRESSION**

1. Durable dysphoria (i.e., for at least 2 weeks)
2. At least four of the following eight symptoms:
   a. Change in weight or appetite (loss or gain)
   b. Sleep disturbance (insomnia, hypersomnolence)
   c. Loss of energy, fatigue
   d. Impaired concentration, indecisiveness
   e. Psychomotor retardation or agitation
   f. Loss of interest or pleasure in usual activities
   g. Feelings of worthlessness, excessive guilt
   h. Recurrent thoughts of death or suicide
3. Not psychotic, bereaved, or clinically demented

**DYSTHYMIA**

1. Depressed mood most days for at least 2 years; asymptomatic periods never exceed 2 months
2. At least two of the following six symptoms:
   a. Poor appetite or overeating
   b. Insomnia or hypersomnia
   c. Low energy or fatigue
   d. Low self-esteem
   e. Poor concentration or difficulty making decisions
   f. Feelings of hopelessness
3. Not caused by organic factors (e.g., antihypertensive medication)

Modified from American Psychiatric Association: *Diagnostic and statistical manual of mental disorders,* ed 3, revised, Washington, DC, 1987, The Association.

---

depression) and, following the traditional therapeutic model, may assume that pharmacologic intervention is not indicated. When the "situation" is a chronic disease, however, distinctions between various types of depression are somewhat irrelevant, and therapeutic decisions are more appropriately made on the basis of the severity and duration of symptoms. Most patients who meet diagnostic criteria for major depression (with or without anxiety or panic disorder) deserve a trial of antidepressant medication. Tricyclic antidepressant agents are the most frequently prescribed class of antidepressants. Fluoxetine (Prozac) is also often used. Selection of a specific drug is generally based on the clinical effect desired, the relative risk of side effects, and the prescribing physician's experience and comfort with a particular preparation.

■ *Tricyclic Antidepressants.* Nortriptyline has been shown to have decisive therapeutic benefits for well-diagnosed depressed patients with COPD (Borson, 1992) and is generally well tolerated even by elderly patients with severe disease. Because they have strong sedative side effects, tricyclic antidepressant agents (TCAs) such as doxepin and amitriptyline may be helpful for patients with agitated depression and profound insomnia. However, anticholinergic side effects and oversedation often limit their usefulness. By contrast, protriptyline has an activating effect, making it useful for the patient whose depression is characterized by psychomotor retardation and hypersomnolence. Table 17-3 presents common TCAs.

■ DOSAGE. The dose of TCA required to achieve an adequate therapeutic response varies greatly between individuals and is best regulated on the basis of clinical response and emergent side effects. A reasonable target dose for nortriptyline is 1 mg/kg of body weight.

■ THERAPEUTIC RESPONSE. Patients usually notice improvement in sleep early in TCA treatment, but significant improvement in mood takes much longer—4 to 6 weeks on average. It is important to advise patients of this expected delay in therapeutic response so that they will not become discouraged and discontinue medication prematurely.

■ SIDE EFFECTS. Common TCA side effects are presented in Table 17-4. Even in severely impaired patients with COPD, most of these can be controlled with the relatively simple measures described (Borson, 1992). TCAs are best tolerated if the patient is started on a low dose, which is increased slowly (i.e., over 2 to 4 weeks) to the target dose. If side effects become troublesome despite preventive measures, the dose may need to be increased more slowly or temporarily reduced. Patients who do not respond or who develop intolerable side effects from one TCA may do better with another (National Institute of Mental Health/National Institutes of Health, 1985).

Abrupt discontinuation of a TCA can cause headache, nausea, malaise, disturbed sleep, and wild dreams (National Institute of Mental Health/National Institutes of Health, 1985). Thus TCA doses should always be tapered slowly. Ideally therapy should be supervised by a psychiatrist who is skilled in treating medically ill patients.

■ *Fluoxetine (Prozac).* Fluoxetine acts by inhibiting serotonin uptake. It is especially recommended for patients with obsessive compulsive symptoms or unwanted weight gain associated with depression and in those who have not responded to or are unable to tolerate the side effects of TCAs. Advantages over TCAs include minimal anticholinergic effects, lack of orthostatic hypotension, minimal sedation, and no prolongation of cardiac conduction time. Disadvantages compared to TCAs are induction of nervousness or anxiety, insomnia, gastrointestinal disturbances, headache, and weight loss. Fluoxetine is considerably more expensive than the TCAs.

The usual dose of fluoxetine is 20 mg daily taken in the morning, although in some patients higher doses (up to 60 mg) may be needed. Doses above 20 mg daily should be divided (i.e., half in the morning and the rest at noon). Because fluoxetine is metabolized by the liver, the dose will need to be lower for patients with impaired liver function. The most common side effects include the following:

- Nausea (25% to 30% of patients); anorexia and weight loss; diarrhea; and dry mouth
- Headache, nervousness, tremor, insomnia, drowsiness; insomnia present in 10% to 20% of patients but can usually be controlled by not giving evening doses
- Excessive sweating (30%)
- Blurred vision (13%)
- Diminished sexual desire or ability (8% of patients)

**Table 17-3**   Tricyclic antidepressants

| Drug | Preparations | Usual adult dose range | Comments |
|---|---|---|---|
| Nortriptyline (Pamelor, Aventyl) | 10, 25, 50, 75 mg capsules; 10 mg/5 ml solution | 75-150 mg daily | A metabolite of amitriptyline but with fewer side effects; less likely to cause postural hypotension; half-life of 18-93 hr |
| Desipramine (Norpramin, Pertofrane) | 10, 25, 50, 75, 100, 150 mg tablets; 25, 50 mg capsules | 75-200 mg daily | Metabolite of imipramine, but with fewer anticholinergic side effects; one of the least sedating |
| Protriptyline (Vivactil) | 5, 10 mg tablets | 5-10 mg tid to qid to maximum of 60 mg qd | Least sedating of all TCAs; may cause overstimulation or insomnia, therefore avoid bedtime administration; also used to treat sleep apnea; longest half-life (54-198 hr) |
| Amoxapine (Asendin) | 25, 50, 100, 125 mg tablets | 100-300 mg daily | Mild anticholinergic effects; may cause tardive dyskinesia or parkinsonian side effects; short half-life (8-30 hr) |
| Imipramine (Tofranil, SK-Pramine) | 10, 25, 50 mg tablets; 75, 100, 125, 150 mg capsules | 75-200 mg daily | Moderate sedative and anticholinergic side effects; *also used to treat childhood enuresis;* short half-life (13-28 hr) |
| Maprotiline (Ludiomil) | 25, 50, 75 mg tablets | 75-150 mg | Similar to imipramine; high incidence of seizures |
| Trazodone (Desyrel) | 50, 100, 150 mg tablets | 150-400 mg daily in divided doses | Moderately sedating but with few anticholinergic side effects; may have ventricular arrhythmogenic effects in patients with cardiac dysfunction, may increase digoxin levels and may cause priapism in males; absorption improved and side effects less if taken just after eating |
| Doxepin (Adapin, Sinequan) | 10, 25, 50, 75, 100, 125 mg capsules; 10 mg/ml solution | 75-300 mg daily | Strong sedative and anticholinergic side effects; short half-life (6-19 hr) |
| Amitriptyline (Elavil) | 10, 25, 50, 75, 100, 150 mg tablets | 50-150 mg daily | Strong sedative and anticholinergic side effects |
| Trimipramine (Surmontil) | 25, 50, 100 mg capsules | 75-200 mg daily | Strong sedative and anticholinergic side effects; also used to treat peptic ulcer disease; short half-life (9-11 hr) |

**Table 17-4**   Management of tricyclic antidepressant therapy side effects

| Side effect | Measures to reduce/prevent |
|---|---|
| **SEDATION (COMMON)** | |
| Beneficial early side effect for sleep | Administer sedating TCAs (i.e., all but protriptyline) in the evening, or divide doses |
| May cause daytime grogginess | |
| **ANTICHOLINERGIC EFFECTS (COMMON)** | |
| Dry mouth | Lemon drops, ice chips, artificial saliva (usually disappears on its own) |
| Constipation | Constipation-prevention regimen (e.g., prunes) |
| Urinary hesitancy (most commonly in men with preexisting prostatic hypertrophy) | Careful monitoring with benign prostatic hypertrophy |
| Blurred vision | Use with caution in glaucoma |
| **POSTURAL HYPOTENSION** | |
| Common only in at-risk patients (i.e., those with preexisting postural hypotension or receiving diuretics) | Instruct patients in slow position changes; monitor blood pressure for postural changes with each dose increase; maintain good hydration; support hose, as needed |
| **CARDIAC EFFECTS** | |
| Slows cardiac conduction | Contraindicated with severe congestive heart failure, a recent myocardial infarction, or significant cardiac conduction defects |
| **CENTRAL NERVOUS SYSTEM AND ADRENERGIC STIMULANT EFFECTS (OCCASIONAL)** | |
| Headache | Use with caution in demented patients |
| Muscle twitching | Careful observation when used in patients with seizure disorder; may need to adjust anticonvulsant dose |
| "Wild dreams" or nightmares | |
| Sweating | |
| Lowered seizure threshold | |

Recent concerns regarding increased suicidal ideation have not borne up under further scrutiny.

■ *Duration of Antidepressant Treatment.* Once a therapeutic effect is obtained, antidepressants should be continued for at least 6 months and the patient followed closely for evidence of relapse or recurrence of symptoms (National Institute of Mental Health/National Institutes of Health, 1985). As a general rule, the longer the duration of the depressive episode, the longer the course of treatment required.

■ *Relapse of Depression.* Relapses are common and are most likely to occur with premature discontinuation of medication, patient noncompliance, intervening medical illness, poor social adaptation, coexisting anxiety, and alcohol or drug dependency (Prien, 1986; Faravelli, 1986). Other risk factors for recurrence include the following:

• Three or more previous depressive episodes
• Depression that has persisted for 2 or more years before treatment
• Presence of residual symptoms following treatment

If the patient experiences a relapse while still taking medication, an increase in the dose may be required. Because the risk of relapse is greatest in the first 8 weeks following discontinuation of medication (Prien, 1986), close contact should be maintained with patients during this period, and patients should be instructed to call if depressive symptoms recur.

## FAMILY DYNAMICS
### Impact of Illness on Family Functioning

Family members also suffer from the impact of the patient's illness and may experience a whole range of emotions, including severe frustration, anger, and guilt. Those close to the patient often wonder if the patient is malingering, or they may view the patient as weak and lacking in drive, motivation, and spirit. They often bear the brunt of hostile or manipulative behavior, without understanding that this reflects the patient's fear or frustration rather than any inadequacies on their part.

Spouses are often responsible for the day-to-day care of the patient and may experience considerable anxiety and stress as the disease progresses. Wives of patients with COPD often add the roles of caretaker, decision maker, finance manager, and errand-doer to their previously assigned roles in the family system, and most are forced—abruptly—to assume responsibilities for which they have had little or no preparation. As a result, they have been found to have more severe symptoms of stress, lower life satisfaction, increased social isolation, and poorer sleep, sexual relations, and self-perceived health than wives of healthy men (Sexton, 1985). They are also much less likely to share their problems and worries with their husbands.

### Supportive Interventions

It is important for the home care nurse to understand the many psychosocial problems faced by patients and their families. Often the mere presence of a sympathetic nurse in the home will help the family mobilize their internal and external resources to find solutions to their problems. The nurse must help the family establish attainable goals and make realistic steps to reach them. Multidisciplinary conferences with the physician, psychiatric social worker, psychiatrist, psychologist,

home health aide, and other members of the home care team may be needed.

If manipulative or angry outbursts become excessive, family members and patients may need help with limit setting. Extreme dependency may respond to measures that slowly desensitize patients to fears of being left alone. For instance, a first step is a planned short absence during which the caregiver is readily available by telephone. Having the patient make telephone contact during the "trial" absence often helps reassure him or her that the system works. Planning the absence to coincide with a favorite television program may help divert the patient's attention from being alone. Another approach is to arrange for a friend or neighbor to visit shortly after the caregiver has left, thereby reassuring the patient that help is close at hand. The telephone and important phone numbers should always be left within easy reach of the patient. Leaving a nebulizer treatment set up and ready may also help prevent a dyspnea-related anxiety attack.

A referral to the home care agency social worker or psychiatric clinical nurse specialist should be considered for any family experiencing a high degree of psychosocial distress. Medicare will reimburse for limited family counseling if it is provided in conjunction with patient counseling.

"Lung clubs" encourage spouses and patients to discuss situations with others who experience similar problems, and some offer spousal support groups. If problems are severe, family members may be referred to private psychiatric or family counselors, community mental health centers, or other resources for ongoing support. Home care staff should maintain a current list of appropriate community counseling resources.

### Respite Care

Periodic respite from the responsibilities of care giving is essential for the primary caregiver and can often be arranged through hourly care agencies or informally through friends, relatives, or volunteers from local churches or community agencies. Family members usually need support and encouragement both to ask for help and to accept it when it is offered. Wives, in particular, tend to lock themselves into the belief that they are abrogating their responsibility if they take time for themselves. It may help to remind a spouse that, unless she can stay healthy herself through careful attention to her own needs and medical problems, she will be unable to continue caring for her husband.

## EFFECTS ON THE HEALTH CARE TEAM

Even with specialized training, caregivers often feel helpless when they are faced with a progressive, debilitating illness. This is especially true when the patient is someone to whom they have grown close over the course of long-term care. These feelings of impotence may be exaggerated by the paucity of expressions of appreciation by respiratory patients. Patients are often so preoccupied with the problems of their disease that they neglect or are unable to give positive feedback to their health care providers. Expressions of appreciation and the rewards of patient progress are the fuels that propel health professionals forward, day to day, through the stresses of providing high-quality patient care. With pulmonary patients, however, the big rewards come in very small steps and result from setting small, attainable goals. Multidisciplinary conferences that focus on patient and family problems and behavior and the care providers' responses may help professional staff regain objectivity, especially with the management of complex patients who are not progressing as hoped.

### REFERENCES

American Psychiatric Association: *Diagnostic and statistical manual of mental disorders*, ed 3 revised, Washington, DC, 1987, The Association.

Beck A et al: An inventory for measuring depression, *Arch Gen Psychiatry* 4:561, 1961.

Benson H: *The relaxation response*, New York, 1975, William Morrow.

Borson S et al: Improvement in mood, physical symptoms, and function with nortriptyline for depression in patients with chronic obstructive pulmonary disease, *Psychosomatics* 33:190, 1992.

Borson S et al: Symptomatic depression in elderly medical outpatients. I. Prevalence, demography and health service utilization, *J Am Geriatr Soc* 34:341, 1986.

Burns BH, Howell JBL: Disproportionately severe breathlessness in chronic bronchitis, *Q J Med* 38:277, 1969.

Dolphin N: Non-personhood: a nursing diagnosis in the psychosocial realm, *Home Health Nurse* 2:16, 1984.

Dudley D et al: Psychosocial concomitants to rehabilitation in chronic obstructive pulmonary disease. II. *Chest* 77:544, 1980.

Faravelli C et al: Depressive relapses and incomplete recovery from index episode, *Am J Psychiatry* 143:888, 1986.

Freedburg PD et al: Effect of progressive muscle relaxation on the objective symptoms and subjective responses associated with asthma, *Heart Lung* 16:24, 1987.

Glassman AH et al: Heavy smokers, smoking cessation and clonidine, *JAMA* 259:2863, 1988.

Grant I et al: Neuropsychological findings in hypoxemic chronic obstructive pulmonary disease, *Arch Intern Med* 142:1470, 1982.

Hughes JR et al: Prevalence of smoking among psychiatric patients, *Am J Psychiatry* 143:993, 1986.

Jacobsen E: *Progressive relaxation*, Chicago, 1938, University of Chicago Press.

Janson-Bjerklie S, Clarke E: The effects of biofeedback training on bronchial diameter in asthma, *Heart Lung* 11:200, 1982.

Janson-Bjerklie S et al: Clinical markers of asthma severity and risk: importance of subjective as well as objective factors, *Heart Lung* 21:265, 1992.

Jellinek M, Goldenheim P, Jenike M: The impact of grief on ventilatory control, *Am J Psychiatry* 142:121, 1985.

Karajgi B et al: The prevalence of anxiety disorders in patients with chronic obstructive pulmonary disease, *Am J Psychiatry* 147:200, 1990.

Katon W: Depression: relationship to somatization and chronic medical illness, *J Clin Psychiatry* 45(3 Sect 2):4, 1984.

Kennedy GJ et al: Hierarchy of characteristics associated with depressive symptoms in an urban elderly sample, *Am J Psychiatry* 146:220, 1989.

Knapp PH, Mathe AA: Psychophysiologic aspects of bronchial asthma. In Weiss EB et al, editors: *Bronchial asthma*, Boston, 1985, Little, Brown.

Light RW et al: Prevalence of depression and anxiety in patients with COPD, *Chest* 87:35, 1985.

McSweeney J et al: Life quality of patients with chronic obstructive pulmonary disease, *Arch Intern Med* 142:1470, 1982.

Morgan A et al: Effect of attitudes and beliefs on exercise tolerance in chronic bronchitis, *Br Med J* 286:171, 1983.

National Institute of Mental Health/National Institutes of Health: Consensus development conference statement: mood disorders—pharmacologic prevention of recurrences, *Am J Psychiatry* 142:469, 1985.

Orme-Johnson D: Medical care utilization and the transcendental meditation program, *Psychosom Med* 49:493, 1987.

Prien RF, Kupfer DJ: Continuation drug therapy for major depressive episodes: how long should it be maintained? *Am J Psychiatry* 143:18, 1986.

Prigitano P et al: Neuropsychological test performance in mildly hypoxemic patients with COPD, *J Consult Clin Psychol* 51:108, 1983.

Radloff LS, Teri L: Uses of the CES-D scale with older adults. In Brink TL, editor: *Clinical gerontology: a guide to assessment and intervention,* Clinical Gerontologist Series, vol 5, nos 1-4, Binghamton, NY, 1986, Haworth Press.

Renfroe KL: Effect of progressive relaxation on dyspnea and state anxiety in patients with chronic obstructive pulmonary disease, *Heart Lung* 17:408, 1988.

Sexton DL: Relaxation techniques and biofeedback. In Hodgkin JE, Petty TL, editors: *COPD: current concepts,* Philadelphia, 1987, WB Saunders.

Sexton DL, Munro BH: Impact of a husband's chronic illness (COPD) on the spouse's life, *Res Nurs Health* 8:83, 1985.

Sheehan DV: *The anxiety disease,* Toronto, 1983, Bantam Books.

Shenkman B: Factors contributing to attrition rates in a pulmonary rehabilitation program, *Heart Lung* 14:53, 1985.

Traver GA: Measures of symptoms and life quality to predict emergent use of institutional health care resources in chronic obstructive airways disease, *Heart Lung* 17(6, Pt 1):689, 1988.

Weissman MM: Advances in psychiatric epidemiology: rates and risks for major depression, *Am J Pub Health* 77:445, 1987.

Yesavage J et al: Development and validation of a geriatric depression screening scale: a preliminary report, *J Psychiatr Res* 17:37, 1983.

Zung WWK: A self-rating depression scale, *Arch Gen Psychiatry* 12:63, 1965.

## SUGGESTED READINGS

Borson S, McDonald GJ: Depression in chronic obstructive pulmonary disease. In Robinson R, Rabins P, editors: *Depression and coexisting disease,* New York, 1989, Igaku Shoin.

Frazier SH, editor: Anxiety and depression, *Med Clin North Am,* vol 72, 1988.

Katon W: Depression: relationship to somatization and chronic medical illness, *J Clin Psychiatry* 45(3 sect 2):4, 1984.

Sandhu HS: Psychosocial issues in COPD, *Clin Chest Med* 7:629, 1986.

Sexton DL, Munro BH: Living with a chronic illness: the experience of women with COPD, *West J Nurse Res* 10:26, 1988.

Shekleton M: Coping with chronic respiratory difficulty, *Nurs Clin North Am* 22:569, 1987.

# CHAPTER 18

# PSYCHOSOCIAL CARE OF FAMILIES AND CHILDREN

ROBIN B. THOMAS • KAY A. WICKS •
MARIJO MILLER-RATCLIFFE • NANCI L. LARTER

The family is the child's most important environment, not only in terms of the child's growth and development, but because the family regulates the child's use of health care systems and compliance with health care advice. Family involvement is essential to the successful treatment of the child's health needs. This chapter focuses on the family's and child's response to special health care needs. Interventions to assist the child and family in their response to chronic illness are discussed.

A chronic condition or special health care need is any anatomic or physiologic impairment that interferes with the individual's ability to function fully in the environment. Chronic conditions are typically characterized by relatively stable periods, interrupted by acute episodes requiring hospitalization or medical attention. The individual's prognosis varies from a normal life span to unpredictable early death. Chronic conditions are rarely cured but are managed through individual and family effort and diligence (Thomas, 1984).

## THE FAMILY

The family's purpose is to provide society with functioning replacement members so that the culture may survive and to maintain existing, or adult, members in operational form so they may continue to contribute to society. It is the only social structure capable of this function. The family essentially functions as society's human resource department. The family is a unique, small social group consisting of individuals varying in age and gender, who are bound together virtually permanently through strong affectionate bonds and who share common traditions, which they expect to transmit to future family members (Thomas, 1986).

Families come in all sizes, shapes, and configurations. The once typical family of two married parents and one or more children is no longer the norm. In fact, this version of the family now represents only about one tenth of all U.S. families (Levitan, Belous, and Gallo, 1988). Increases in the divorce rate (from 9% in 1960 to 21% in 1987) and more out of wedlock births (from 5% in 1960 to 22% in 1985) add to the variety of family structures providers will see (Levitan, Belous, and Gallo, 1988). The important fact about family structures is that generally any and all of them work. In a recent study by McCubbin, no differences were found in a child's outcome for children with chronic conditions when single-parent and two-parent families were compared (McCubbin, 1988). This study and others clearly emphasized that families' capacity to care for their children cannot be judged on their structure alone. Many family styles seem unusual and may even make providers uncomfortable because they do not meet the providers' expectations of family life. Especially in home health care, providers are offered a view of the most intimate family interactions. It is wise to remember that unless the family abuses or neglects the child, the provider has no right to intervene in family dynamics. It is often difficult for caring, involved providers to limit their interactions with the child and family when family interactions appear painful or unsatisfying. However, unless the family requests further assistance or responds favorably to tactfully stated offers of help, the providers should not pressure the family to change their functioning. Caring for a child in the family's home can be a difficult role.

Care of a chronically ill child requires an enormous amount of knowledge and patience by parents. Hymovich (1976) believes that mothers or caretakers must accomplish the following three tasks to cope with a child's illness:

- Understand and manage the child's illness
- Assist the child in coping with and understanding the illness
- Meet the needs of all family members, including their own and those of the ill child

A variety of factors need to be evaluated when assessing the home health care treatment being provided by a family. Many health care providers find it much easier to give didactic information and explain procedures than to explore and deal with family dynamics, routines, and emotional problems. Yet these issues have a dramatic impact on the child's care and outcome. From a nursing perspective, the focus should be on assisting the parents to function at their best, given any family constraints. Once problems have been identified, a long-term perspective is necessary. An immediate solution may not be available for all problems; however, prioritization and mutual goal setting by parents and health care providers become imperative. A primary focus for home care staff during this transition phase is to build confidence as the parents assume increasing responsibility for all aspects of their child's care.

Reviewing the parents' understanding and perception of their child's respiratory illness is a primary step in evaluating the care they provide at home. Most families attempt to normalize their child into the home or social environment based on these perceptions. This helps them to reduce their own concerns and society's negative perceptions of the child. Another strategy useful to a family in adjusting to home health care requirements is to share the burden of the illness through support systems. Ideally, this involves other family members, but regardless of its composition, the support system should provide intermember communication and decision making, role flexibility, and a mutual consensus that all members are contributing, and therefore all are important.

The nurse is encouraged to work with the family to assess its strengths and needs. For example, the nurse and family could take the child's health care plan, review each required activity (such as aerosol treatments), and discuss who within the family will be responsible for the treatments, how much time it will take, whether the financial costs are a problem for the family, and what must be eliminated or changed in the family's daily living to allow for the treatment time. In the process of identifying each additional task the family must perform for the child, it is appropriate to discuss whether the activity places a strain on the family. A request for respite care to avoid fatigue on the part of the family is an example of the kind of issue the nurse and family might discuss. Any concerns on the part of the nurse that are relevant to the child's care could be raised in the context of this assessment.

It is useful for the nurse to know about community-based family support groups that exist in almost every state or region of the United States and other countries. A referral to an appropriate family support group is often helpful to the family. These groups can be located through local chapters of the American Lung Association (e.g., asthma programs), hospitals, crisis lines, United Way referral agencies, or the Cystic Fibrosis Foundation.

## THE CHILD

In addition to evaluating a parent's understanding of the disease, treatments, and support systems available, the child's perception should be probed when he or she is verbally expressive. Cognitive maturation primarily determines a child's understanding of an illness. In general, a child under 7 years of age reasons in a very finalistic manner, equating illness with misbehavior or some type of wrongdoing. From about the age of 7 to approximately 10 years, most children are capable of understanding that the cause of an illness is separate from their own actions or thoughts (i.e., germs can cause illness). After 9 to 10 years of age, illness is recognized as having multiple causes, including infections and the lack of ability to fight infections; in addition, children at this age may perceive that they may have caused or contributed to their own illness (Brewster, 1982). It therefore becomes important to analyze the child's cognitive understanding of his or her illness before expecting cooperation with treatment. What may appear to be sabotage on the child's part may merely be an indication of the child's perceived solution. Reassurance and explanations must also take into account the child's cognitive abilities.

The child's response to a chronic condition has been inconsistently presented in the literature. Historically, researchers took the position that children with chronic conditions were seriously disturbed as a result of their physical impairment. This perspective has shifted to the view that the majority of children deal positively with their impairment. A variety of factors intertwine and affect a child's adjustment. It is the disability (physical consequences of the impairment), the handicap (social consequences of the impairment), and the extended family's response to those factors that have the greatest impact on the child's adjustment.

When the child requires technologic assistance (e.g., ventilator, tracheostomy tube, intravenous line), stress increases within the home. A child is likely to have more difficulty adjusting to these care interventions if they are the result of a sudden catastrophic illness or injury. The child's age, involvement in social activities, and potential for independence and the degree of parental nurturing will affect the child's response. The ventilator-dependent adolescent must struggle with the need to rely on parents and nurses when peers are developing greater independence. The disability sets the adolescent apart from peers and may produce feelings of unattractiveness and inferiority that may lead to depression and isolation. The home health care nurse has the opportunity to monitor the adolescent's or child's psychosocial status so that problems can be identified early. Interventions can then be planned and administered by the family, health care providers, and mental health specialists.

## HOME CARE

The ultimate goal of home care for a child with a chronic respiratory illness is that the child and family lead as normal a life as possible in a supportive, nonisolating environment. Caring for a child with chronic respiratory illness can be both a frustrating and a satisfying experience for any caregiver. Satisfaction on the part of both the caregiver and the patient must be measured differently from that associated with most illnesses. Satisfaction (sometimes viewed as a "soft" outcome) has been shown to be related to compliance with necessary home treatments and quite possibly could be a crucial variable leading to an improved medical outcome.

### Treatment Administration

The administration of treatments such as chest physiotherapy and nebulized or oral medications can lead to parent-child conflicts at home. Both parents and children need to understand the amount of flexibility available in this area. If the treatment or medication is imperative, the parents must assume a matter-of-fact attitude regarding its administration, be consistent in their behavior regarding its performance, and reward the child with something they view as positive after completion (e.g., reading a book together, holding, hugging, having a favorite breakfast food). All parents need support initially and at intervals whenever they are being asked to do something their child resists. Observations of parent-child interactions during treatments at home provide insight into their relationship, allow for assessment of the parent's delivery technique and effectiveness of the treatment, and assist the health care team in planning care.

Another important consideration involves the frequency of treatments required of parents in the home setting. Periodically, the necessity for on-going treatments and medications should be reviewed to eliminate unnecessary home procedures (Schulman, 1983). As home health care has become more common and necessary, health care providers have become increasingly tolerant of the large workloads required of parents caring for the chronically ill child at home. Parents must learn a variety of new procedures and troubleshoot equipment such as monitors, feeding pumps, nebulizers, or gastrostomy tubes. In addition, they may be asked to assess their child's respiratory status and problem solve correctly, based on their assessments. All this is in addition to attending to normal well child needs and caring for other siblings, partners, and those household responsibilities that are required 24 hours a day, 7 days a week. Tasks that must be performed four or more times a day are difficult for any parent to maintain over a period of time. The compliance problem that may ensue may belong not to the parents but to the health care team who expect such superhuman feats.

## ADAPTATION

Research and clinical papers offer an inconsistent perspective of family experiences when a child has a chronic condition. Older publications portray a family in extreme difficulty, with marital disruption inevitable and family functioning ineffective, whereas more recent research emphasizes family strengths and describes family growth as a result of the child's condition. Chronic conditions occurring in childhood are significant stressors for the family. However, families in this situation can generally be viewed as normal families coping with an abnormal situation.

Although families generally tend to adapt well to the strain of caring for a child with a special health care need, occasionally the family's approach to parenting their child may have less than positive effects.

## Overprotection

Preconceived notions of abilities and expectations influence a child's capacities. Lower expectations for behavior result in the expected behavior, a self-fulfilling prophecy. These social expectations are held by both parents and society, resulting in childrearing practices that discourage the child's experiences and the experimentation ordinarily helpful to development of the child's inherent abilities. Overprotection is an excess of attention on the child with a chronic condition; specifically, attention is directed at the impairment rather than the child. Activities are restricted and with them the opportunity to learn, especially to learn independence and mastery of the environment. Thus the child is restricted from experiences that "healthy" children encounter. Hence the child is often handicapped more by the attitudes of those around him or her, or by his or her own attitudes (a learned response), than by the condition.

## Rejection

Parental refusal to accept the child's diagnosis or handicapping condition can lead the child to believe that he or she is unworthy of the parent's love and affection. This may be demonstrated in many ways: unrealistic parental expectations for the child with the chronic condition; increased attention given to nonimpaired siblings; abandonment (physically or psychologically) of the affected child; or conditional love, which is given when the "ill" child acts or responds according to parental needs. Rejection of the child instills feelings of worthlessness in the child and promotes low self-esteem.

One major problem between families and health care providers is that each sees the world differently (i.e., with their own perspective or world view). Each person's perspective embodies a basic set of assumptions or beliefs through which all perception is filtered and on which all behavior is based. Perspectives are developed as a result of real world experience and learning.

An important finding of a study of family perception of the health care system was the differences in views between families and health care providers when a child had a chronic condition (Thomas, 1986). The discrepancy in perspectives was significant. For example, health care providers tended to be future oriented and viewed movement toward long-term goals for the child as reason enough to engage in uncomfortable treatments. For parents, it was exceedingly difficult to see the child in pain or distress. This is not to say the providers were insensitive to the child's distress, only that they were better able to see the distress in light of the eventual good the treatment or procedure might offer the child.

## Control Issues

Traditionally, health care providers are accustomed to having control over their environment and considerable control over children under their care. Before recent advances in medical technology, children with severe chronic conditions either recovered or died. Currently many of these children return home. Their families have both the desire and the opportunity to regain their role as independent care providers for their child.

In a study of family and health care provider relationships, the struggle for control over care of the child with a chronic condition—and over other aspects of the family's life-styles—was a major concern for families (Thomas, 1986). It was the one aspect of health care provider and family interaction that engendered the most anger on the part of families. In general, families who have a child with a chronic condition interact with the health care environment over long periods. The families become expert in their child's care needs and specific idiosyncratic responses to treatment. Most families eventually wish to contribute their knowledge to the health care decision-making process. A problem may arise if health care providers (some of whom may be socialized to believe they should control the child's care) resist the change in the family's role from that of recipient to that of active participant in the health care process.

In the home setting the provider should recognize and affirm the parents' knowledge about the changes they have made to cope with necessary treatments. Many families deal with conflicts and alterations in life-style, such as physical changes in the house, oxygen tanks, suction machines, housekeeping changes, financial strain, frequent physician and hospital visits (requiring transportation of both child and all the necessary accompanying equipment to care for the child), and changes in social life events. It would be very easy for families to view these as severe self-deprivations without an accompanying feeling of purpose and satisfaction.

Predicting and preventing future stresses can facilitate family stabilization and coping. Predictable conflicts in most families who have children with chronic respiratory problems center on nutrition, medications, and other physical treatments. Most parents have been taught the important relationship between caloric intake and chronic respiratory disease; however, children quickly learn that they gain increased attention by refusing to eat. Their parents, in desperate attempts to get calories into them, may promise unusual treats or cajole and bribe their children. Offering a variety of calorically dense foods and additives to a child's known favorite foods can prevent some difficult meals and minimize control issues. In addition, some children may need supplemental tube (nasogastric or gastrostomy) feedings to promote growth and decrease feeding control issues. Parents may need help in recognizing the kinds of behavior that begin a cycle of frustration for all involved. A knowledge of normal eating habits for a child's stage of development can be helpful (e.g., toddlers rarely eat "meals" or may have "food jags" for days at a time).

## EDUCATIONAL SYSTEM

Of equal importance to the response of health care providers is the educational system's compliance with legal requirements that guarantee a child's right to an education in a barrier-free environment. Attitudes of educators influence both their interpretation of the law and their daily interaction with the child. Education plays a major role in molding the adjustment of the child with a chronic illness. Communication between teachers and school-based nurses, families, home care nurses, and the primary care provider is important (Thomas, 1986). Most school nurses desire to be more involved in the process of supporting families who have children with special health care needs. They can offer the child assistance in attending school on a regular basis by supervising medications, educating the child's peers and teachers regarding the condition, and supporting the child's participation in regular school activities, as appropriate. This kind of support can be made available to the child and family through regular communication between home care providers and school-based nurses and teachers. To forge such an alliance, the family's permission to share privileged information must be obtained and the family kept involved in all goals and activities.

Caring for a child with special health care needs can be a rewarding experience for the family and home care providers. Anticipation of the expected stress points in conjunction with the appropriate solutions can provide additional support for a family. Goals must be mutually supported by the child, family, and health care team to promote safe and effective community-based home care.

## REFERENCES

Brewster A: Chronically ill hospitalized children's concepts of their illness, *Pediatrics* 69:355, 1982.

Hymovich D: Parents of sick children: their needs and tasks, *Pediatr Nurs* 2:9, 1976.

Levitan S, Belous R, Gallo F: *What's happening to the American family?* Baltimore, 1988, Johns Hopkins University Press.

McCubbin M: Family stress, resources, and family types: chronic illness in children, *Fam Relations* 37:203, 1988.

Schulman J: Coping with major disease: child, family, pediatrician, *J Pediatr* 102:988, 1983.

Thomas R: *Cognitive development in children with chronic conditions,* Unpublished manuscript, 1984, University of Washington, Seattle.

Thomas R: *Ventilator dependency consequences for child and family,* doctoral dissertation, Seattle, 1986, University of Washington.

## SUGGESTED READINGS

Cardoso P: A parent's perspective: family-centered care, *Child Health Care* 20:258, 1991.

Rose MH, Thomas RB, editors: *Children with chronic conditions: nursing in a family and community context,* New York, 1987, Grune & Stratton.

# CHAPTER 19

# SEXUALITY

SALLY CRIM TIBBALS

Sexuality is an important component of healthy living. Chronic illness and the losses associated with aging can influence sexual function in many ways. Sexuality has a profound influence on the overall emotional adjustment of patients and is one of the factors of most concern to them (Anderson, 1986). Ample evidence exists that chronic lung disease adversely affects sexual functioning. Male impotence has been shown to increase with a decline in pulmonary function in men with chronic obstructive pulmonary disease (COPD) (Fletcher, 1982). Chronic respiratory disease has been reported to have a significant detrimental effect on the sexual component of marriage (Hanson, 1982). Over half of the wives of men with COPD in one survey reported that they no longer had marital relations; this is in contrast to 10% in a matched control population (Sexton, 1985).

Problems with sexuality are not confined to older patients with COPD. Young people with cystic fibrosis must deal with especially burdensome issues relating to sexuality and generativity. Patients with asthma may experience significant wheezing with sexual activity (Andrews, 1985), reinforcing negative feelings about intimacy. Adults in their thirties and forties with hereditary emphysema often find that sexual activity leads to significant respiratory distress.

Despite these factors, health care professionals have paid little attention to this important aspect of human functioning. Assessment and education about sexual functioning are often omitted from pulmonary rehabilitation and home care programs. Home care staff can play an important role in helping respiratory patients enhance their sexuality and resume more normal and fulfilling sexual relations with their partners. This chapter discusses the etiologic factors, assessment of, and nursing interventions for problems with sexuality experienced by respiratory home care patients.

## ETIOLOGY

Many factors are commonly associated with diminished sexual activity in patients with chronic lung disease. These factors include the physiologic impact of lung disease and its treatment, aging, psychosocial problems, and coexisting illnesses.

## Factors Associated with Cardiopulmonary Dysfunction
### Dyspnea

Dyspnea in association with sexual intercourse is a common complaint for patients with chronic lung disease. The physical requirements in terms of oxygen consumption, cardiovascular function, and respiratory workload may be so taxing that coitus is considered to be impossible. Oppressive dyspnea and the accompanying fear and panic that prevent satisfactory intercourse may lead to a sense of frustration, despair, and dejection.

Orgasm is accompanied by respiratory rates that may exceed 40 breaths per minute, heart rates that may exceed 180 beats per minute, and hypertension (Masters, 1966). This physiologic burden increases dyspnea and may well be difficult for patients with end-stage cardiopulmonary dysfunction. Orthopnea may limit positions for lovemaking. Complaints of a smothering sensation may be increased in a situation that involves physical closeness with another person. The need for a cool environment and intolerance of odors may also contribute to the sensation of dyspnea with sexual activity.

### Coughing, Sputum Production, and Wheezing

Frequent coughing and sputum production may interrupt or disrupt lovemaking. Exercise-induced wheezing may be frightening for both partners.

### Hypoxemia

Male potency requires at least three hormones for normal functioning, the secretion of which may be affected by hypoxemia. The neurotransmitter function within the brain also begins to fail under the stress of decreased oxyhemoglobin saturation, interfering with normal penile erection (Petty, 1986). Symptoms of hypoxemia such as anxiety, irritability, agitation, skeletal muscle tremor, insomnia, and headache may also act as deterrents to intimacy.

### Psychosocial Factors

■ *Young Adults. Teenagers with asthma or cystic fibrosis are often dependent on others for treatments and may be overprotected by their parents (Waechter, 1985). Breathing problems may also limit the adolescent's social experience and skills, making it more difficult to compete with healthy peers for dates with the most desirable partners. Chronically ill teenagers often feel insecure and inadequate in their sex roles and may have been treated as asexual beings by parents, health care professionals, and society (Waechter, 1985).*

*Physical attractiveness and athletic prowess are important to adolescents—so, too, is the need to be and think like everyone else. However, teen-agers with cystic fibrosis are often short and thin and have delayed development of secondary sex characteristics. They cough up thick sputum and have malodorous bowel movements and significant clubbing of fingers and toes. These factors contribute to a poor body image and may invite ridicule from healthier peers.*

For those with cystic fibrosis who marry, the financial burden of expensive health care, a complex daily treatment regimen, physical limitations, frequent illness, and the specter of premature death can cause tremendous stress that spills over into all aspects of the couple's marital relationship. Most men with cystic fibrosis are infertile, and women with cystic fibrosis may have difficulty conceiving or bearing a child. Adoption is more difficult because of the patient's disease. If a women with cystic fibrosis decides to bear a child, she risks stressing an already compromised cardiopulmonary system. In addition, the couple must cope with the fact that any children they might have will carry the cystic fibrosis gene and that the affected parent may not live to see the children grow up.

■ *Adults.* Adult-onset asthma and hereditary emphysema ($\alpha_1$-antitrypsin deficiency) are seen in adults under 50 years of age. Many of these patients must cope with the necessity for significant lifestyle changes, including altered family relationships, increasing disability, and alteration of their self-image. During this usually active period of life, they must change or eliminate many activities.

Patterns of communication between patients and their families are often dramatically altered as a result of a chronic illness and may break down altogether, further compromising intimacy. Partners are often hesitant to engage in sexual activity for fear that it will be too physically taxing for the patient or that the resulting dyspnea and distress will be harmful. The partner may also feel guilty for being interested in sex when the other person is not. Partners must deal with their own frustration and grief over losses associated with the ill partner's declining physical condition.

Chronic illness also threatens the patient's ability to fulfill the traditional stereotyped gender roles that are still the norm for most couples over 50 years of age and often results in role reversal. For example, the wife becomes the breadwinner, while the patient is confined to tasks in the home more usually thought to be "women's work." These changes are particularly intolerable for men whose self-esteem is based on earning capacity and masculine pursuits. Comparable losses and propensity to depression probably occur in women with COPD, but this has not been studied.

### Other Factors Affecting Sexuality

■ *Aging.* The incidence of organic impotence in older males is more common than was formerly believed (Timms, 1982). Men over 50 years of age may notice changes in the frequency, strength, and duration of erections and sex drive, leading to concerns related to their masculinity. Secondary impotence (impotence occurring after a male has already established a pattern of successful sexual relationships) is more related to lack of understanding, inaccurate information, fear of performance, disuse, and other factors than to a natural component of aging. Decreased vaginal lubrication is a common manifestation of menopause and may result in dyspareunia. Orgasmic dysfunction and dyspareunia are common sexual problems for older women.

■ *Coexisting Illness and Medications.* Coexisting chronic illnesses such as diabetes mellitus, arteriosclerosis, and prostatic hypertrophy can have profound effects on erectile power and potency. Many chronic illnesses impair orgasmic responsiveness indirectly by affecting libido and general health. Medications—notably antihypertensive agents, muscle relaxants, and tranquilizers—can also contribute to impotence.

■ *Alcohol Abuse.* Alcohol is a central nervous system depressant that interferes with the nerve pathways of reflex transmission necessary for sexual arousal. Male chronic alcohol abusers display decreased libido and may be impotent or have ejaculatory difficulties. Women alcohol abusers may have difficulty with arousal and a reduction in the intensity or frequency of orgasm. Peripheral neuropathy associated with alcoholism also contributes to sexual dysfunction.

■ *Poor Communication and Emotional Issues.* Lack of clear, honest communication appears to be a causal factor for most people reporting dissatisfaction with their sexual relationships. People tend to avoid the topic of sex, thereby limiting opportunities for frank discussion. Half-truths and myths often increase anxiety over sexual performance and can lead to further sexual dysfunction. Sexual functioning is highly responsive to stress and emotional tensions. Specific emotions that may inhibit sexual performance and response include depression, anxiety, grief, embarrassment, fear, doubt, anger, and guilt. Conversely, impaired sexual function may be a factor in precipitating feelings of anxiety and depression.

## ASSESSMENT

The assessment of sexual dysfunction must be based on the history obtained from the patient and partner. It is difficult, however, to separate the assessment from therapeutic intervention because the sexual history itself may be a therapeutic intervention. During the interview the nurse provides an opportunity for the patient and partner to discuss their concerns, contributes information and suggestions, and validates the normalcy and acceptability of concerns and practices.

### Sexual History

A complete assessment of sexual health should include information on past sexual attitudes and functioning, as well as current effects of the patient's chronic lung disease on interpersonal relationships, behavior, intimacy, and sexual function. Obtaining the sexual history early in the therapeutic relationship allows the integration of concepts of sexuality throughout the relationship. When addressed as part of total physical and emotional functioning, questions about sexuality convey the message that this is a legitimate component of health.

Initial questions regarding sexuality are best integrated into the baseline history, usually among questions about dyspnea-related changes in the activity level. If the patient acknowledges concerns about sexuality, the door is opened for further open-ended questions.

A detailed discussion of sexual concerns may be appropriate on a first visit, but it is more typically deferred until the nurse and patient have had time to establish a rapport. If sexual function is identified on the first visit as an area that will be addressed in the future, the patient will be prepared for later questions.

Because chronic respiratory disorders can negatively affect the psychosociosexual functioning of both partners, the assessment should ideally involve both partners. Interviewing the couple both together and separately is helpful. A joint interview allows observation of their interactions and responses to one another. However, different information is often obtained from talking with each partner separately. Partners may be uncomfortable about revealing their true feelings in the other person's presence or may fear being misunderstood or causing hurt to the other. It is also important to know whether the patient and partner have congruent goals regarding sexual functioning. For example, the patient may desire a more active sex life, whereas the spouse is relieved "to be done with it." When interviewing the patient and partner separately, it is important to assure both that their responses will remain confidential.

## Use of Interview Guides and Questionnaires

The following interview guide, incorporating generic questions from the work of Masters and Johnson with questions specific to respiratory disease, may help to organize the sexual history:
*Generic questions*
- Are you currently sexually active? If so, what is the approximate frequency of sexual activity?
- Are you satisfied with your sex life? If not, please explain.
- (For men) Do you have difficulty achieving or maintaining an erection? Do you have any difficulty with control of ejaculation?
- (For women) Do you have any difficulty becoming sexually aroused? Do you ever experience pain during intercourse? Do you have difficulties reaching orgasm?

- Do you have questions or problems related to sex that you would like to discuss?

*Questions specific to patients with respiratory disease*
- Have you noticed any change in your interest in sexual activities since the onset of your breathing problems?
- Have you noticed any change in your partner's response to your sexual overtures since your breathing problems began?
- Do you ever have to stop in the middle of sexual activities because of shortness of breath or weakness?
- Do you ever avoid sexual activity you would otherwise have engaged in because it may cause your breathing to get worse? Because you are just too tired or weak? Because you are disinterested?
- Do you ever try to rush intercourse to reach orgasm quickly before you get too tired or short of breath?
- If you use oxygen at home, do you use it during sexual activity?
- What position do you and your partner use for intercourse? Has this changed since your breathing problem developed?
- Have you noticed any change in your moods, behaviors, or feelings since your breathing problem developed?

Even when patients deny problems with sexuality, they often bring the subject up at a later date: "Remember when you asked me all those questions about sex? Well, there *are* a few things I would like to discuss with you." Patients have been given permission to talk about their concerns.

Information on sexual concerns can also be obtained by adding questions to a self-reported health history or by leaving a sexual history questionnaire with the patient and a respiratory partner questionnaire (Fig. 19-1) with the spouse to be completed before the next home visit. Questionnaires cut down on interview time, may be a less embarrassing way for patients and their partners to impart necessary information, can provide the couple with time to think about their responses, and may even prompt some interim discussion between them.

**Partner assessment of sexual function since onset of patient's respiratory symptoms**

1. Age: _____ Sex: _____ Respiratory patient's age: _____

2. Do you have any major health problems?    Yes _____ No _____
   If yes, please explain _____
   _____
   _____

3. What year did you first begin to notice your partner's breathing problem, i.e., shortness of breath, cough, etc.? _____

4. Have you noticed any change in your sexual relationship since the onset of your partner's breathing problem?    Yes _____ No _____
   If yes, please explain briefly: _____
   _____
   _____

5. When was the last time you and your partner engaged in pleasurable sexual intercourse?
   (a) 1-7 days ago _____      (c) 14-30 days ago _____      (e) 60-365 days ago _____
   (b) 7-14 days ago _____      (d) 30-60 days ago _____      (f) over 1 year ago _____

6. Have you ever noticed an increase in your partner's physical distress during or after sex?
   Yes _____ No _____    If yes, how do you react to or handle this? _____
   _____
   How does your partner handle this? _____
   _____

7. Do you ever hesitate to initiate sexual activity because you are concerned that it might make your partner's breathing worse or cause your partner other physical distress?
   Yes _____ No _____

8. Do you ever discourage your partner's interest in sexual activity because you feel it may cause your partner physical distress?    Yes _____ No _____

9. Have you noticed any change in your partner's personality, behavior, or emotions since the onset of his or her breathing problems?    Yes _____ No _____    If yes, does this change ever affect your ability to respond to your partner sexually? _____
   _____

10. Would you be interested in talking with a health professional regarding any question you might have related to sexuality?    Yes _____ No _____

**Fig. 19-1**    Respiratory Partner Questionnaire.

When questionnaires are used, it is important to allow plenty of time during the next home visit to review and discuss the couple's responses. Interestingly, men, whether patient or partner, nearly always report more frequent and more recent sexual relations than do their partners.

## Assessing the Efficacy of Sexual Counseling

For some, marked improvement in sexual functioning can be attained with a few simple suggestions for reducing dyspnea and fatigue. For others, progress toward a more effective sexual relationship is slow. The success of interventions is determined by the degree to which expected outcomes have been met. As changes occur or more information is obtained, new interventions may be needed. If interventions have been successful, the patient and significant other will be able to accomplish the following, as appropriate:

- Communicate sexual concerns and problems
- Identify stresses involved in their life-style that impair sexuality
- Discuss feelings, likes, dislikes, and alternative sexual activities with their significant other and, if indicated, with the counselor
- Verbalize plans for enhancing sexual activity
- Identify comfortable alternative positions for sexual activity that are acceptable to both partners
- Participate in pleasurable sexual activities without significant dyspnea, discomfort, or panic
- Maintain a relationship conducive to sexual functioning
- Express sexuality in a manner comfortable and rewarding to patient and partner
- Express sexual feelings in a manner consistent with personal values and beliefs

## NURSING INTERVENTIONS

Because home care nurses provide one-on-one care over time, they often develop a relationship in which clients feel safe in raising questions about sexuality. Nurses should be prepared to meet these needs through counseling or, for more complex problems, by referral to appropriate community resources.

## Counseling the Adolescent and the Young Adult

*Teenagers often feel more comfortable confiding in someone other than a parent about sexual issues and may raise questions or casually hint at concerns when talking with the nurse in private. These concerns need to be acknowledged and explored. Issues may focus on anxieties about dating and anticipated first sexual experiences. As for all individuals, patients who are or soon plan to be sexually active need information on birth control and sexually transmitted diseases. They may also need advice on where to obtain the necessary supplies and encouragement to follow through.*

## Genetic Counseling in Cystic Fibrosis

Genetic counseling is extremely important for the parents of a child with cystic fibrosis and for the young adult who is contemplating marriage and a family. It is important for the home health care nurse to have at least a general understanding of the genetic implications of cystic fibrosis and to encourage and be able to direct the patient or family members to appropriate counseling resources. Genetic counseling is provided as part of the usual care through cystic fibrosis centers affiliated with the National Cystic Fibrosis Foundation (1-800-344-4823).

### Issues for the Parents of a Child with Cystic Fibrosis

As known carriers of the cystic fibrosis gene, parents must know that, with each pregnancy, they face a 25% chance of having a child with cystic fibrosis, and a 50% chance of having a child who is a carrier. They must decide whether they are willing to take this risk.

### Issues for Siblings of People with Cystic Fibrosis

Well siblings of someone with cystic fibrosis may or may not be carriers of the gene, but they can be tested to determine carrier state. Currently available carrier testing can identify about 85% of carriers.

### Issues for the Young Adult with Cystic Fibrosis

Cystic fibrosis is the most common autosomal recessive genetic disorder affecting whites. Because 1 in every 25 whites is a carrier, the chances of someone with cystic fibrosis marrying a carrier are substantial. Should this happen, and should the couple decide to have children, they face a 50% chance of producing a child with cystic fibrosis with each pregnancy and the certainty that each child will be, at minimum, a carrier. This concern is added to the potential risk to the mother's health of carrying a child to term. Increasingly, relatively healthy young women with cystic fibrosis are choosing to have children and, with vigilant prenatal care, are doing well. However, it is a decision that should be made with full awareness of the potential problems.

## The PLISSIT Model: A Framework for Limited Sexual Counseling

The PLISSIT model developed by Annon and associates provides a framework for limited sexual counseling (Annon, 1976; Kravitz, 1982). It has the following components:

- Giving *P*ermission to talk about sexual function
- Offering *L*imited *I*nformation by way of a direct answer to the question
- Providing *S*pecific *S*uggestions relevant to the problems (e.g., "Try using your bronchodilator 30 minutes before sexual activity.")
- Referring for *I*ntensive *T*herapy

The authors of the PLISSIT therapeutic model maintain that up to 90% of all sexual problems and dysfunction can be handled by personnel with a minimal background in sexual counseling, with only 10% of problems requiring intensive therapy by a certified sex counselor or therapist.

### Providing "Limited Information"

In the process of providing information the nurse can dispel sexual myths and furnish concrete, ac-

curate information appropriate to that individual (e.g., sexual changes that occur with aging). Four specific questions that pulmonary patients often ask about sex are the following (Kravetz, 1980).

1. *How will my breathing be affected by having sex?* The patient should be reassured that a moderate increase in dyspnea associated with sex is not harmful, and should be provided with information on measures to improve exercise tolerance and control of breathing.

2. *How much can I exert myself sexually?* Patients should be reassured that (in the absence of a recent life-threatening cardiac event) their body is well able to tolerate the increase in heart rate, blood pressure, and respiratory rate associated with sex. However, they must allow time during foreplay for the body to adjust to the increased oxygen and circulatory demands.

3. *What effect will my medications have on my sexual functioning?* The male patient should be told whether any of the medications he is taking could interfere with sexual performance, so that he does not confuse medication-induced dysfunction with primary erectile dysfunction.

4. *What changes in sexual function should I expect at my age?* Older adults may attribute changes in sexual response to their breathing problems rather than to normal changes associated with aging. They should be given enough information to recognize age-predictable changes in erections, ejaculation, refractory period, and duration of stimulation needed to reach orgasm. Women over 50 years of age need information about decreased lubrication and size of the vaginal barrel and ways to overcome discomfort associated with penetration.

## Specific Suggestions for Reducing Dyspnea

To reduce symptoms and enhance sexual enjoyment, the patient can be encouraged to do the following:

- Use an inhaled bronchodilator 30 to 45 minutes before planned sexual activity. Include additional bronchial hygiene measures if copious or thick secretions interfere with activities.

- Plan sexual activity for the "best breathing" time of the day. Wait at least 2 to 3 hours after meals.
- Choose a position that avoids pressure on the chest and abdomen and eliminates the need to support oneself on the arms. The traditional "male superior" position may be extremely difficult for either partner. A side-lying position, either face to face (Fig. 19-2) or with the male behind the female (Fig. 19-3), allows for lovemaking without the additional strain of propping oneself up on elbows and knees. The side-lying position also relieves the potentially suffocating feeling of having the partner's body weight on the patient's chest. Try different positions: a position that permits the patient's upper body to be propped up will be more comfortable for the person with mild orthopnea. For example, the female patient can sit, with the male kneeling or standing (Fig. 19-4), or the male can semirecline against the headboard or sit in a chair with the female sitting atop (Figs. 19-5 and 19-6).
- Use oxygen during sexual activity if home oxygen therapy has been prescribed. The oxygen flow rate should be the same as that prescribed for exercise.
- Try a waterbed to aid in thrusting.
- If dyspnea becomes severe during lovemaking, slow down or stop, use relaxation techniques, perhaps share a glass of wine, and try to regain control of dyspnea. If these measures do not work, suggest postponing further activity but reinforce one's enjoyment of the closeness.
- Try touching, cuddling, talking about likes and dislikes, and exploring each other's bodies. A rewarding sexual relationship is more encompassing than merely reaching orgasm.
- Implement a graduated exercise program or enroll in a formal pulmonary rehabilitation program to increase muscle strength and endurance. This increases capacity for all activities of daily living, including lovemaking.
- Use massage to relax tense muscles. The patient's partner can be taught to massage tense shoulder girdle muscles to reduce dyspnea,

tension, and anxiety. Massage has many benefits, not the least of which is touching and working together. The use of massage and coaching of pursed lip breathing and relaxation may also set the stage for spontaneous experimentation with gentle foreplay.
- Allow extra time for foreplay to allow the body to adapt gradually to increased oxygen and circulatory demands. Slow, relaxed foreplay during the arousal and plateau phase reduces emotional and physical stress.

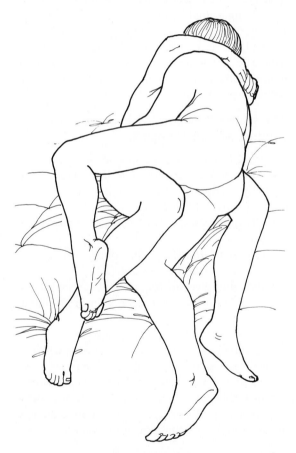

**Fig. 19-2** Initially this position may be a more acceptable modification and promotes feelings of closeness.

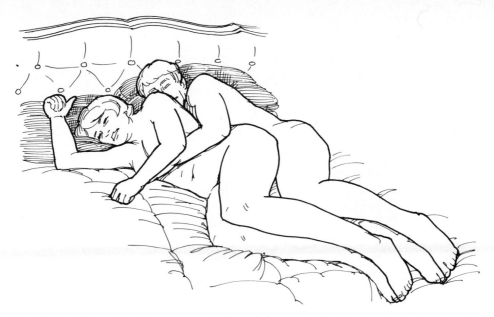

**Fig. 19-3** This position also promotes feelings of closeness and minimizes smothering sensations.

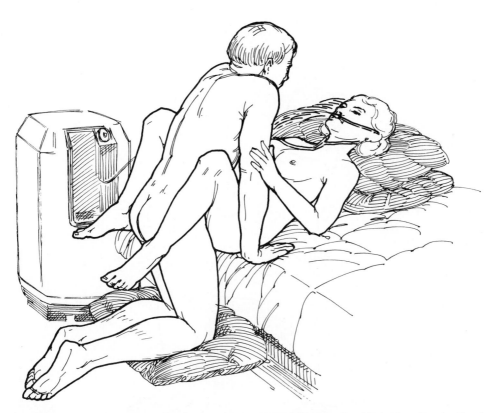

**Fig. 19-4** For the male patient, elevation of shoulders reduces work of breathing. For the female patient, reclining against pillows on a couch, chair or bed may facilitate breathing.

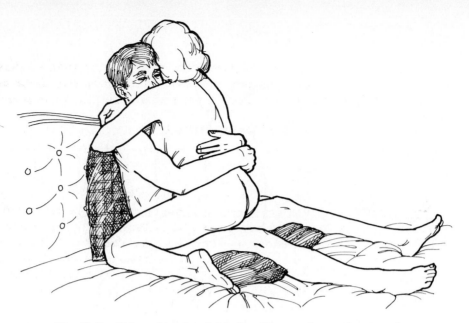

**Fig. 19-5**  This position is suitable for either a male or a female patient.

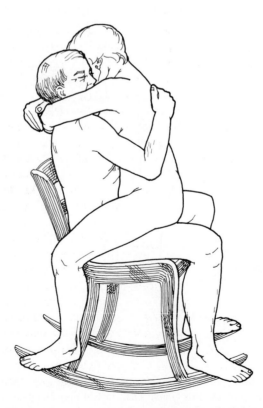

**Fig. 19-6**  This position has been suggested for patients when both have breathing problems.

## Sensate Routine

For patients who have not successfully achieved orgasm for some time or for those whose cardio-pulmonary status is very impaired, the following sensate routine may be integrated into a broader pulmonary rehabilitation program:

- Encourage the patient to progress gradually from noncoital experiences to sexual intercourse. Initially, couples may begin with mutual holding, touching, and caressing, without stimulation of the genitals.
- As the couple becomes comfortable with this, they can proceed to mutual stimulation of breasts and genitalia.
- If acceptable, self-pleasuring, oral-genital sexuality, or both may be added.
- Finally, when physically and emotionally ready, the couple may proceed to intercourse.

Emphasis is placed on giving and receiving pleasure, enjoying sensuous exercises, and learning to communicate likes and dislikes. Experimentation and the use of humor are encouraged, reinforcing the philosophy, "If it feels good to you both, then do it!"

## Use of Patient Education Materials

Patient education materials can reinforce points made in counseling sessions. The patient education handout (see box at right) and the pamphlets, books, and videotapes included in the patient education resources listed in the box on p. 336 address issues of sexuality specific to the pulmonary patient and can be used either to introduce the topic of sexuality or to reinforce counseling. Videotapes are often available through local pulmonary rehabilitation programs, lung clubs, or patient education libraries.

## Cultural Issues Relevant to Sexual Counseling

Cultural norms dictate what types of sexual behavior are acceptable and who may perform them. Because nurses provide care for patients from all socioeconomic, religious, and ethnic backgrounds, they must be sensitive to the impact these factors

---

### How to Enjoy Sex More— Helpful Hints

1. Build up your general body strength by a gradual conditioning program such as walking.
2. Learn and practice relaxation techniques.
3. Choose the best breathing time of the day for sexual activity.
4. Never have sex after a heavy meal or large amounts of alcohol.
5. Keep the room cool and well ventilated.
6. Be rested.
7. Use your bronchodilator inhaler about 30 minutes before sex.
8. Start sex slowly. Spend more time in foreplay, enjoying each other. If you begin to get anxious, stop, relax, cuddle, and maybe have a little wine together.
9. Find a comfortable position that does not put pressure on your chest or abdomen and that does not require you to support yourself on your arms.
10. If you breathe better with your head elevated, experiment with positions that allow you to be sitting up or in a semireclining position.
11. If you normally use oxygen, continue to use it during sex.
12. Experiment with each other.

Do what makes you feel relaxed
and comfortable.
Whatever you do, do not work at it.
Enjoy each other.

---

may have on the patient's value system. For example, it would be a serious breach of etiquette to discuss sexuality with a traditional Asian couple before a good rapport had been established and "bad luck" to discuss sexual issues when a women is pregnant or during the Asian holidays.

Expected behavior of males and females within a culture often differs, as does behavior of older couples compared to younger couples. Examples include positions for intercourse, active or passive

## Patient Education Resources

Barrow MH, Hull NR: *To air is human: a manual for people with chronic lung disease,* Atlanta, 1989, Pritchett & Hull.
- A patient education booklet with an excellent section on sexuality. Call 1-800-241-4925 to order.

*Being close,* Denver, 1987, National Jewish Center for Immunology and Respiratory Medicine.
- A helpful pamphlet about intimacy for people with respiratory disorders; free of charge. Call 1-800-222-LUNG to order.

Butler R, Lewis M: *Love and sex after sixty,* New York, 1977, Harper & Row.
- Discusses normal physical changes with aging, the common medical problems affecting an older age group, and the impact of the loss of one's partner.

Dickinson P: *The fires of autumn: sexual activity in the middle and later years,* New York, 1977, Sterling Publishing.

Petty TL, Nett LM: *Enjoying life with emphysema,* Philadelphia, 1984, Lea & Febiger.
- An outstanding self-care booklet for the patient with COPD; Chapter 10 deals with sexuality.

**AUDIOVISUAL TEACHING RESOURCES**

*You can do it: living with a breathing problem—pulmonary self-care: a program for patients* (1980), Chicago, Encyclopaedia Britannica Educational Corporation.
- An excellent videotape, 25 minutes in length; deals with all aspects of coping with COPD, including sexuality.

Kravetz, HM: *A visit with Harry* (1981) and *A visit with Helen* (1982).
- Excellent slide/cassette tapes appropriate for men or women with COPD. Available from Howard Kravetz, MD, Prescott, AZ.

roles, frequency of sexual activity, duration of intercourse, and the variety of methods considered appropriate for sexual stimulation and for contraception. Many older women experience internal conflicts between the more liberal current sexual behaviors and the attitudes and values they learned in their earlier sociocultural environment.

When working with patients from different social, ethnic, or cultural backgrounds, it is important to determine in advance whether there are cultural proscriptions regarding sexual counseling. University programs in transcultural nursing and churches or community service groups working with immigrant, ethnic, religious, or other special populations are excellent resources for such information.

## Developing Professional Skills in Sexual Counseling

It is difficult for many nurses to discuss sexual matters with patients and to teach and counsel them appropriately. Nurses must have a sincere feeling of comfort with their own sexuality to discuss sexual functioning with patients. A nonjudgmental attitude is also imperative; otherwise, the nonverbal messages projected will prevent patients from raising a sexual concern no matter how important the question is for them.

Workshops, courses on sexuality, and other health professionals with expertise in sexual counseling are excellent resources for factual information. Such resources can also assist the nurse to recognize attitudes and emotions that inhibit effective communication with patients.

**REFERENCES**

Anderson BJ, Wolf FM: Chronic physical illness and sexual behavior: psychological issues, *J Consult Clin Psychol* 54:168, 1986.

Andrews JL: Sex and asthma. In Weiss EB et al, editors: *Bronchial asthma,* Boston, 1985, Little, Brown.

Annon JS: The PLISSIT model: a proposed conceptual scheme for the behavioral treatment of sexual problems, *J Sex Educ Ther* 2:1, 1976.

Fletcher EC, Martin RJ: Sexual dysfunction and erectile impotence in chronic obstructive pulmonary disease, *Chest* 81:413, 1982.

Hanson EI: Effects of chronic lung disease on life in general and on sexuality: perceptions of adult patients, *Heart Lung* 11:435, 1982.

Kravetz HM: Sexual counseling for the COPD patient, *Clin Challenge Cardiopulm Med* No 1 vol 4:1, 1982, American College of Chest Physicians.

Kravetz H, Weiss M, Meadows R: *Sexual counseling for pulmonary patients* (slide-tape presentation), Prescott, Ariz, 1980.

Masters WH, Johnson VE: *Human sexual response*, Boston, 1966, Little, Brown.

Petty TL: Health, sex and better quality of life for your COPD patient, *Med Aspects Hum Sexuality* 20:70, 1986.

Sexton DL, Munro BH: Impact of a husband's chronic illness (COPD) on the spouse's life, *Res Nurs Health* 8:83, 1985.

Timms RM: Sexual dysfunction and chronic obstructive pulmonary disease, *Chest* 81:398, 1982.

Waechter EH, Phillips J, Holaday B: *Nursing care of children,* Philadelphia, 1985, JB Lippincott.

## SUGGESTED READINGS

Butterworth MJE et al: Sexual dysfunction in the elderly male, *J Am Geriatr Soc* 35:1014, 1987.

Della Bella L: Sexuality and the pulmonary patient. In Hodgkin JE, Zorn EG, Connors GL, editors: *Pulmonary rehabilitation: guidelines to success,* Boston, 1984, Butterworth.

Patient education resources, as previously listed.

# CHAPTER 20

# SMOKING BEHAVIOR

LOUISE M. NETT

Reports of the harmful effects of smoking became well known with the Surgeon General's Report of 1964. Many people have chosen to ignore the warnings or do not feel that the warnings apply to them. Once people are addicted to smoking, quitting often seems impossible. This chapter discusses the effects of smoking, the etiologic factors and assessment of nicotine addiction, and important nursing interventions to help patients to stop smoking.

## HARMFUL EFFECTS OF SMOKING

There is clear evidence that smoking causes emphysema, chronic bronchitis, and lung cancer, exacerbates asthma, increases the incidence of childhood respiratory illnesses, increases the risk for cardiovascular disease, and impairs fetal health. The many deleterious effects of smoking are summarized in Table 20-1.

### Medication Interactions

Serum levels of several medications are markedly altered by smoking. Most often, smoking increases the rate of metabolism of a drug, resulting in the need for a higher dose to achieve a therapeutic level. If the patient subsequently stops smoking abruptly and without reducing the drug dosage, toxic reactions may result. Conversely, someone who was abstinent, then relapsed, may experience symptoms of an inadequate drug dose.

### Socioeconomic Impact of Smoking

Smoking is increasingly viewed as a socially undesirable behavior. It stains fingers and teeth and leaves breath, hair, and clothes foul smelling. It impairs acuity of taste and smell. It is also expensive, costing over $100 a month for a two-pack-a-day smoker, depending on the state of residence. This can be a significant percentage of monthly disposable income for someone living on a low, fixed income.

### Secondhand Smoke

Research has clearly demonstrated the harmful effects of secondhand smoke on nonsmokers (Lefcoe, 1983). Effects that begin in utero and continue throughout childhood and adulthood include the following:
- Increased levels of carboxyhemoglobin in the bloodstream
- Nicotine levels in saliva, urine, and amniotic fluid equivalent to those of a light smoker
- Frequent complaints of airway and eye irritation, cough, headache, and nasal symptoms
- Increased risk of respiratory tract infection, greater likelihood of wheezing and asthma, shorter stature, and a threefold increase in mortality in children (Frequent infections in childhood increase the risk of developing respiratory symptoms and illness later in childhood or adulthood.)

**Table 20-1**   Harmful effects of smoking

| Pathophysiologic changes | Clinical impact |
| --- | --- |
| **EFFECTS ON PULMONARY SYSTEM** | |
| Airway irritation leading to inflammation, ulceration, fibrosis, squamous metaplasia, and increases in mucus-producing goblet cells | Increased cough, sputum production |
| | Impaired mucociliary clearance |
| Increase in inflammatory cells (macrophages, neutrophils) in lung parenchyma | In susceptible individuals (10%-20% of population), accelerated declines in expiratory flow rate, associated with small airway collapse, hyperinflation (i.e., emphysema) |
| Destruction and reduced motility of cilia | Increased incidence of respiratory infections, both in smokers and those exposed to smoke |
| Inhibition of protective lung enzymes (e.g., $\alpha_1$-antitrypsin), predisposing to loss of elastase | Increased incidence of COPD, and lung, mouth, laryngeal, and esophageal cancer |
| | Exacerbation of symptoms of asthma |
| **EFFECTS ON CARDIOVASCULAR SYSTEM** | |
| Sympathetic nervous system stimulation (nicotine effect) leading to increases in myocardial oxygen demand | Increased blood pressure, heart rate, cardiac output; increased coronary blood flow, countered by increases in myocardial oxygen demand |
| Displacement of oxygen by carbon monoxide on Hgb molecule leading to decreased oxygen transport | Potentiates tissue hypoxia; increased potential for arrhythmias |
| Shift of oxyhemoglobin dissociation curve to left, leading to decreased oxygen unloading at tissue level | Increased risk for atherosclerosis; predisposes to thrombus formation, leading to increased risk for stroke, angina, myocardial infarction |
| Peripheral vasoconstriction (nicotine effect) | Impaired peripheral circulation leading to peripheral vascular disease which causes increased risk for gangrene and other complications of peripheral vascular disease |
| Increase in erythropoietin secretion (CO effect), leading to increases in hematocrit and blood viscosity | |
| Decrease in high-density lipoprotein (the "good" lipid); increase in low-density lipoprotein, free fatty acids, and total cholesterol | Reduced placental circulation leading to increased risk for miscarriage, stillbirths, low birthweight babies, and retarded child development |
| Increased platelet aggregation and adhesiveness, reduced platelet survival, increased plasma fibrinogen, reduced clotting time; may change vessel walls to favor lipid deposit | |

Modified from National Institutes of Health: *Clinical opportunities for smoking intervention*, NIH Pub No 86-2170, Washington, DC, 1986, US Government Printing Office.

- Increased risk of chronic lung disease and lung cancer in adults. (The risk of secondhand smoke appears to be dose related. Compared with wives of nonsmokers, the risk of lung cancer was 2.4 times greater in wives of moderate smokers and 3.4 times greater in wives of heavy smokers [Trichopoulos, 1981].)

## PREVALENCE OF SMOKING

The encouraging decrease in the overall prevalence of smoking is somewhat masked by the large number of people who continue to smoke and the high incidence of smoking among adolescents. It is true that the percentage of people who smoke has decreased from 42% of the population in 1964 to below 30% currently. However, we are still faced with 51 million smokers in America (U.S. Surgeon General, 1988). One in seven smokers, 400,000 people, will die prematurely as a result of smoking (U.S. Surgeon General, 1989). These premature deaths and associated expenses cost the country approximately 65 billion dollars a year (Staff memo, 1985).

## MARIJUANA

Marijuana smoke is highly irritating and can trigger bronchospasm in persons with irritable airways. Of particular concern is the manner in which marijuana is smoked. Inhalation tends to be deep and is followed by prolonged breath holding, which permits greater deposition of smoke and particulates within the peripheral airways. Wu and associates noted a fivefold increase in blood carboxyhemoglobin levels, a threefold increase in tar inhalation, and a 33% increase in inhaled tar retention from smoking marijuana, as compared with smoking a comparable quantity of tobacco (Wu, 1988).

## ETIOLOGY
### Profile of the Smoker

Currently, the average cigarette smoker tends to be from the lowest income levels and most often has never married or is divorced. He or she is not likely to be a college graduate. Although more black men smoke than do white men, the reverse is true among women. Blue- and pink-collar workers form the largest occupational group of smokers. Smoking prevalence is highest for men who are construction workers, maintenance men, truck drivers, and laborers; for women the highest prevalence is among waitresses, cashiers, assemblers, and nurses' aides (U.S. Surgeon General, 1985).

### Acquiring the Habit

Understanding why and how an individual acquires the smoking habit can provide valuable insight for the health professional charged with helping that person quit. Smoking is a ritual deeply entrenched in our culture. Most individuals begin to smoke as adolescents. Their reasons for doing so are complex. Typically they are copying their parents or other role models, but many youths also see smoking as an expression of independence from adults or as a means of being nonconformist. Factors associated with adolescent smoking include the following*:

- Truancy
- Drinking alcohol
- Inability to resist peer pressure to smoke
- Friends who smoke
- Parents in lower income groups
- Parents in lower education groups
- Single-parent households
- Parental smoking
- Parental acceptance of smoking experimentation
- Older sibling who smokes
- Being a student who works
- Lower education aspirations
- Lack of acceptance of health risks of smoking
- Type A personality trait
- Extroversion personality trait
- Risk-taking orientation
- Anger

In vigorous efforts to recruit new smokers, cigarette advertisers create an image of smokers as attractive, energetic, successful young people. By

---

*Modified from Risser N: *Semin Oncol Nurs* 3:228, 1987.

spending billions of dollars on such advertising, they have succeeded in attracting thousands of youth each year to this highly addictive habit. Indeed, the present trend in smoking among adolescents is toward starting at a younger age than ever before, with the greatest increase in smoking prevalence found among teenage girls.

## Smoking as an Addiction

Smoking is now recognized to be a true physiologic addiction (U.S. Surgeon General, 1988). The development of the smoking habit generally takes 3 to 4 years and in many respects is strikingly similar to that of other addictive substances.

- The drug (nicotine) acts on the brain and nervous system (and does so within seconds, providing a remarkably fast feedback loop that enhances its addictive properties).
- There is gradual tolerance leading to daily use, a need for increased dose of nicotine, and a desire for repeated administration.
- Deprivation causes drug-seeking behavior.
- Withdrawal symptoms develop on acute cessation.
- Relapse rates are high.

The 1988 report of the U.S. Surgeon General noted that physiologic withdrawal symptoms occurring after cessation may be as severe as, and in many cases may last longer than, the withdrawal symptoms experienced by people who are addicted to cocaine or heroin.

Smokers also become psychologically dependent on the smoking habit. Many smoke because they simply enjoy the taste and experience of smoking. Smoking may help them relax or may add a pleasant "finishing touch" to a good meal or conversation. Others, especially women, smoke as a means of controlling unwanted weight gain. Young people most often continue to smoke because they like the sophisticated or liberated image they believe it portrays or because they want to emulate others who smoke. Tense or high-strung individuals often find satisfaction in handling smoking materials. Cigarettes may reduce an individual's negative feelings about himself or his situation, or they may simply

satisfy a habit or craving. Whatever reason an individual may have to continue smoking, however, the addiction to nicotine must be assumed to be the primary and overriding factor.

## ASSESSMENT
### Smoking History

A smoking history should be incorporated into the baseline assessment of any patient referred for home health care and should include the following questions:

- At what age did the patient start smoking? At what age did the patient become a regular smoker?
- How much is the patient smoking now? What brand is smoked? What is the usual pattern of inhalation?
- Why does the patient smoke? What pleasurable events and activities does the patient connect with smoking? What "good" things does smoking do?
- Who else in the family smokes?
- Has the patient ever tried to quit? How many times and for how long? What caused the patient to start smoking again? Were withdrawal symptoms experienced?
- What is the patient's usual way of handling stress and anger? How much stress is the patient experiencing at present? Is there a history of depression, alcohol abuse, or both?
- What is the patient's usual caffeine intake?
- Are there contraindications to the use of nicotine substitutes?

The smoking history questionnaire presented in Fig. 20-1 can be used as an interview guide or left with the patient for completion before the next home visit. Lifetime cigarette dosage is typically expressed as the "pack-year history." Calculation of the pack-year history is noted in Chapter 1.

A detailed smoking history reveals the degree to which smoking is an integral part of family and work life, how important it is to celebrations, and how often nicotine is used as a drug of comfort for the patient. Questions concerning stress, history of depression, and alcohol abuse are important be-

A. Use of cigarettes
   1. Age _____
   2. Age started regular smoking (1 or more cigs/day) _____
   3. Current number smoked/day _____
         Maximum ever smoked/day _____
         Average smoked/day _____
   4. Cigarette brand smoked _____
   5. Usual pattern of inhalation _____
   6. What are your reasons for smoking? _____
      _____

B. Past efforts to change or stop smoking
   1. Previous quit attempts?                          YES        NO
      If yes:
         What was the reason you tried? _____
         _____
         How many attempts and how long did each attempt last? _____
         _____
         When was the most recent? _____
         What method was used? _____
         _____
         Why do you think you started smoking again? _____
         _____
         _____

   2. Do you feel you could be successful if
      you were to decide to stop smoking now?          YES        NO

C. Environmental factors
   1. Live with spouse or friend?                      YES        NO
      If yes:
         Does she/he currently smoke?                  YES        NO
         Is she/he currently wanting to quit?          YES        NO        NA
         Is she/he interested in your quitting?        YES        NO
   2. Number of cups caffeinated beverages/day? _____
   3. Alcohol use:  Average _____
                    Maximum _____
   4. Current life stress (0 = no stress to 10 = high stress) _____

D. Do you want to quit?                   YES        NO        UNCERTAIN
   If "yes" or "uncertain":
   What are your reasons for wanting to quit? _____
   _____
   _____
   _____
   _____

- - - - - - - - - - - - - - - - - - - - - - - - - - - - - - - - - - - - - - - - -

To be completed by the clinician:
   Pack/years history:
   Current estimated daily intake of:
      Carbon monoxide
      Tar
      Nicotine

**Fig. 20-1**    Smoking history.

cause quitting is more difficult during periods of high stress and for individuals who have experienced a depressive disorder (Glassman, 1988) or have other addictive problems. Information on caffeine intake is important because smoking is often associated with cues such as having a cup of coffee and because caffeine is likely to cause more withdrawal symptoms with cessation.

In obtaining the smoking history, it is important to show genuine interest in the characteristics of the habit and to be as open and nonjudgmental as possible. Remember that most older patients with chronic obstructive pulmonary disease (COPD) began their smoking careers when smoking was the socially accepted norm, and many actually believed the effects were beneficial.

## Recognizing the Addicted Smoker

Smokers typically move through stages in their smoking careers—from casual use to a psychologic dependency and finally to a true physiologic addiction. Identification of those who are physiologically addicted is important in planning cessation strategies because these individuals are more likely to experience withdrawal symptoms and are at high risk for relapse. However, they are also more responsive to pharmacologic interventions (e.g., nicotine substitutes) than are nonaddicted smokers. Diagnostic criteria for tobacco addiction, as defined by the American Psychiatric Association (1980), include the following:

- Use of tobacco continually for a period of at least 1 month
- At least one of the following:
  Previous unsuccessful serious attempts to quit or reduce smoking
  Withdrawal symptoms occurring with previous attempts to quit
  Continued tobacco use despite a serious medical disorder known to be exacerbated by tobacco use

The Fagerström Nicotine Tolerance Scale (Fagerström, 1978) is a simple tool that can help assess the severity of the physiologic addiction to nicotine (Fig. 20-2).

## Recognizing Nicotine Withdrawal Symptoms

Common symptoms of nicotine withdrawal include the following (Schneider, 1985):

- Craving for tobacco
- Nervousness, restlessness, anxiety, tremulousness
- Impatience, irritability
- Difficulty concentrating
- Fatigue, loss of energy
- Somatic complaints: headache, gastrointestinal disturbances, hunger, eating, light-headedness
- Frequent and lengthy sleep awakenings, drowsiness

The presence and severity of withdrawal symptoms vary greatly between people, with some heavy smokers experiencing severe symptoms and others experiencing few or none. The dose of nicotine is probably the greatest determinant of the severity of symptoms, but individual tolerance for discomfort, heavy caffeine use, and other drug interactions may play a role.

Tobacco withdrawal symptoms appear within hours of abstinence and seem to peak between 36 and 72 hours. Symptoms decline gradually over the next 1 to 2 weeks, although they can last up to 6 weeks. Occasionally smokers complain of withdrawal symptoms for several months.

## NURSING INTERVENTIONS

Home health care personnel have a responsibility to the patient who smokes, and the nurse is in a particularly good position to assist patients and family members in their efforts to stop smoking. Because care is provided in the patient's home and often continues over several weeks, health habits are observable and patients tend to be more relaxed and have time to develop a sense of trust in their care providers. This often facilitates more open discussion of issues such as smoking cessation.

## Motivating the Smoker to Quit

The patient who continues to smoke despite significant lung disease is likely to need considerable

| | | A = 0 points | B = 1 point | C = 2 points | Score |
|---|---|---|---|---|---|
| 1. | How soon after you wake up do you smoke your first cigarette? | After 30 min | Within 30 min | — | |
| 2. | Do you find it difficult to refrain from smoking in places where it is forbidden, such as the library, theater, doctor's office? | No | Yes | — | |
| 3. | Which of all the cigarettes you smoke in a day is the most satisfying? | Any other than the first one in the morning | The first one in the morning | — | |
| 4. | How many cigarettes a day do you smoke? | 1-15 | 16-25 | More than 26 | |
| 5. | Do you smoke more during the morning than during the rest of the day? | No | Yes | — | |
| 6. | Do you smoke when you are so ill that you are in bed most of the day? | No | Yes | — | |
| 7. | Does the brand you smoke have a low, medium, or high nicotine content? | Low | Medium | High | |
| 8. | How often do you inhale the smoke from your cigarette? | Never | Sometimes | Always | |

Assign no points for each answer in column A, 1 point for each answer in column B, and 2 points for each answer in column C (note that not all questions have an answer in column C). Then, total the number of points to arrive at the Fagerström score. The highest possible score is 11.

Consider patients who score 7 or more to be highly dependent on nicotine; patients who score less than 6 have low nicotine dependence. Bear in mind that a low score does not rule out the use of nicotine chewing gum or other therapy based on physiologic nicotine addiction. In general, however, the higher the score, the better the result of such therapy.

**Fig. 20-2**  Fagerström nicotine tolerance scale. (From Fagerström KO: *Addict Behav* 3:235, 1978.)

education, compassion, and help to quit. The following approaches may help provide the necessary motivation.

- *Make it a priority.* Do not assume that anyone has discussed the benefits of quitting with the patient. Make this a priority on your start list. Ask the patient directly if he or she has thought about quitting or wants to quit. The response will suggest the direction that the subsequent discussion should take.
- *Explore and reinforce the benefits.* Explore all the benefits with the patient. The list can and should be long. Write these out as you and the patient develop the list together. Guide the patient away from negative comments and from fears that he cannot quit; for the moment, focus only on the positive benefits of quitting. For some people a letter clearly describing the benefits of quitting may increase the impact of the verbal message. The seriousness of the message may be reinforced by asking patients to sign the letter, acknowledging that they have read it. A copy should be retained by the patient and may be referred to again in future discussions.
- *Help the patient find a personal reason to quit.* If the smoker does not assume personal responsibility for quitting, the chances of success are minimal.
- *Recognize the subtle clues.* Most patients with respiratory disease have already had some introduction to the idea of giving up smoking and are ambivalent about their addiction. Conflicting thoughts and attitudes include the desire to quit smoking, resistance to giving up the "pleasures" of tobacco, and reluctance to subject themselves to the painful process of quitting. For some, the problem is not that there are no motivations for quitting, but that these have not been translated into a dominant, conscious commitment to quitting.

  Look at the smoker's tobacco history and current smoking practice for clues to some precognitive readiness to quit. If the patient has recently switched brands or changed the pattern in which he or she buys cigarettes (e.g., switched from purchasing cartons to purchasing individual packs), the patient may be demonstrating a tentative commitment to quitting.

- *Build on previous attempts to quit.* Ask the patient to describe any previous attempts to quit and build on them. It is extremely important to dispel any feelings of hopelessness concerning failed quit attempts. Instead, reinforce the idea that previous quit attempts actually *increase* one's chance of being successful the next time. Many people quit six or seven times before they are finally able to remain abstinent.
- *Reinforce the patient's strengths.* Help the patient identify positive health behaviors he or she has already adopted, such as success in controlling alcohol abuse. Use prior successes to reassure the patient that he or she has the necessary strength of character to stop smoking.

Such discussions may take place in the course of one visit or over several visits, but they should lead finally to the question, "Do you want to change your smoking habits?" Having the patient write out his or her reasons for wanting to quit may reinforce the patient's motivation.

## Benefits of Quitting

The many benefits of smoking cessation far outweigh the discomforts and difficulties of stopping (Samet, 1990). If an individual quits early enough, the risks of death and disability from lung, heart, and vascular disease are greatly reduced. These beneficial effects are realized regardless of the age at which a person quits. Figs. 20-3 and 20-4 can be used to encourage smokers who have not yet developed smoking-related disease to more seriously consider quitting.

Elimination of the exposure to secondhand smoke greatly reduces fetal risk and improves the symptoms of asthmatic children and vulnerable adults. Enhanced taste and smell increase the enjoyment of meals and may improve nutritional status. Social benefits include greater social accep-

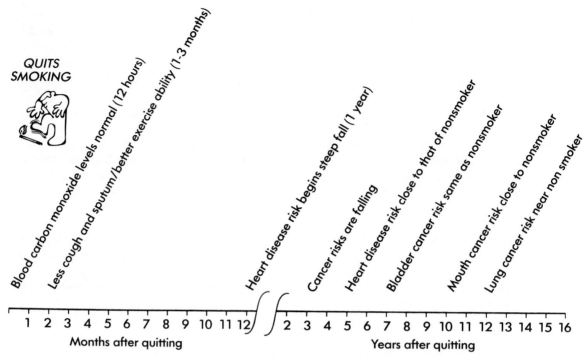

**Fig. 20-3** Benefits of quitting smoking. (From Risser N: *Semin Oncol Nurs* 3:228, 1987.)

tance, at least by the growing number of friends and acquaintances who do not smoke, and gradual disappearance of unsightly staining of fingers and teeth.

### Benefits of Quitting for People with Chronic Lung Disease

When patients with chronic lung disease stop smoking, the following additional improvements in physiologic functioning and quality of life may result:

- Less nasal stuffiness and morning phlegm
- Decreased exertional dyspnea
- General feeling of being "fitter"
- Less cough, sputum, wheezing, and chest tightness (symptoms may disappear altogether)
- Increased exercise tolerance, usually within 1 to 3 months of quitting
- Enough improvement in arterial oxygen saturation in candidates for home oxygen therapy

($Pao_2$ less than 55 mm Hg) that supplemental oxygen may no longer be needed (Openbrier, 1987)
- A beneficial reduction in packed red blood cell volume in response to long-term oxygen that is not seen in patients receiving supplemental oxygen who continue to smoke (Calverley, 1982)

### Using Medical Information to Encourage Quitting

Research findings can be used to support the benefits of smoking cessation, especially if the studies described are directly relevant to the individual being counseled (e.g., studies of smoking's effects on the fetus when counseling a pregnant asthmatic). Providing feedback from lung tests is another effective way to personalize the negative effects of smoking. Examples of such tests are discussed in the following.

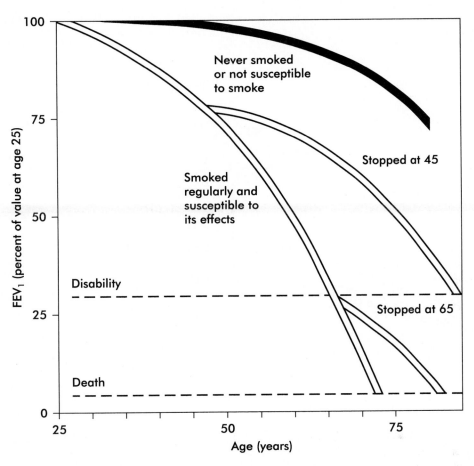

**Fig. 20-4**  Risks for men with varying susceptibility to cigarette smoke, and effect of smoking cessation. (From Fletcher CM, Peto R: *Br Med J* 1:1645-1648, 1977.)

### Calculating Lung Age

Lung function nomograms list normal values under the heading of age, height, and gender. Using the nomogram displayed in Fig. 20-5, a 72-inch, 56-year-old man should have a vital capacity (VC) of 5 L and a forced expiratory volume in 1 second ($FEV_1$) of 3.6 L. If actual values obtained by spirometry are lower than the predicted values, one can plot the lower $FEV_1$ on the nomogram, noting the age that corresponds to the lower value (Morris, 1985). For example, if the patient described above had an $FEV_1$ of 3.12 L instead of his predicted $FEV_1$ of 3.6, he would have "the lungs of a 70-year-old." Patients tend to take notice when their lungs are "older" than their chronologic age.

### Exhaled Carbon Monoxide Testing

The level of CO in exhaled air is a reliable measure of carboxyhemoglobin and is a good indication of how much someone has smoked in the previous 36 hours (Grabowski, 1983). The exhaled carbon monoxide test is simple and inexpensive and can be performed in the hospital, home, or work setting (Risser, 1986). Results are instantaneous, giving powerful feedback to the patient about the effect of smoking on the body. CO levels always are

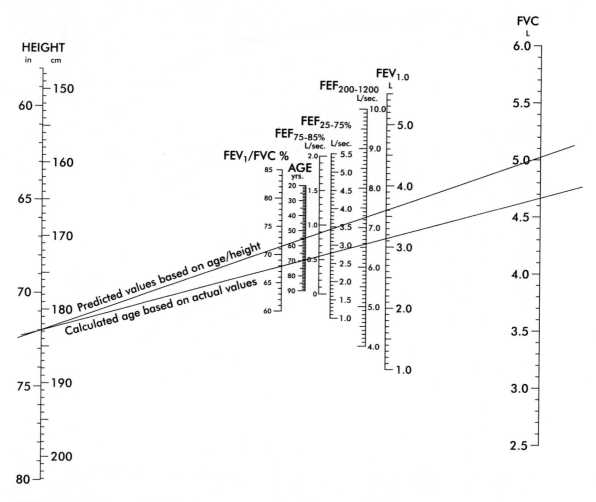

FEF200-1200=Average flow between 200 and 1200 ml of the FVC
FEF25-75%=Forced midexpiratory flow

FEF75-85%=Forced end-expiratory flow
FEV₁=One-second forced expiratory volume
FVC=Forced vital capacity

**Fig. 20-5**   Calculation of "lung age" using a prediction nomogram for normal men. Nomogram is from Morris et al: *West J Med* 125:110, 1976. Nomogram used to calculate "lung age" in a smoker is from Morris JF, Temple W: *Prev Med* 14:655, 1985. A similar nomogram is available for normal women.

elevated (above 10 ppm) in a chronic smoker and spike immediately after smoking. Levels of 20 to 30 ppm are common in a healthy, young, one-pack-a-day smoker and are even higher in someone with chronic lung disease. It takes approximately 36 hours of abstinence for values to return to normal. Exhaled CO results are shared with the patient along with an explanation of how CO displaces

oxygen from the hemoglobin molecule, reducing exercise capacity by reducing the amount of oxygen available to the tissues.

Expressing the results of pulmonary function tests in terms of "lung age" or comparing results of spirometry and exhaled CO with predicted normal values has been shown to result in quit rates as high as 20% (Morris, 1985; Risser, 1986).

# Dealing with the Rationalizations for Not Quitting

## Fear of Weight Gain

Many people gain and maintain an extra 8 to 10 lb when they quit smoking. This is due to (1) a reduced metabolic rate associated with the discontinuation of nicotine and (2) a postcessation increase in appetite and craving for sweets (Fagerström, 1978). For undernourished patients this is beneficial. Undesirable weight gain can be minimized by implementing a regular exercise program and restricting caloric intake at the time of cessation. Reading the American Lung Association's pamphlet, *Stop Smoking, Stay Trim,* referral to a nutritionist, or both may also be helpful. Use of a nicotine substitute may delay but does not prevent postcessation weight gain (Fisher, 1990).

## Too Much Stress

Most patients with chronic lung disease live with continual stress and may feel that they need their cigarettes to relax. Nicotine is known to stimulate specific brain receptors, producing euphoric and possibly sedative and anxiolytic effects (Fisher, 1990). With cessation, smokers experience not only the loss of these pleasurable effects but the distress of withdrawal symptoms. Patients need support and encouragement through the period of withdrawal, as well as reassurance that after a few weeks of not smoking they will feel less nervous. Prior instruction in controlled breathing and relaxation techniques may increase the patient's confidence concerning his or her ability to get through this difficult period (see Chapter 8).

## "The Damage Is Already Done"

Many patients with end-stage lung disease question the point of quitting when smoking is one of the "few pleasures" they have left in life. This rationale may have validity for the person who is truly at the end-stage of disease. However, a prediction of life expectancy is at best a guess. Thus the benefits of quitting even when patients are severely disabled by COPD (reduction in symptoms, improvement in oxygenation, and increased safety with use of oxygen) should be reinforced.

# Counseling Adolescents

*Adolescents (even those with chronic lung disease) may view themselves as invincible. They do not personalize warnings of the long-term health consequences of smoking. Discussing how smoking limits endurance for sports, makes breath and hair smell bad, and "turns off" potential dates is more effective than warnings about diseases that may develop 30 years hence. Antismoking messages are generally more effective if they come from peer leaders than from health care providers.*

# Approaches to Quitting

## Setting the Quit Date

Once motivated, the patient is encouraged to set a quit date. This should fit into a reasonable personal schedule and allow time to prepare for quitting. Quitting during periods of high stress is not advisable. A support person should be prepared and available to help during the first weeks and months of cessation. The smoker should be taught specific behavioral and cognitive coping skills to prevent early and late relapse.

## Self-Help Resources

Most of the 38 million ex-smokers in the United States quit more or less on their own. The educated self-quitter is one who has sought out and used self-help resources such as commercially available pamphlets, books, videos, and audiotapes. Uneducated quitters have no particular cessation strategy. They tend to tough out the urge for a cigarette rather than consciously using coping skills to deal with potential relapse situations. Relapse is more common in this group, but it can be reduced by encouraging conscious use of coping strategies and providing literature that deals with relapse prevention.

Several excellent publications are available from the local offices of the American Lung Association:

*Freedom from Smoking in 20 Days*
*Freedom from Smoking for You and Your Family*
*Freedom from Smoking for You and Your Baby*

Self-help videotapes are also available from the American Lung Association and the American Cancer Society to help with cessation and maintenance and for health professionals needing more information on cessation methods.

Two good commercially available self-help books are Weatherall's *Quit: Read This Book and Stop Smoking* and Ferguson's *The Smoker's Book of Health*. Weatherall's book is the exact size of a pack of cigarettes and is meant to be kept in the space where the new ex-smoker formerly carried his or her cigarettes. Tips for remaining abstinent are short and to the point. The Ferguson book was written after the author interviewed hundreds of smokers, ex-smokers, and smoking cessation researchers. It is permissive in allowing the smoker to make his or her own decision to quit and appeals to smokers who want a lot of background on smoking and quitting.

### Specific Smoking-Cessation Interventions

If self-help methods and the support, encouragement, and guidance of family, friends, and health providers have not succeeded, the patient may need a more structured smoking cessation program. Programs vary widely in the educational approaches and methods used and in their stated efficacy (Schwartz, 1987). The lack of biologic verification of quitting in many of the programs makes it difficult to compare the efficacy of one program with another. However, multicomponent programs appear to be the most successful (Kottke, 1988). Tests to increase self-awareness and discussions that focus on quitting and coping skills and the importance of diet, exercise, and a support person are common components. Specific smoking cessation interventions are summarized in Table 20-2.

Behavioral strategies are likely to be most effective when they are keyed to the reasons patients smoke. The National Institutes of Health questionnaire, "Why do you smoke?" (1980), may help to identify an individual's specific reasons for smoking (Fig. 20-6). It is available without charge from the U.S. Department of Health and Human Services. Frequent reasons for smoking and behavioral strategies to break these patterns are described in the following:

- Stimulation—The smoker who uses cigarettes for stimulation can substitute alternatives such as splashing ice water on his face or walking up a flight of stairs.
- Handling—The "handler" can fiddle with objects such as a pen, a pencil, safety pins, paper clips, or toothpicks in place of cigarettes. Un-

**Table 20-2**   Smoking cessation interventions

| Intervention | Approach |
|---|---|
| Hypnosis | Carried out in single- or multiple-individual sessions or in groups; tends to be most successful when combined with other cessation strategies |
| Acupuncture | Therapists use two sites for treatment: site at nose intended to cause disgust of tobacco, and site at ear allows use of staples or needles and is thought to affect the neurovegetative system |
| Aversion therapy | Repeated 15- to 20-min sessions of deep, rapid smoking in way that exaggerates the unpleasant sensations (e.g., foul taste, dizziness, nausea); often combines rapid smoking with noxious stimuli such as electric impulse to forearm; reported high success with initial quitting, but when used alone, does not assist long-term habit change or skill development; has been shown to be safe for smokers with mild to moderate cardiopulmonary disease (Hall, 1984) |
| Quitting by mail (Schneider, 1984) or computer interactive programs (Schneider, 1986) | Home or office computers can be used to access personalized information on smoking cessation that has previously been entered by client; may be useful for homebound patient |

## Why do you smoke?

Here are some statements made by people to describe what they get out of smoking cigarettes. How often do you feel this way when smoking?

Circle one number for each statement. Important: *Answer every question.*

| | Always | Fre-quently | Occa-sionally | Seldom | Never |
|---|---|---|---|---|---|
| A. I smoke cigarettes in order to keep myself from slowing down. | 5 | 4 | 3 | 2 | 1 |
| B. Handling a cigarette is part of the enjoyment of smoking it. | 5 | 4 | 3 | 2 | 1 |
| C. Smoking cigarettes is pleasant and relaxing. | 5 | 4 | 3 | 2 | 1 |
| D. I light up a cigarette when I feel angry about something. | 5 | 4 | 3 | 2 | 1 |
| E. When I have run out of cigarettes I find it almost unbearable until I can get them. | 5 | 4 | 3 | 2 | 1 |
| F. I smoke cigarettes automatically without even being aware of it. | 5 | 4 | 3 | 2 | 1 |
| G. I smoke cigarettes to stimulate me, to perk myself up. | 5 | 4 | 3 | 2 | 1 |
| H. Part of the enjoyment of smoking a ciga-rette comes from the steps I take to light up. | 5 | 4 | 3 | 2 | 1 |
| I. I find cigarettes pleasurable. | 5 | 4 | 3 | 2 | 1 |
| J. When I feel uncomfortable or upset about something, I light up a cigarette. | 5 | 4 | 3 | 2 | 1 |
| K. I am very much aware of the fact when I am not smoking a cigarette. | 5 | 4 | 3 | 2 | 1 |
| L. I light up a cigarette without realizing I still have one burning in the ashtray. | 5 | 4 | 3 | 2 | 1 |
| M. I smoke cigarettes to give me a "lift." | 5 | 4 | 3 | 2 | 1 |
| N. When I smoke a cigarette, part of the enjoy-ment is watching the smoke as I exhale it. | 5 | 4 | 3 | 2 | 1 |
| O. I want a cigarette most when I am comfortable and relaxed. | 5 | 4 | 3 | 2 | 1 |
| P. When I feel "blue" or want to take my mind off cares and worries, I smoke cigarettes. | 5 | 4 | 3 | 2 | 1 |
| Q. I get a real gnawing hunger for a cigarette when I haven't smoked for a while. | 5 | 4 | 3 | 2 | 1 |
| R. I've found a cigarette in my mouth and didn't remember putting it there. | 5 | 4 | 3 | 2 | 1 |

**Fig. 20-6** Why do people smoke? (From Horn DH: US Dept of Health and Human Services, Washington, DC, National Institutes of Health Pub No 80-1822-A, 1980.)

*Continued.*

**How to score**

1. Enter the number you have circled for each question in the spaces below, putting the number you have circled to question A over line A, to question B over line B, etc.

2. Add the three scores on each line to get your totals. For example, the sum of your scores over lines A, G, and M gives you your score on Stimulation—lines B, H, and N give the score on Handling, etc.

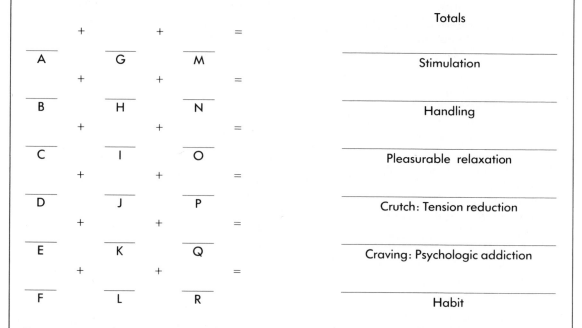

Scores can vary from 3 to 15. Any score 11 and above is high; any score 7 and below is low.

**Fig. 20-6, cont'd.** Why do people smoke? (From Horn DH: US Dept of Health and Human Services, Washington, DC, National Institutes of Health Pub No 80-1822-A, 1980.)

shelled sunflower seeds can keep hands busy and help to satisfy oral cravings.

- Pleasurable relaxation—Cigarettes are often associated with breaks in the usual routine and are part of the permission to stop, sit back, and relax from usual activities. Cognitive self-talk, combined with planned breaks in which other activities (e.g., painting fingernails, working crosswords, reading the sports page) are performed, can often fill the void for the ex-smoker.

- Stress reduction—Replacing cigarettes that were used to reduce stress and tension may require the mastery of techniques of visualization or meditation and the effective use of humor.

- Cravings—A person who has a high score for craving or psychologic addiction may also have a high score on the Fagerström Scale (Fig. 20-2) and is a good candidate for nicotine substitutes. Other approaches include physical changes in body position, taking 10 slow deep inhalations through the mouth, total body tensing and relaxing (see Jacobsen method in Chapter 8), or rubber band pings to the ankle or wrist to interrupt the cravings. Being ill with a cold or influenza may provide an opportunity to go "cold turkey." Because patients are often referred for home health care following an acute exacerbation and hospitalization, they may have been abstinent from cigarettes for several days when the home care nurse makes the initial visit. This presents a unique opportunity for the nurse to reinforce and encourage continued cessation. Physiologic withdrawal symptoms will be reduced or absent by this time, and patients can be reminded that they are already well on their way to complete cessation.

- Habit—Habit breaking takes time and is best done by eliminating cues and completely changing old routines. Measures that make it inconvenient to smoke (e.g., removing all cigarettes from the house or wrapping them in several layers of plastic wrap and storing them in the freezer) may also help by making the unconscious use of cigarettes impossible.

## Pharmacologic Interventions

Nicotine replacement (and reduction) therapy is the only therapeutic approach for the treatment of nicotine dependence approved and recognized by the Food and Drug Administration. Studies that differentiate smokers by levels of dependence show that the dependent smoker is more successful when given adequate nicotine replacement.

Nicotine polacrilex (gum) has been used to treat smokers since 1982. Multiple studies indicate it is safe and effective when used correctly (Blöndal, 1989; Tonnesen, 1988). Key factors in the correct use of the gum include a smoker who is committed to quitting, education for behavior change, adequate dosage, and avoidance of acidic oral products at the time of use.

Nicotine therapy via a transdermal patch has been available in the United States since late 1991. Three companies manufacture patches, and others are awaiting approval. The transdermal patches are

safe and efficacious. Double-blind placebo-controlled trials indicate the patches' effectiveness compared with placebos (Daughton, 1991; Transdermal Nicotine Study Group, 1991; Fiore et al, 1992). The transdermal patches should be used for a minimum of 6 weeks and a maximum of 12 weeks. They should be used with caution when certain medical conditions are involved. The reader is advised to check the manufacturer's label for information on contraindications.

The transdermal patch has several advantages over polacrilex gum. A more consistent blood level provides more satisfying nicotine replacement. Patient compliance is improved because the patch requires once a day therapy, there is less need to acknowledge therapy socially, and fewer gastrointestinal side effects occur.

The cost disadvantage of treatment should be weighed against the cost of continued smoking. Whereas the transdermal patch is more expensive than cigarettes during a 3-month period, the total treatment cost is less than the cost of a year's supply of cigarettes. Although the patches come in dosage packages, the pharmacist has the option of dispensing enough for 1 week at a time. Nicotine reduction therapy is summarized in Table 20-3.

### Built-In Rewards for Abstinence

Having a pleasurable goal or reward for successful abstinence (e.g., renting a videotape, buying a special book or a piece of furniture) may provide additional motivation for some people. Money saved by not smoking can be earmarked for chosen rewards, which need not be large but should be frequent and concrete.

## Predicting Success in Quitting

Although there is no one test that will help to determine which smokers will successfully quit, factors that suggest a positive result are the following (Tunstall, 1985):

Women
    Living with nonsmokers
    Low alcohol and coffee consumption
    Low tobacco consumption (few cigarettes, lower nicotine brands)

**Table 20-3**  Nicotine reduction therapy

| Agent | Action | Dosage | Use | Contraindications |
|---|---|---|---|---|
| Nicotine polacrilex | Maintains serum nicotine level | One piece gum to each two cigarettes previously smoked; chew slowly and gently until tingling sensation felt in mouth, then "park" between gums and teeth; used on and off in this manner for 30 min | For at least 3 mo, up to 2 yr; wean over several weeks | Angina; gastric ulcers, gastroesophageal reflux; temporal mandibular joint disease; gingivitis; dentures (sticks to them) |
| Nicotine patch | Maintains serum nicotine level | Nicoderm and Habitrol: 21 mg patch, qd × 4-6 wk; 14 mg patch × 2-4 wk; 7 mg patch × 2-4 wk— for total of 10-12 wk; Prostep: 22 mg patch × 6-8 wk, with option of 11 mg patch for additional 2-4 wk | Wear patch 24 hr per day for 6-12 wk of therapy | Continuing smoker; pregnant women; immediate cardiac event; serious cardiac arrhythmia; hepatic or renal insufficiency; skin allergy or nicotine-sensitive skin |

Expectation of success
At least one previous easy quit attempt
Presence of social support system
Introversion personality traits
Low level of stress
Diagnosis of cancer, emphysema, or heart disease
No previous history of major depression
Men
    Older age
    Higher education and income level

## Preventing Relapse

Spontaneous first-time quitters are successful approximately 20% of the time (i.e., they are still abstinent at the end of 1 year). However, most smokers need to make repeated attempts at quitting for success to last. The likelihood of success tends to increase with each attempt. The smoker may learn new coping maneuvers with each attempt, or perhaps the resolve to be abstinent becomes more intense. The important thing is to regard each attempt as a positive move, even if cessation was short. This helps the smoker maintain a good attitude about trying again.

The most critical relapse time is within the first 3 months; new ex-smokers need to be cautious during this time. Once a smoker is completely off cigarettes for a year, the chance of relapse is less. Mental rehearsal before any new, potential high-risk situation may help prevent relapse. Common causes of relapse include the following (National Institutes of Health, 1986):

- Increased stress in one's life
- Feeling depressed, angry, or anxious
- Loss of motivation to quit
- Weight gain (or fear of weight gain)
- Cravings for cigarettes, withdrawal symptoms
- Social celebrations or situations commonly associated with smoking (e.g., family parties)
- Alcohol consumption
- Habitual smoking cues (e.g., habitual cigarette after dinner or with morning coffee)
- Social pressure from peers

## Role of Spouse in Quitting

The spouse should be included in smoking cessation education, whether done in the home or in the clinic. The support of friends and family is especially important in helping to maintain abstinence during the early months of quitting. A supportive spouse can be a skilled interventionist in the smoking cessation process, giving helpful suggestions rather than negative, nagging comments and reminding the patient of the cognitive and behavioral skills he or she possesses. The cessation process is encouraged by a home environment that is devoid of tobacco reminders. The supportive spouse knows that every situation experienced as a nonsmoker tests the coping skills of the new ex-smoker and can suggest specific behavioral coping strategies (e.g., walking away from the urge or taking deep breaths) and self-talk strategies (e.g., "I'm stronger than a cigarette," "I never liked those lousy, smelly weeds," "My lungs are better off with fresh air"). However, the supportive spouse must continue to place ultimate responsibility for quitting where it belongs—on the shoulders of the smoker.

## Role of Health Care Providers

People are more likely to quit smoking and stay abstinent if they receive a direct, face-to-face message from their health care providers and if that message comes from both physician and nonphysician counselors. A greater number and duration of reinforcing sessions also improve 6-month quit rates.

Home health care staff can help prevent relapse by collaborating with physicians to reinforce the stop-smoking messages, providing positive reinforcement for continuing abstinence, reviewing with patients the short- and long-term benefits they can expect, and pointing out physiologic improvements, such as reduced frequency of infections, improved peak flow rates, or reduced volume of sputum. Home care staff also can refer patients to community maintenance programs or ex-smokers' hot lines and can prepare patients to deal with the short-term sequelae of smoking cessation, such as weight gain and withdrawal symptoms. The special

bond that often develops between a patient and the home health care nurse can be used effectively to reinforce desirable behaviors.

## Smoking Cessation for the Oxygen-Dependent Patient

Because there is a high risk for facial burns and house fires when an oxygen-dependent patient smokes, vigorous efforts must be made to help such patients quit smoking. In some countries physicians refuse to prescribe long-term oxygen therapy when patients continue to smoke. A more tolerant approach is generally taken in the United States. However, if an oxygen-dependent patient is unable to stop smoking even after persistent and supportive measures have been taken to achieve this goal, home health care staff must seek an agreement with the patient that he or she will turn off the oxygen while smoking and will *never* smoke in bed or try to light a cigarette with oxygen flowing through the tubing. A signed patient contract may add strength to the agreement and help ensure compliance with this minimal goal (see Chapter 21).

## Other Important Home Health Care Nursing Considerations
### Medication Interactions

Nurses must be aware of interactions between prescribed medications and smoking behavior as noted earlier. It is important to observe the patient carefully for signs of toxicity or less than therapeutic doses whenever smoking behavior is abruptly changed.

### Impact of Secondhand Smoke

The impact of secondhand smoke on children and adults with chronic lung disease living in households where others continue to smoke is of particular concern for the home health care nurse. These individuals are already exceptionally vulnerable to the harmful effects of secondhand smoke and need to be protected from further respiratory insult. Family members who are unable or unwilling to stop smoking should be counseled to smoke outside and not to smoke in the car. At the very least, they must limit their smoking to a part of the home that is separate from the patient. Most family members are concerned enough about the well-being of the patient that they willingly adhere to these requests. For the few who do not, home health care nurses must use their understanding of family dynamics and all their counseling skills to encourage the desired behavior change.

## REFERENCES

American Psychiatric Association: *Diagnostic and statistical manual,* ed 3, Washington, DC, 1980, The Association.

Blöndal T: Controlled trial of nicotine polacrilax gum with supportive measures, *Arch Intern Med* 149:1818, 1989.

Calverley PMA et al: Cigarette smoking and secondary polycythemia in hypoxic cor pulmonale, *Am Rev Respir Dis* 125:507, 1982.

Daughton DM, Heatley SA, Prendergast JJ, et al: Effect of transdermal nicotine delivery as an adjunct to low-intervention smoking cessation therapy, *Arch Intern Med* 151:749, 1991.

Fagerström KO: Measuring degree of physical dependence to tobacco smoking with reference to individualization of treatment, *Addict Behav* 3:235, 1978.

Ferguson T: *The smoker's book of health,* Austin, 1989, GP Putnam Self-Care Productions.

Fiore MC et al: Tobacco dependence and the nicotine patch, *JAMA* 268:2687, 1992.

Fisher EB et al: Smoking and smoking cessation, *Am Rev Respir Dis* 142:702, 1990.

Glassman AH et al: Heavy smokers, smoking cessation and clonidine, *JAMA* 259:2863, 1988.

Grabowski J, Bell CS: *Measurement in the analysis and treatment of smoking behavior,* NIDA Research Monograph 48, Pub No (ADM) 83-1285, Washington, DC, 1983, US Government Printing Office.

Hall RG: Two year efficacy and safety of rapid smoking therapy in patients with cardiac and pulmonary disease, *J Consult Clin Psych* 52(4):574, 1984.

Kottke TE et al: Attributes of successful smoking cessation intervention in medical practice, *JAMA* 259:2883, 1988.

Lefcoe NM et al: The health risks of passive smoking, *Chest* 84:90, 1983.

Morris JF, Temple W: Spirometric "lung age" estimation for motivating smoking cessation, *Prevent Med* 14:655, 1985.

National Institutes of Health: *Why do you smoke?,* NIH Pub No 80-1822-A, Washington, DC, 1980, US Department of Health, Education, and Welfare.

National Institutes of Health: *Clinical opportunities for smoking intervention,* NIH Pub No 86-2170, Washington, DC, 1986, US Government Printing Office.

Openbrier DR: Smoking cessation results in significant improvement in $PaO_2$ in home oxygen therapy candidates, *Am Rev Respir Dis* 135:A354, 1987 (abstract).

Risser N, Belcher DW: Personalizing the risk of smoking using spirometry, expired carbon monoxide measurements and a symptom questionnaire improves smoking cessation rates, *Am Rev Respir Dis* 133:A64, 1986 (abstract).

Risser N: The key to prevention of lung cancer: stop smoking, *Semin Oncol Nurs* 3:228, 1987.

Samet JM: The 1990 report of the Surgeon General: the health benefits of smoking cessation, *Am Rev Respir Dis* 142:993, 1990 (editorial).

Schneider NG, Murray JE: *Nicotine gum vs placebo gum: comparisons of withdrawal symptoms and success rates,* NIDA Monograph 53, DHHS Pub No (ADM) 85-1333:83, Washington, DC, 1985, US Government Printing Office.

Schneider SJ, Benya A: Computerized direct mail to treat smokers who avoid treatment, *Comput Biomed Res* 17:409, 1984.

Schneider SJ, Tooley J: Self help computer conferencing, *Comput Biomed Res* 19:274, 1986.

Schwartz JL: *Review and evaluation of smoking cessation methods: the United States and Canada, 1978-1985,* National Cancer Institute, NIH Pub No 87-2940, Washington, DC, 1987, US Government Printing Office.

Staff memo: Smoking related deaths and financial costs, Office of Technological Assessment, 1985, US Congress.

Tonnesen P et al: Effect of nicotine chewing gum in combination with group counseling on the cessation of smoking, *N Engl J Med* 318:15, 1988.

Transdermal Nicotine Study Group: Transdermal nicotine for smoking cessation, *JAMA* 266:3133, 1991.

Trichopoulos D et al: Lung cancer and passive smoking, *Int J Cancer* 177:1, 1981.

Tunstall CD, Ginsberg D, Hall SM: Quitting smoking, *Int J Addict* 20:1089, 1985.

US Surgeon General: *Report of the US Surgeon General: the health consequences of smoking—cancer and chronic lung disease in the workplace,* Pub No (PHS) 85-50207, Washington, DC, 1985, US Government Printing Office.

US Surgeon General: *Report of the US Surgeon General: the health consequences of smoking—nicotine addiction,* Pub No (CDC) 88-8406, Washington, DC, 1988, US Government Printing Office.

US Surgeon General: *Report of the US Surgeon General: reducing the health consequences of smoking—25 years of progress,* DHHS Pub No (CDC) 89-8411, Washington, DC, 1989, US Government Printing Office.

Weatherall CF: *Quit: read this book and stop smoking,* Minneapolis, 1979, Weatherall Publishing.

Wu T et al: Pulmonary hazards of smoking marijuana as compared with tobacco, *N Engl J Med* 318:347, 1988.

## SUGGESTED READINGS

Fiore M, guest editor: Cigarette smoking, *Med Clin North Am* 76:1, 1992.

Samet JM, Coultas DB, guest editors: Smoking cessation, *Clin Chest Med* 12:1, 1991.

# CHAPTER 21

# PATIENT COMPLIANCE

JOAN TURNER

Patient compliance or adherence is defined as "the extent to which a person's behavior coincides with medical or health advice" (Haynes, 1979). Issues about compliance with therapeutic regimens in patients with chronic lung disease are presented in this chapter. The discussion may be applied to many aspects of health care advice, including medications, diets, exercise prescriptions, and life-style changes. Whenever home health care nurses work with patients on compliance issues, they must be certain that the prescribed therapy is appropriate and more likely to benefit than harm the patient and that the patient or parent is willing to follow the prescription.

In general, adult and pediatric patient compliance with prescribed therapy tends to be only about 50%, with error rates as high as 58% (i.e., errors such as overuse, underuse, scheduling errors) (Parker, 1988; Rapoff, 1991). Complicated, long-term regimens of oral and inhaled medications are frequently prescribed for patients with chronic lung disease, and compliance tends to be poor in the few studies that have been reported in the literature (Dolce, 1991). Compliance with home nebulizer therapy was only 51% in one study, even with home visits every month by a nurse or respiratory therapist to educate the patient and reinforce the importance of the therapy (Turner, 1985). Adults and children with asthma have been shown to have poor rates of compliance with oral and inhaled medications, increasing the incidence of exacerbations and emergency room visits (Parker, 1988).

## ETIOLOGY

Compliance may be affected by many factors, including type of regimen, disease process, patient's personality, or other psychosocial factors.

### Type of Regimen

It is well documented that compliance tends to be reduced when several drugs are prescribed at frequent intervals, when therapy is of long duration, and when the cost is high (Krall, 1991). Patients with asthma have been shown to comply better with twice daily (bid) inhaled steroids than with four times daily (qid) dosing (Mann et al, 1992). Safety lock containers may adversely affect compliance because some patients have difficulty opening them. The adverse effects of therapy and the patient's perception that there is no benefit or relief of symptoms may be reasons for noncompliance. Complicated treatment procedures or equipment maintenance may also adversely affect compliance unless the patient is highly motivated and has the energy and the economic resources to comply.

Patients may have particular difficulty complying with such regimens as postural drainage with percussion and vibration. One of the biggest problems is that chest physical therapy usually requires the assistance of another person. Other problems are that the regimens are time consuming, may cause discomfort, require special positions that necessitate privacy, and are generally distasteful for some patients (Currie, 1986).

## Type or Severity of Disease

In general, the type of disease does not have a significant effect on patient compliance. However, patients with psychiatric problems such as schizophrenia, paranoia, and personality disorders tend to be less compliant. Increasing symptoms may have an adverse effect, although increasing disability has had a positive effect in some studies (Parker, 1988). In one study patients with chronic obstructive pulmonary disease (COPD) who were more short of breath and who had lower forced expiratory volume in 1 second ($FEV_1$) values were more likely to comply with home nebulizer therapy than were others who were less ill (Turner, 1985). These patients were more disabled because of their disease and may have received more professional supervision and encouragement to comply. In another study of patients with COPD, compliance with home oxygen therapy increased in the 3 months before death when the patients were more ill (Aegeret, 1986).

## Emotional, Personality, and Intellectual Factors

There is evidence that personality and emotional and intellectual factors influence compliance. Hypoxemia causes difficulty in processing information (Wilson, 1985). Patients with hypoxemia who are not treated may not understand instructions or may forget to take medications. Concomitant medications may also cause confusion and lead to compliance problems. Depressed patients may feel that "nothing matters" and lack the emotional energy to comply with therapy. In severely depressed patients, noncompliance may be a manifestation of suicidal behavior.

*Parents of ventilator-dependent children may be exhausted and lack the energy to comply with therapy for the child, especially if the therapy is complicated. These parents generally benefit from respite care for the child so that they can be temporarily relieved from the emotional and physical demands of providing care.*

Patients who fear discomfort and feel helpless and unable to cope may tend to overuse medications or demand increased medical support. Patients who feel that they have something to gain from the sick role and want to remain symptomatic may be noncompliant. Others may deny their illness and not use prescribed therapy, particularly if the therapy represents sickness to them. *Teenagers may discontinue medications and treatments in an effort to deny their illness because they do not want to be different from healthy peers.*

An external locus of control may also be a reason for noncompliance. Patients with an external locus of control often perceive that their lives are controlled by outside forces such as God or the physician and that their own actions are meaningless. By contrast, patients with an internal locus of control are more likely to comply because they feel that they have control over their lives and that their actions have a meaningful impact on the present and the future (Rotter, 1966).

## Sociodemographic Factors

Social factors may enhance or inhibit patient compliance. The influence of family and friends has generally been shown to have a positive effect on patient use of prescribed therapy, whereas social isolation has had an adverse effect. Significant others who strive to meet the emotional needs of the sick person generally reinforce behaviors that are necessary for compliance.

Younger, nonwhite patients and those with more disruption in their homes and family lives tend to be less compliant (Turner, 1985). Although sociodemographic factors such as age, education, race, sex, and marital status have not been shown to have a significant effect on compliance in general, they may be significant when the therapeutic regimen requires life-style changes. In one study, older patients with COPD who were white, better educated, and married were more likely to comply with home nebulizer therapy, a therapy that requires life-style changes (Turner, 1985). Poorly educated patients may not understand basic principles about disease and the rationale for therapy. In addition, they may not have had enough experience to be familiar with the concept of therapy and may reject it because it is foreign.

If there are significant financial problems, health

care may have a lower priority than basic necessities. The patient or family also may not have adequate financial resources to pay for the therapy or prescribed medications.

## Cultural Beliefs

Views of health, causes of illness, the meaning of symptoms, and the responsibilities of patients, families, and health care workers may vary according to the patient's culture and social class (Clark, 1983). These and other cultural and class issues may significantly affect patients' compliance with prescribed therapy. A full discussion of various cultural beliefs is beyond the scope of this chapter, and beliefs constantly change as people are assimilated into Western society; however, it is important for the home care provider to consider cultural issues when evaluating patient compliance problems.

## Patient Perceptions

The Health Belief Model (Fig. 21-1) and a hypothesized model for mothers' compliance (Fig. 21-2) are frameworks that attempt to explain and predict the acceptance of health care recommendations. The models are based on basic perceptions of the threat of illness and the benefit of therapy (Becker, 1975). A threat may be a motivating factor for compliance with patients and parents if it is relevant to them and is presented along with ways to cope with the perceived danger. The Health Belief Model applies when the patient or parent knows that treatment effectively controls disease. In general, patients who perceive that they have significant disease and that there might be adverse effects of stopping their medication are more likely to comply with treatment than others; however, some will not comply, even though they appear to obtain relief of symptoms with treatment. Lack of satisfaction with medical care and lack of faith in the physician prescribing the therapy may lead to noncompliance (Eraker, 1984).

## Personal Habits

Personal habits may have a negative or positive impact on compliance. Patients with COPD who

smoked and drank alcohol were less compliant with home nebulizer therapy than others (Turner, 1985). Habitual behavior may enhance compliance with long-term regimens, diets, and exercise programs in that patients are likely to remain compliant once they incorporate a therapy into their life-styles.

## Pediatric Regimens

*Compliance considerations in pediatrics are more complicated because they involve the parent or caregiver as well as the child. Issues that have been shown to be related to noncompliance in the child are the following\*:*
*Patient and family factors*
- *Low patient self-esteem*
- *Family dysfunction or disharmony, conflicts, and poor parental coping*
- *Increased family size*
- *Limited parental supervision of regimen*
- *Intent to adhere (on patient's or parent's part)*
- *Developmental stage and abilities*

*Disease factors*
- *Patient asymptomatic or in remission*
- *Type of disease being treated (acute versus chronic)*
- *Disease severity, as perceived by family*

*Regimen factors*
- *Longer duration of or more frequent treatments*
- *Complex regimens*
- *Costly treatments*
- *Types of regimens (e.g., regimens that require life-style changes)*
- *Lack of continuity of care*
- *Limited provider supervision of regimen*
- *Pharmacy errors (incorrect filling of prescriptions)*
- *Regimen adverse reactions (e.g., pain when exercising)*

---

\*From Rapoff MA, Barnard MU: Compliance with pediatric regimens. In Cramer JA, Spilker B, editors: *Patient compliance in medical practice and clinical trials*, New York, 1991, Raven Press.

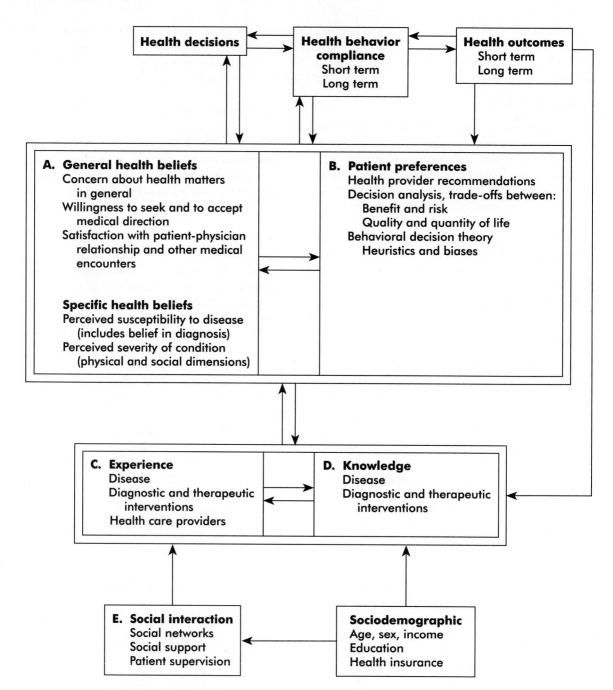

**Fig. 21-1**  Health Belief Model. (From Becker MH, Maiman LA: *Med Care* 13:12, 1975.)

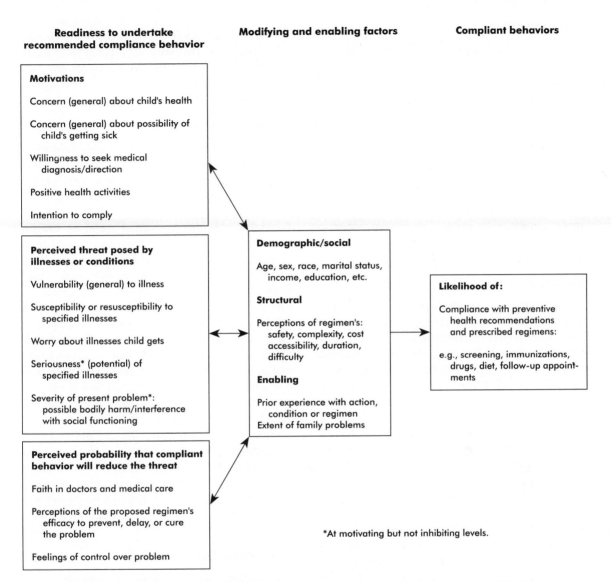

**Fig. 21-2** Hypothesized model for predicting and explaining mothers' compliance behaviors (From Becker MH et al: Patient perceptions and compliance: recent studies of the Health Belief Model. In Haynes RB et al: *Compliance in health care*, Baltimore, 1979, Johns Hopkins University Press, pp 79-80.)

## ASSESSMENT

Assessing the level of compliance is important to evaluate the effectiveness of prescribed therapy. If compliance cannot be determined, it is difficult to know if the lack of a therapy's efficacy is due to noncompliance or inappropriate therapy. For instance, if an infection persists, it might be because the patient is not taking the antibiotic properly, rather than not responding to it. It is difficult to assess the actual level of compliance with certainty, however; compliance can only be inferred. Estimates of compliance may be determined by patient reports, medication counts, physiologic determinations, health care provider estimates, and other assessments.

### Patient Reports

Patients may take their medications as prescribed; however, they generally tend to overestimate their degree of compliance. They may be forgetful, eager to please, or afraid to admit that they have not been following the prescription properly. On the other hand, patients are usually accurate if they admit to being noncompliant (Eraker, 1984).

A trusting relationship with the home health care provider usually helps the patient or parent to be open about difficulties complying with therapy. It may help for the nurse to preface compliance questions with a statement that it can be difficult for some people to take all of their medication as prescribed (Hilbert, 1985). Questions should be non-threatening, encourage the patient to be open, be phrased in words that are understood, and not prejudice patient responses. Only one specific question should be asked at a time. Usually, more information is obtained if questions cannot be answered with a yes or no. An opening statement might be, "Sometimes people have trouble taking every dose of their medication. Tell me how you have been doing." If the desired information is not obtained, specific questions can follow, such as "How many times a day do you think you have missed a dose?" Family reports may be helpful to augment patient reports, but they should not be used in a threatening or divisive way. Some patients keep diaries to help them remember that they have taken their medications or treatments and to document any side effects. Such diaries can be helpful when assessing compliance.

### Medication Counts

Pill counts, measurements of liquid medication, or weights of metered dose inhalers may be more accurate than patient reports (Backes, 1991). However, it is necessary to know the exact amount of medication the patient received and the date it was first taken. If other household members use the same medication or if supplies are obtained from more than one source, it will be difficult to determine how much the patient actually took. Pharmacists may also dispense less medication than was ordered. Records of prescription and oxygen tank refills also may provide useful estimates of patient compliance. Cronologs or elapsed time meters may be built into oxygen concentrators, oxygen tanks, and nebulizers to record the time the device is in operation. Microchips may be attached to metered dose inhalers to record the number of times the device is activated (Spector, 1991). However, most of these types of electronic devices are used only in research settings, are costly, and are usually unavailable for routine management. Such devices also document only that the oxygen or nebulizer was turned on or that the metered dose inhaler was activated, not that they were actually used by the patient.

### Physiologic Determinations

Physiologic determinations of compliance are more accurate than patient reports or medication counts; however, the levels must be carefully interpreted. Saliva, blood, or urine samples may be analyzed for drug or drug metabolite levels or levels of markers that can be added to drugs. Appropriate or therapeutic physiologic levels document adequate patient medication compliance; however, low levels do not always indicate noncompliance. There can be significant variation among patients in the absorption, body distribution, metabolism, and excretion of drugs (Backes, 1991). Therefore the standard medication dosage may not result in therapeutic drug levels for all patients, even if compliance is ideal. It is important to estimate the level of compliance before increasing the dose of a drug when physiologic determinations reveal inadequate levels. If low drug levels are likely to be the result of poor compliance, drug levels should be measured again after compliance is improved before the dosage is increased. The dosage should be increased only if the physiologic levels are low despite patient compliance with the regimen. Concomitant medications, personal habits, diet, and other disease states may also affect the physiologic levels of certain drugs. The home care nurse should be aware of such potential interactions.

Whenever physiologic samples are obtained for drug or metabolite levels, the time of the drug ingestion must be known relative to the time the sample is obtained to interpret the results correctly. The sample must be obtained when sufficient amounts of the drug, metabolite, or marker are present in the body and can be measured. Low levels could be due to clearance of the drug from the body before the sample was obtained.

### Health Care Provider Estimates

Physicians generally tend to overestimate the level of compliance. The home health care nurse or therapist is in a unique position to assess it more accurately because of observations that can be made in the home. For example, cigarettes, full ashtrays, bottles of unopened pills, and dirty respiratory therapy equipment are evidence of poor patient compliance with health care advice.

### Other Compliance Assessments

Compliance with medications cannot always be inferred from compliance with other aspects of health care, such as appointment keeping. However, there is evidence that certain types of people tend to be more compliant in general than others. These characteristics were discussed previously under personality, psychosocial, and sociodemographic factors.

Clinical outcomes may suggest medication compliance but cannot be related to it with certainty. Improvement may be related to associated factors such as diet, other drugs, reassurance and attention from the provider, or a reduction in allergen and irritant levels and not to the medication or treatment in question. Because of idiosyncratic responses, a patient may also recover after taking less medication than what was actually prescribed. In addition, side effects do not indicate compliance with any certainty because they may be the result of other medications or conditions, rather than sensitivity of the patient to the drug's effect.

### Summary of Patient Compliance Assessments

There are no certain assessment tools of patient compliance with health care advice. Generally, patient and family reports, medication or exercise diaries, and pill counts are the most practical and least expensive ways to infer compliance. Physiologic determinations are often expensive and not always available, but they can augment information obtained from other compliance assessments.

## NURSING INTERVENTIONS

Many strategies have been shown to enhance compliance. Patient and family education, simplifying the regimen, and helping patients incorporate it into their life-styles may be the most important. Other strategies include compliance contracts, written instructions, medication calendars, special medication preparations, special attention, and behavior modification techniques.

### Patient and Family Education

The home health care nurse plays a vital role in helping the patient or parent understand the nature of the disease and the rationale for therapy. There are two primary objectives of the teaching: (1) to provide the patient or parent with sufficient information to make a decision about therapy and (2) to enable the patient or parent to develop the skills necessary for carrying out the prescribed treatment.

It is important to remember that teaching is an

ongoing process and is usually a component of every home visit. The teaching can be verbal, written, or provided by demonstration and practice. There are several advantages of patient teaching in the home: (1) the teaching can be geared to the specific needs of the patient and family; (2) specific materials and resources available in the home can be incorporated into the teaching plan; and (3) the teaching program can readily be evaluated during follow-up visits and reinforced or altered as appropriate.

### Skills of the Provider

The nurse must possess the following knowledge and skills to effectively provide health education:

- Basic understanding of the disease process and the material being taught
- Knowledge to assess patient readiness and ability to learn
- Ability to help the patient or parent determine realistic goals for therapy
- Ability to communicate effectively and present information appropriate to the learner's level of understanding
- Ability to evaluate the effectiveness of teaching and to alter the approach when appropriate

### Assessing the Knowledge Base

It is important to assess how much the patient or parent already knows about the disease and the therapy before establishing a teaching plan. Much of the baseline knowledge may be determined while the nurse is taking the initial history and reviewing the medications and treatments. It is generally not necessary to administer a written pretest.

### Assessing Readiness and Ability to Learn

Certain questions should be answered before the teaching plan is developed: Is the patient or parent motivated to learn? How much does he or she want to know? How much does he or she need to know in order to carry out the prescribed therapy? What do the disease and treatment mean to the patient and family? Does the parent or patient perceive a benefit from the teaching? Does he or she possess the necessary intellectual and physical skills to learn and use the information provided? Can he or she read and understand written materials? Are there factors in the home environment that would interfere with the educational goals? Is it possible to set aside time when there are no distractions so that learning can take place? Are there language or cultural barriers to the teaching or learning?

Adults with chronic lung disease who are hypoxemic often have mild organic brain disorders (Prigatano, 1983) and acquire new information with difficulty. The results of aging and the COPD process may make them irritable, inflexible, and unable to see that certain behaviors may aggravate their lung condition. More serious dysfunctions such as paranoia and apathy are also possible. *Parents or caregivers of small children may have learning problems because of anxieties and fatigue.* Patients cannot learn effectively when they are acutely dyspneic, experiencing an acute exacerbation, or anxious or depressed.

### Educational Objectives

Measurable objectives should always be established before the teaching program is initiated. They should be written clearly and well documented in the patient record for legal purposes and to ensure third-party reimbursement. The objectives should be appropriate for the patient's level of understanding, perceived needs, and desires. The objectives should be realistic and established in conjunction with the patient or parent. The content should also be relevant and meaningful for the patient. For instance, an exercise program will be more successful if it is geared toward an activity that is important to the patient. Activities that can be planned with others may also be more successful than those that the patient performs alone. A teaching program will not be successful if the patient can never accomplish the goal or does not feel that it is important. Some patients may not want or understand information about the disease and the rationale for treatment. They may feel that it is the role of the physician, nurse, or therapist to tell them what they should do. Others may be intellectually curious and want information to help them understand the disease and therapy.

The home care teaching plan should include the following:

- The basic disease processes, signs, and symptoms of exacerbations
- Rationale and benefits of therapy
- How and when the therapy should be used
- Signs and symptoms of adverse effects and what to do about them
- How to troubleshoot equipment and get help if necessary
- How to obtain refills and equipment supplies
- Sources and limits of insurance reimbursement

## Teaching Resources

Booklets, audiovisual aids such as flip charts, television cassettes, and tape recordings are available through the local chapters of the American Lung Association and Cystic Fibrosis Foundation, hospitals, or other community resources. Pulmonary rehabilitation programs and support groups for patients with COPD, programs for children and adults with asthma, and other group programs may be available locally and provide important resources for education and social support. The home care nurse can then individualize the teaching to the home setting.

## Teaching Strategies

Learning takes place most effectively when more than one sense is stimulated simultaneously. Demonstration and practice can be used in the home because of the 1:1 teacher/learner ratio. The home care nurse demonstrates a given procedure with the equipment the patient will use in the home. The patient or parent practices the demonstration until he or she feels ready to perform it independently. A repeat demonstration should be scheduled a few days later to be sure the procedure is being performed properly. It is important to pace the teaching so that the learner is not overwhelmed with too much information at once.

Verbal instructions should always be reinforced

with clear, simple written instructions. Instruction sheets should be developed that can be given to the patient. Generally, one should provide only the information that is necessary for the patient or parent to perform the necessary task. Once the task is mastered, more information may be imparted as indicated. Many patient education materials are geared to a level beyond patients' understanding. Grade levels that have been reached in school are probably the best predictor of reading ability, although they may not be completely accurate (Redman, 1992). As a general rule, teaching materials should be prepared for an eighth grade level of understanding. A "formal" teaching program with pretests and posttests may be a more successful approach for some patients. Such programs may give the patients an enhanced sense of the importance of what they are learning.

Open communication and rapport between the provider, patient, family, and physician is essential for a successful teaching program. If possible, the same nurse should conduct the teaching visits. The nurse must respect the patient and provide information in a sincere, warm, tactful, nonthreatening manner, and the teaching sessions should be scheduled when the patient is rested and feeling relatively well. The teaching program should be coordinated with the hospital or rehabilitation program staff when it is appropriate.

## Teaching Children

*The ability of children to learn depends on their stage of intellectual growth and development (Redman, 1992). Trust is most important until the age of 2 years, whereas imagination is important between 3½ and 7 years. During the school years, children become industrious and pay attention to the outside world, and during adolescence, they begin to learn to think and behave as adults.*

■ *Preschool Children. Preschool children have a short attention span and cannot comprehend what they cannot see. They believe that people cause illness and that illnesses may be their fault. They may think that medical treatments are punishment for being bad. They learn primarily by play.*

■ *Children 7 to 9 Years of Age. Children between the ages of 7 and 9 years can begin to learn about the causes of illness and the reason for treatment. They are able to talk about feelings and can cooperate with treatments because they can think before they act. They can begin to problem solve and think logically. At this age, they can also follow several consecutive commands, a skill that is necessary for them to begin self-management.*

■ *Children 9 to 11 Years of Age. Children between 9 and 11 years of age can begin to understand relationships between things and make associations. They can understand abstract concepts, hypotheses, and theories, such as those of germs and bodily resistance to disease.*

■ *Adolescents. Adolescents learn in relationship to peers and are developing sexual identity. They may be shy and full of self-doubt and are struggling to learn the roles they will play as adults. A higher percentage of adolescents with cystic fibrosis were more compliant when they learned to use the following coping skills: (1) understanding the severity of illness; (2) responsibility for medications at home; (3) information seeking about the illness; (4) future goal orientation; (5) involvement in school or work; and (6) openness with peers about their illness (Czajkowski, 1986).*

### Evaluating Education

Determine whether teaching goals have been met (i.e., objectives successfully completed) by observing the patient or parent perform the necessary actions and by asking questions about what he or she is doing. Ask the patient or parent how he or she feels about the material that was presented in the teaching program and if they are ready to perform the task independently.

If it is obvious that the teaching plan has not been successful, several questions should be asked. Were the educational goals appropriate? Were the objectives realistic? Would another teaching strategy be more appropriate? Is it possible for the patient or parent to carry out the necessary activities? Is additional home care support indicated?

It is important to document the success of the teaching program in the patient record. One way of doing this is to attach a copy of the patient learning objectives that indicate when the objective was accomplished.

## Simplification of the Regimen

Any strategy that simplifies the therapy is likely to enhance compliance. Sustained release tablets that allow less frequent doses are better than preparations that need to be taken more often. Unit-dose packaging of liquid medications for nebulizers may enhance compliance by simplifying medication preparation. Similarly, cards with bubble packets for each tablet help patients see that the appropriate doses have been taken. Such special packaging is expensive, however, and may not always be available. Pills can also be placed in envelopes or medicine cups and clearly marked with the date and time they are to be taken. Plastic containers with separate compartments for multiple doses of tablets or capsules are available in sizes that hold medications for 1 to 7 days. Such containers are especially useful when patients have several pills to take at different times. Patients can also see that they have taken their previous doses of medication when the compartments are empty. This helps to prevent accidental overdoses when patients decide that they may have forgotten a dose and take another "just to be sure." Multidose containers are useful for all patients who are receiving several medications, not just those who tend to be foregetful. They are available in most pharmacies.

Patients or family members can usually be taught to prepare the medications. However, if a patient and family are clearly unable to manage, the nurse may have to make special arrangements for preparation of medications. It may be possible for a friend or neighbor to assist the patient. Funds may be available from state, local, or private resources to pay for private duty nurses to supervise the patient and prepare the medications. It may also be possible to administer some drugs parenterally if compliance problems with oral medications cannot be resolved.

## Compliance Contracts

It may be appropriate to formalize a plan to resolve compliance problems with the patient by preparing a written or verbal contract. The contract can be any written statement of the agreement to resolve the compliance problem. It should be signed by the patient and the caregiver. Having a witness sign the contract is also helpful. Copies are retained by the patient and the caregiver. It is important that family members, the physician, and others in the home environment be supportive of the plan. Any contract must contain realistic goals and steps to resolve the compliance problem or it will not be effective. It is important to include the rewards for successful resolution of the problem and the penalty for not following through with the contract. Usually the patient should select the rewards and penalties so that they will be meaningful.

## Written Instructions, Medication Calendars, and Electronic Reminders

Written instructions are effective in enhancing compliance with short-term, but not long-term, regimens. The name of the medication, the dosage, the frequency of administration, and special instructions, such as "take with meals," must be written clearly in words that the patient can understand. The home care nurse should have a fat felt-tip pen and a pad of paper available for writing instructions. It may be helpful to post a medication calendar and a pencil in a strategic location, such as the bathroom mirror or the refrigerator door, and have the patient check off each dose as it is taken (Fig. 21-3). The medication calendar should include simple instructions that are geared to the patient's usual daily routine.

Patients can set alarms to remind themselves that it is time to take medication; and voice mail and computer terminals can be used to remind patients to refill prescriptions (Levy, 1991). Computers can also be used to collect data about symptoms and alert patients that it is time to take medications (Dahlstrom, 1991).

## Special Attention

*Parental encouragement has been shown to enhance compliance in children* (Weinstein, 1985). Adults have also been shown to respond to special attention from physicians, nurses, friends, and family. It is important for the home health care provider to check on the patient's progress with any plan that is adopted to enhance compliance. It is important to reinforce appropriate patient actions and to help the patient find new solutions if there are continuing problems. Telephone calls and notes may be helpful if home visits must be limited.

## Behavior Modification Techniques

In behavior modification, desired behaviors are reinforced with reminders, self-monitoring techniques, and rewards to help the patient establish the habit of compliance.

Organizing or tailoring medication and treatment times according to established daily activities, such as meals or work schedules, will reinforce compliance. Treatments that are prescribed three times daily may be taken in the morning, early evening, and bedtime (instead of morning, noon, and night) if it is more convenient and does not compromise control of symptoms.

Self-monitoring may also be used effectively. Peak flow meters may be used to document the efficacy of inhaled bronchodilator therapy. Serum theophylline levels can be reported to patients and caregivers to reinforce compliance. Patients can be taught to take their pulse to monitor their heart rate in response to exercise. Pulse oximetry can also provide feedback on the effects of oxygen therapy.

Special rewards that are important to the patient can be used to reinforce compliance. Conversely, penalties such as monetary fines can be assessed if the patient is noncompliant. Such rewards and penalties usually require close supervision by another person unless patients are exceptionally motivated and self-disciplined. Most often, positive reinforcement is thought to be superior to punishment or negative reinforcement. Behavior modification techniques may be especially helpful with smoking cessation interventions.

Name: John Doe                                          Week of: May 3-9

| Sunday | Monday | Tuesday | Wednesday | Thursday | Friday | Saturday |
|---|---|---|---|---|---|---|
| **9 am** Prednisone 40 mg (2 20 mg tabs) | | | **9 am** Prednisone 20 mg (1 20 mg tab) | | | |
| Septra DS (1 tab) | | | | | | |
| Albuterol 2 to 4 puffs from inhaler (repeat every 1 to 2 hours as needed) | | | | | | |
| **9 pm** Septra DS (1 tab) | | | | | | |

**Fig. 21-3**   Medication calendar.

## Other Compliance Enhancement Techniques

Cost containment strategies may be effective in improving compliance if cost is a factor. It may be possible to use less expensive generic drug preparations, if efficacy is not altered by the preparation, and to shop around for a less expensive pharmacy. Sometimes mail order programs are less expensive than local pharmacies. The patient may be eligible for government aid programs that pay for medications. Saline diluent for aerosolized medications can be made at home with salt and water if the cost of bottled saline is prohibitive.

Other solutions to compliance problems include teaching attendants or home health aides to clean respiratory therapy equipment, using oxygen to treat cognitive impairments related to hypoxemia, treating depression, and allaying anxieties. There may be many solutions to compliance problems if the patient and family are motivated and the provider is willing and able to help them.

The home health care nurse must always be aware of patient and family psychosocial problems that may adversely affect patient compliance. A referral to a family guidance counselor, social worker, psychologist, or psychiatrist may be indicated for significant dysfunction.

## Medicare Documentation

Teaching or training should be appropriate to the medical condition and capabilities of the patient, complexity of medications and treatment, and treatment goals. Medicare reimburses for patient teaching visits if one of the following situations is documented in the patient record:

- Teaching or training by a skilled nurse is necessary for treatment of the illness; may include teaching of nonskilled services such as cleaning equipment
- Need for skilled nurse to teach effectiveness and safety of new medications or treatments
- Skilled nursing required to train family or caregiver to manage patient treatment regimen
- Reinforcement of previous teaching required

because of one of the following:
  New issues about safety or effectiveness; modifications of therapy
  Gaps in knowledge of patient or caregiver
  Need to adapt hospital-based teaching to home environment
  Patient or caregiver not properly carrying out regimen

Continued home visits for skilled nursing instruction are not reasonable and will not be reimbursed by Medicare if the patient or caregiver is unable or unwilling to be taught.

### REFERENCES

Aergeret C et al: Compliance of COPD patients with long-term oxygen therapy, *Eur J Respir Dis* 69(suppl 146):421, 1986.

Backes JM, Schentag JJ: Partial compliance as a source of variance in pharmacokinetics and therapeutic drug monitoring. In Cramer JA, Spilker B, editors: *Patient compliance in medical practice and clinical trials,* New York, 1991, Raven Press.

Becker MH, Maiman LA: Sociobehavioral determinants of compliance with health and medical care recommendations, *Med Care* 13:10, 1975.

Clark MM, editor: Cross-cultural medicine, *West J Med* 139:806, 1983.

Currie DC et al: Practice, problems and compliance with postural drainage: a survey of chronic sputum producers, *Br J Dis Chest* 80:249, 1986.

Czajkowski DR, Koocher GP: Medical compliance and coping with cystic fibrosis, *J Child Psychol Psychiatry* 28:311, 1987.

Dahlstrom B, Eckernas SA: Patient computers to enhance compliance with completing questionnaires: a challenge for the 1990s. In Cramer JA, Spilker B, editors: *Patient compliance in medical practice and clinical trials,* New York, 1991, Raven Press.

Dolce JJ et al: Medication adherence patterns in chronic obstructive pulmonary disease, *Chest* 99:837, 1991.

Eraker SA et al: Understanding and improving patient compliance, *Ann Intern Med* 100:258, 1984.

Haynes RB et al: *Compliance in health care,* Baltimore, 1979, Johns Hopkins University Press.

Hilbert GA: Accuracy of self-reported measures of compliance, *Nurs Res* 34:319, 1985.

Krall RL: Interaction of compliance and patient safety. In Cramer JA, Spilker B, editors: *Patient compliance in medical practice and clinical trials,* New York, 1991, Raven Press.

Levy RA: Failure to refill prescriptions: incidence, reasons, and remedies. In Cramer JA, Spilker B, editors: *Patient compliance in medical practice and clinical trials,* New York, 1991, Raven Press.

Mann M et al: A comparison of the effects of bid and qid dosing on compliance with inhaled flunisolide, *Chest* 101:496, 1992.

Parker SR, Lenfant C: Educational and behavioral approaches to the prevention and control of lung disease. In Murray JF, Nadel JA, editors: *Textbook of respiratory medicine,* Philadelphia, 1988, WB Saunders.

Prigatano GP et al: Neuropsychological test performance in mildly hypoxemic patients with chronic obstructive pulmonary disease, *J Consult Clin Psychol* 51:108, 1983.

Rapoff MA, Barnard MU: Compliance with pediatric regimens. In Cramer JA, Spilker B, editors: *Patient compliance in medical practice and clinical trials,* New York, 1991, Raven Press.

Redman BK: *The process of patient education,* ed 7, St Louis, 1992, Mosby.

Rotter JB: Generalized expectancies for internal versus external control of reinforcement, *Psychol Mono* 80 (1), 1966.

Spector SL, Mawhinney H: Aerosol inhaler monitoring of asthmatic medication. In Cramer JA, Spilker B, editors: *Patient compliance in medical practice and clinical trials,* New York, 1991, Raven Press.

Turner J et al: Patient compliance with long-term home nebulizer therapy for chronic obstructive pulmonary disease, *Am Rev Respir Dis* 131:A166, 1985 (abstract).

Weinstein AG, Cuskey W: Theophylline compliance in asthmatic children, *Ann Allegy* 54:19, 1985.

Wilson DK et al: Acute effects of oxygen treatment upon information processing in hypoxemic COPD patients, *Chest* 88:239, 1985.

## SUGGESTED READINGS

Cramer JA, Spilker B, editors: *Patient compliance in medical practice and clinical trials,* New York, 1991, Raven Press.

Gessner BA, Armstrong ML, guest editors: Patient teaching, *Nurs Clin North Am* 24:583, 1989.

# CHAPTER 22

# The Dying Patient

CAROL M. TAYLOR

Severe chronic lung disease eventually takes the patient on a downward course toward the terminal phase of illness. Many patients tire of the long struggle to breathe and welcome death as a release from years of suffering and disability. Many choose to die at home rather than in a hospital.

A plethora of literature is available on hospice care and care of the dying, and home health care nurses are encouraged to explore this information in more detail. The purpose of this chapter is to focus on the typical experiences and problems faced by patients with end-stage respiratory disease and their families as death approaches. The chapter addresses the importance of anticipatory planning for death, presents practical approaches to assessing and managing symptoms, and discusses psychosocial, spiritual, and legal issues surrounding a planned death at home.

## EVENTS PRECIPITATING DEATH

Typical diagnoses that may result in death at home from respiratory failure include chronic obstructive pulmonary disease (COPD), cystic fibrosis, pulmonary fibrosis, lung cancer, human immunodeficiency virus infections, and amyotrophic lateral sclerosis. These are all chronic diseases for which there is no cure; they are characterized by an inevitable downhill course, even though treatable exacerbations are common. The most common cause of death in patients with chronic lung disease is acute respiratory failure, often complicated by

heart failure. However, death may also occur as a result of complications or events associated with the underlying disease process. Potential problems associated with specific end-stage lung diseases that have implications for care are presented in the box on p. 372.

## ASSESSMENT OF APPROACHING DEATH

The clinical signs and symptoms of rapidly worsening end-stage lung disease are initially those of severe hypoxemia, but eventually they also include hypercapnia, leading to $CO_2$ narcosis, and possibly biventricular failure. Signs and symptoms of hypoxemia and $CO_2$ narcosis are presented in the boxes on p. 373. Those of cardiac failure are described in Chapter 10. Anorexia, malnutrition, wasting, and skin breakdown are common in dying patients. Symptoms unique to the underlying disease may also be present, as summarized in the box on p. 372.

## NURSING INTERVENTIONS

The patient's inner coping strengths, patterns of behavior, social and family supports, and spiritual beliefs provide the framework for the delivery of supportive care in the home. The needs most often articulated by the dying person are the following (Blues, 1984):

- Respect for one's wishes; autonomy
- Control of pain and shortness of breath

## Potential Complications Associated with Specific End-Stage Respiratory Problems

**CHRONIC OBSTRUCTIVE PULMONARY DISEASE (COPD)**

Progressive respiratory failure caused by loss of alveolar and capillary surface area, chronic inflammation, and other changes
Respiratory infection or pneumonia resulting from marked impairment in secretion clearance
$CO_2$ narcosis
Sudden death resulting from cardiac arrhythmia

**LUNG CANCER**

Respiratory failure caused by pneumonia, pleural effusion, or encroachment of tumor
Pulmonary hemorrhage resulting from erosion of tumor into blood vessel
Intractable chest pain caused by tumor pressure
Severe dyspnea, which may or may not be associated with hypoxemia; present in up to 70% of patients with terminal cancer, including those without pulmonary involvement (Foote, 1986)
Pathologic fractures as the result of bony metastases:
    Rib fractures causing chest pain
    Vertebral compression fractures leading to myopathies, loss of bowel and bladder control, and possibly paralysis

**PULMONARY FIBROSIS**

Intolerable dyspnea with respiratory rate in excess of 50 breaths per minute, leading to hypocapnia
Profound hypoxemia requiring high (up to 15 L/min) oxygen flow rates

**CYSTIC FIBROSIS**

Respiratory failure caused by diffuse bronchiectasis and airway obstruction with unusually thick purulent secretions
Pulmonary hemorrhage resulting from erosion of bronchial arteries through airway walls (can occur at any time in the course of the disease, usually in association with infection and inflammation, and can result in sudden, unexpected death)

**HUMAN IMMUNODEFICIENCY VIRUS (HIV)**

Multisystem involvement
Opportunistic infections caused by impaired immune system
    Respiratory failure as the result of *Pneumocystis carinii* pneumonia
    High incidence of *Mycobacterium avium* infection
    Painful oral lesions caused by candidiasis, herpes
Kaposi's sarcoma, leading to pulmonary infiltrates and oral lesions
Drenching night sweats
Neurologic involvement (memory lapses, peripheral neuropathies, confusion, seizures) in 60% of patients, with progressive dementia in 10% to 20%
Intractable diarrhea or gastrointestinal malabsorption

**AMYOTROPHIC LATERAL SCLEROSIS (ALS)**

Progressive loss of muscle function including respiratory muscles, leading to reduced cough intensity and, ultimately, respiratory failure
Dysphagia, causing aspiration pneumonia
Impaired communication resulting from vocal cord weakness

---

### Signs and Symptoms of CO₂ Narcosis

**SYMPTOMS**

Headache

Lethargy → drowsiness → coma

**SIGNS**

Redness of skin, sclera, and conjunctiva from increased cutaneous blood flow

Sweating

Hypertension and increased heart rate

Tremulousness or asterixis

Inappropriate response or lack of response to verbal questioning

Blank stare into space

---

Modified from Kersten LD: *Comprehensive respiratory nursing,* Philadelphia, 1989, WB Saunders.

---

### Signs and Symptoms of Hypoxemia

**RESPIRATORY**

Dyspnea

Tachypnea

**CARDIOVASCULAR**

Increased heart rate (HR)

Cardiac arrhythmias

Acute hypertension with increased HR (sympathetic response)

Hypotension with decreased HR

Paleness or cyanosis

**CENTRAL NERVOUS SYSTEM**

Impaired judgment

Disorientation

Restlessness

Combativeness

Motor incoordination

Personality change or paranoia

Delirium

Coma

**OTHER**

General fatigue

Gradual increase in blood hemoglobin and hematocrit values

---

Modified from Kersten LD: *Comprehensive respiratory nursing,* Philadelphia, 1989, WB Saunders.

---

- Normal family relationships or a redefinition of them in agreeable terms

The skills most needed by the home health care nurse are those of "active listening and silent presence" and the ability to clarify the patient's choices and to maintain a balance between patient advocacy and coercion. Home health care nurses have a wealth of clinical expertise, resources, and compassion to share with patients and families as they face the terminal stage of illness.

## Identification of the Terminal Stage of Illness

A diagnosis of "end-stage" COPD tells us little about how imminent death is. Many patients with COPD live a revolving door existence between hospital and home, gradually losing function and requiring frequent hospitalizations for acute exacerbations. When initially assessing a debilitated patient with "end-stage" COPD at home, the caregiver must distinguish between the patient for whom terminal care is appropriate and the patient who may appear to be terminally ill but who in truth is suffering depression, general deconditioning, or debilitation.

The home health care nurse's role in assisting the patient to "live until he dies" cannot be overestimated. Knowing how to integrate the threads of hope with the realities of planning for the end of life comes from listening to the patient's perception of illness. Home health care nurses develop an almost instinctual knowledge (based on professional experiences and on having worked closely with a patient) that dictates when the approach should change from a rehabilitative focus to one of support for the process of dying. Proactive nursing and anticipatory guidance are extremely important (Blues, 1984). These skills require knowledge of problems that commonly occur as a result of a particular disease process.

## Management of Shortness of Breath

Managing the sensation of dyspnea is of paramount concern both to patients and to those around them (see Chapter 8). Patients dying from lung cancer have described the sensation of dyspnea in many ways and have described a number of coping strategies (Brown, 1986). Interventions that may reduce intolerable dyspnea, regardless of the underlying diagnosis, are discussed in the following sections.

### Positioning

Severely dyspneic patients are usually most comfortable in a high- or semi-Fowler's position. A hospital bed is the most effective means of maintaining this optimal position. However, a restful position can be achieved with firm cushions. Arms can be elevated and supported with pillows or an overbed table placed at chest height. A high-backed chair with armrests or a recliner will also support patients in a comfortable position. Patients dying of cystic fibrosis often fold themselves into a modified fetal position. The physiologic advantage of this position is unclear, but it seems to be their position of greatest comfort.

### Breathing Control

Use of pursed lip or abdominal diaphragmatic breathing may help patients with COPD control panic and anxiety and decrease air trapping. If spouses or significant others are taught how to coach pursed lip breathing, they can often help anxious patients who are unable to follow through on their own. Pacing of activities is also important. Pursed lip breathing may function as a short-term relaxation and panic control strategy, even for patients with interstitial pulmonary fibrosis, in which it has no physiologic basis for efficacy.

### Oxygen Therapy

Oxygen therapy is clearly indicated in the presence of hypoxemia. However, patients with lung cancer often experience severe dyspnea in the last few days of life that is not associated with hypoxemia. Despite this lack of physiologic justification for oxygen therapy, it appears to provide some subjective relief and is often provided. However, it must be understood that home oxygen therapy, when prescribed for shortness of breath without documented hypoxemia, will not be covered by Medicare, at least under current oxygen reimbursement guidelines.

The unusually high flow rates required by patients with pulmonary fibrosis may cause nose and throat irritation and often require innovative combinations of oxygen delivery systems (e.g., liquid oxygen bled into an oxygen concentrator) to control costs and reduce the frequency with which oxygen deliveries to the home are needed. Oxygen delivery systems are discussed in Chapter 15.

### Use of Fans

The feeling of air hunger can sometimes be minimized by directing a fan toward the patient. Although the mechanism by which a fan provides relief is unclear, it probably has a physiologic basis (Schwartzstein, 1987).

### Inhaled Bronchodilators

Inhaled bronchodilators may be helpful for patients for whom bronchospasm or retained secretions contribute to dyspnea and discomfort. The benefit of treatments in relieving dyspnea must be weighed against the fatigue that may result from taking the treatment. Mask attachments deliver medication more quickly and with less fatigue, but they may precipitate feelings of claustrophobia with some patients. Bronchodilator therapy is discussed in Chapter 6.

### Corticosteroids

Corticosteroid therapy may be indicated for bronchospasm and pulmonary inflammation and, for patients with lung cancer, to decrease inflammation and edema around the tumor (White, 1987). Corticosteroid therapy is discussed in Chapter 6. A beneficial side effect for many terminally ill patients is stimulation of appetite.

### Narcotics and Sedatives

Narcotics and sedatives are used to suppress cough and alleviate the sensation of dyspnea. Narcotics are available in oral (tablets and solutions), sublingual, suppository, and injectable or intravenous forms. The many preparations available allow the caregiver to tailor the therapy to the patient's needs. Long-acting oral narcotics can help patients and families sleep at night. Short-acting drugs (e.g., sublingual morphine) are effective for acute severe breathlessness, breakthrough pain, or when more medication is needed to manage increased activity. Hydroxyzine pamoate (Vistaril) and diphenhydramine (Benadryl) may also reduce breathlessness and apprehension without significant respiratory depression. Doses of 25 mg every 4 to 6 hours are usually effective. These drugs can also enhance the effectiveness of narcotics and have antiemetic properties. The use of narcotic and nonnarcotic medications to control symptoms is discussed in the section on pain control.

## Management of Respiratory Tract Secretions

Many lung diseases are associated with increased secretion production, airway inflammation and edema, and impaired mucociliary clearance. Neuromuscular deficits and weakness inhibit effective coughing. Airway clearance is discussed in Chapter 7. In patients with terminal illness, adequate oral hydration should be maintained as much as possible to keep secretions from becoming too thick. Chest physical therapy should be instituted only if the patient finds it helpful and tolerates the procedure without evidence of bronchospasm or positional hypoxemia. Treatment of underlying pneumonia and pleural effusions should be consistent with the patient's wishes. Symptom relief from suctioning should be weighed against the trauma and stimulation of increased secretions that may result from suctioning. Small bulb syringes or Yankauer tip suctions may be helpful to clear oral secretions.

## Management of Pain

In the past decade many advances have been made in the management of pain. Pain is defined by the patient, with the individual response being based on the type, duration, and severity of the pain and other psychosocial, environmental, cultural, and spiritual factors.

The home health care nurse has a unique opportunity to assess how the patient and family cope with the effects of pain and can, in conjunction with the physician, orchestrate pharmacologic and nonpharmacologic methods of achieving pain control if the patient desires. Not all patients want pain relief; for some, experiencing the pain means that they are alive (McCaffrey, 1979). It is important to determine the patient's desire for pain control before implementing pain control measures.

### Nonpharmacologic Modalities for Pain Relief

A number of nonpharmacologic interventions may be used to control the patient's perception of pain. Basic to all of these is the establishment of a therapeutic nurse-patient relationship.

■ *Cutaneous Stimulation or Pressure Measures.* Cutaneous stimulation or pressure can eliminate or decrease the intensity of the pain. Potential methods include the following:

- Selective application of heat or cold
- Massage—has the beneficial effects of muscle relaxation and sedation (Patients with hyperesthesias, however, may not tolerate massage. Caution should be used in patients who are undergoing radiation therapy to the chest or back because those areas may be sensitive. Foot massage may be a good alternative.)
- Shiatsu—a Japanese art that incorporates the use of gentle range of motion exercises with finger and hand pressure on the body's energy meridians (Lawrence, 1986); an important option to offer patients who may be culturally opposed to traditional Western options

- Acupressure—a Chinese art; differs from Shiatsu in that range of motion and stretching exercises are excluded
- External analgesics—ointments, lotions, gels, liniments, and balms; may have a mild anesthetic effect and may be useful for the relief of painful muscles and joints (If the patient is undergoing radiation therapy, such measures should not be used without prior consultation with the physician or radiologist.)

■ *Relaxation.* Relaxation is defined as "a state of freedom from anxiety and skeletal muscle tension, either of which can cause or aggravate existing pain" (McCaffrey, 1989). Strategies that enhance relaxation are thought to counteract the autonomic nervous system hyperactivity that accompanies (and often exacerbates) acute pain. Relaxation techniques are discussed in Chapters 8 and 17. Progressive muscle relaxation has been shown to be effective in reducing pain and the associated distress in patients with cancer (Graffam, 1987).

■ *Guided Imagery.* In guided imagery the patient uses his or her imagination to develop sensory images that decrease the intensity of the pain experience. Tapes approximately 15 minutes long can be made that focus on the patient's needs or experiences—for example, "You are walking through the forest when you come upon a pleasant meadow. You lie down to rest; the sun is warm on your skin. You can hear the chirping of birds nearby. Your arms and legs feel heavy and warm. You close your eyes and take a deep breath. Blow it out slowly and feel yourself relax. Concentrate on breathing slowly and deeply from your abdomen. Breathe with this slow, steady rhythm for a few moments. Now, as you breathe in, imagine a flow of warm, healing energy coming into your body. Then as you blow out, all the discomfort that you feel in your lungs flows out with it . . . "

■ *Distraction Techniques.* Distraction techniques involve focusing attention on stimuli other than the pain. They usually help increase tolerance of pain, but the effect lasts only while the distraction is being used. Examples are music, humor, rhythmic massage (effluage), and concentration on a specific object.

■ *Deep Hypnosis.* Deep hypnosis, administered by an experienced hypnotherapist, may be helpful to some patients with pain.

## Pharmacologic Modalities for Pain Relief

Several principles govern the pharmacologic management of pain in terminally ill patients. It is important that pain medication be individualized and evaluated on an ongoing basis. Analgesic agents should be given routinely around the clock and not on an as needed (prn) basis. The goal is to achieve a plateau of comfort rather than the peaks and valleys that occur when pain is allowed to escalate in intensity and medication is given only when the pain becomes severe.

■ *Nonnarcotic Pain Medication.* Acetylsalicylic acid (ASA) and other nonsteroidal antiinflammatory drugs (NSAIDs) are used frequently in the management of cancer pain. They are administered for mild pain or as adjunctive therapy with narcotic agents in the treatment of bone pain. The belief is that NSAIDs decrease the inflammatory reaction and inhibit prostaglandin synthesis. Prostaglandins have a role in sensitizing receptors at the sites of bone metastases. ASA, 650 mg every 4 hours, may be helpful in relieving the pain of bony metastases.

■ *Narcotics.* Patients often say that they do not like to take pills or express a fear of becoming addicted to narcotic agents. They equate the use of these medications with the psychic craving found in narcotic abusers. In pain associated with terminal illness, drug dependence does not occur when a narcotic is taken at regular intervals and in individually tailored dosages. Once the patient's goals in the dying process are understood, the nurse and physician can collaborate to develop strategies for pain management. The nurse can then teach the patient and family about the medication, expected actions, and potential side effects. It is important to evaluate the effectiveness of pain control measures frequently. The goal is to provide optimal pain relief with a minimum of side effects. Dosages are titrated according to the patient's degree of pain, mental status, and respiratory rate (Blues, 1984). Pain should be controlled without excessive sedation and with a respiratory rate of at least 10 breaths per minute.

Oral agents are the route of choice for most patients who can swallow. Breakthrough pain can be managed by titrating the usual oral dosage upward, by administering an injection, or by using a sublingual form of the drug if available. Because pain cocktails consist of two or more drugs in solution, they may have toxic effects if the dose must be titrated upward. For this reason they are seldom used for pain relief (Blues, 1984). Bowel programs should be established at the same time narcotics are initiated to avoid problems with constipation.

■ *Chemotherapy and Radiation Therapy.* By shrinking tumors that cause pain, chemotherapy and radiation therapy may also serve as palliative measures.

## Management of Pulmonary Hemorrhage

Although relatively rare, pulmonary hemorrhage may occur if a tumor erodes into blood vessels. Patients with severe bronchiectasis (including non–terminally ill patients with cystic fibrosis) can also experience sudden massive hemoptysis resulting from the erosion of distended tortuous bronchial arteries through airway walls. This usually occurs in association with a respiratory tract infection and inflammation. Many terminally ill patients are at increased risk for bleeding because of impaired synthesis of prothrombin and a reduction in platelets (Blues, 1984). Patients with cystic fibrosis are at increased risk because of impaired vitamin K production associated with antibiotic therapy and may need vitamin K supplements while taking antibiotics. Pulmonary hemorrhage in the terminally ill patient may be managed as follows:

- Maintain calm at the bedside.
- Sedate the patient to control apprehension and restlessness.
- Provide analgesia if accumulated blood is causing pressure on pain-sensitive structures.
- Apply ice and pressure over bleeding sites if indicated.

- Use disposable tissues and towels to soak up blood; remove these quickly to minimize psychologic distress. Red blankets may be useful (Blues, 1984).

Death resulting from hemorrhage can occur peacefully with a gradual loss of consciousness. Nonetheless, it is difficult for caregivers to watch a patient bleed to death. If hemorrhage is a predictable complication, it is helpful for the home health care nurse to talk with the family ahead of time about how they might handle the situation. Patients and family should always be offered the option of hospitalization if they feel they cannot manage the situation at home.

Pulmonary hemorrhage in the *nonterminally* ill patient with bronchiectasis is a medical emergency. Anyone who expectorates more than about one-quarter cup of frank blood should be transported immediately to an emergency room and is usually hospitalized for observation. Usual interventions include the following:

- Discontinuation of chest physical therapy
- Avoidance of forced expiratory maneuvers (e.g., spirometry)
- Cough suppressants; sedation
- Vitamin K
- Possibly bronchial artery embolization

## Management of Other Physical Problems

Other manifestations of end-stage disease include slowly progressive but profound nutritional deficits, problems with skin integrity, and problems with elimination. Nutrition is discussed in Chapter 11 and constipation in Chapter 13.

### Diarrhea

If diarrhea occurs, reevaluate the bowel program that was instituted when pain control measures were begun and make any necessary adjustments. Medications such as diphenoxylate with atropine (Lomotil), 2.5 to 5 mg, or loperamide (Imodium), 2 to 4 mg, every 4 to 6 hours, may be needed to control diarrhea. Use of disposable briefs (e.g., Attends) may decrease the patient's and family's distress and reduce the need for frequent bed changes. Adult-sized cloth diapers may be a more environmentally sound solution and are a natural extension of existing diaper services. The nurse should refer to agency body substance precautions for guidelines regarding proper disposal of disposable briefs and bed pads.

### Skin Breakdown

Problems with skin breakdown occur when immobility and weakness result in prolonged bed rest. Skin breakdown is also aggravated by the nutritional deficiencies that are inevitably present. Strategies include the following:

- Assist the patient to turn every 2 hours as tolerated.
- Place a small pillow under the patient's hip (alternating hips every 2 hours) to relieve pressure on the sacrococcygeal areas.
- Use a pressure reduction or foam Egg-Crate mattress.
- Massage pressure areas frequently, and provide passive range of motion to enhance circulation.

It is important to realize that, when a person is near death, the development of decubiti does not necessarily reflect inadequate care. The predominant goal in caring for a terminally ill patient is comfort. If the patient is comfortable in only one position, providing comfort is more important than preventing decubiti.

Ulcerating metastatic lesions may have purulent drainage and a foul odor. Nursing interventions are geared toward minimizing odor, infection, and bleeding. Proper cleansing of the wound and use of charcoal-backed dressings or other odor antagonists are essential for the patient's physical and psychologic benefit.

### Management of Imminent Death

As the patient nears death, demystifying the signs and symptoms that may be exhibited is often helpful. These signs and symptoms, along with strategies for managing them, are presented in the box on p. 379. It is important to counsel the patient and family that not all of these symptoms will be present and some may never appear.

When a peaceful death at home is the goal, it is helpful to review the rationale for *not* calling emergency services when signs and symptoms of imminent death appear. Various models for delivering terminal care services are used by home health care agencies; those that include 24-hour on-call services often provide a critical link of support. Family members should be encouraged to call the on-call home health care nurse if they start to panic. The nurse can usually give supportive guidance, reducing the likelihood that patients will be resuscitated against their will.

### Facilitating Anticipatory Planning

Helping the patient and significant others prepare for death is based on a philosophy of care that fear of the unknown is always greater than fear of the known. Some anxieties may be relieved when the patient discusses business and financial matters with the family and puts his or her will in order. This is especially important in relationships in which the remaining spouse has never handled the family finances. Other issues that may need to be discussed include the following:

- Does the patient have any specific questions or fears about dying? Many patients are terrified that dyspnea will become unbearable and they will suffocate. It is often comforting for them to hear that death itself is usually peaceful because of the increased somnolence associated with carbon dioxide narcosis.
- Does the patient want to be in the hospital or at home for the actual moment of death?
- Does the spouse have any specific questions or fears about caring for a dying partner, if the choice is to die at home?
- Has the patient made a clear decision about mechanical ventilation?

### Decisions Regarding Mechanical Ventilation

In an ideal world patients and families have time to gather information, work through issues of grief and loss, and make rational decisions regarding the initiation or withholding of mechanical ventilatory support. Patients with end-stage lung disease seldom opt for ventilator support in the home. When

## Information for Families Concerning Imminent Death

**SIGNS OF APPROACHING DEATH**

The arms and legs of the patient may become cool to the touch, and you may notice the underside of the patient's body becoming much darker in color. These are signs of blood circulation slowing down.

The patient will gradually spend more and more time sleeping during the day and at times will be difficult to arouse. This sign is a result of a change in the body's metabolism.

The patient may become increasingly confused about time, place, and identity of close and familiar people. Again, this is a result of change in body metabolism.

Incontinence (loss of control) of urine and bowel movements may become a problem during the final days.

Oral secretions may become more profuse and collect in the back of the throat. You may have heard friends refer to a "death rattle." This sign is a result of the patient's inability to cough up normal saliva.

Clarity of hearing and vision decrease slightly.

You may notice the patient becoming restless, pulling at bed linen, and having visions of people or things that do not exist. These signs are a result of a decrease in the oxygen circulation to the brain and a change in body metabolism.

The patient will have decreased desire for food and drink because the body will naturally begin to conserve energy that would otherwise be expended in eating and drinking.

During sleep, at first, you will notice the patient's breathing patterns changing to an irregular pace and there may be 10- to 30-second periods of no breathing. Your physician and nurse refer to this as periods of "apnea." This sign is common and indicates a decrease in circulation and a buildup of waste products in the blood.

You will notice that the amount of urine will decrease as death grows near.

**WHAT TO DO ABOUT THESE SIGNS**

Keep warm blankets on the patient to prevent him or her from feeling too cold. Electric blankets should be used with caution so that burns do not occur.

Plan your times with the patient for occasions when he or she seems most alert.

Remind the patient frequently about what day it is, what time it is, who is in the room, and who is talking.

Consult with your nurse about obtaining pads to place under the incontinent patient and other techniques to ensure cleanliness.

If and when oral secretions build up, elevating the head of the bed with pillows will make breathing easier.

Ice chips and cool, moist wash cloths will relieve feelings of dehydration.

Keep lights on in the room when vision decreases and never assume that the patient cannot hear you. Hearing is the last of the five senses to be lost.

Talk calmly and assuredly with a confused person so as not to startle or frighten him or her.

Developed by the Seattle/King County Visiting Nurse Services, Seattle, Wash.

given a choice, most choose to allow the natural onset of $CO_2$ narcosis to occur. Others may want nocturnal ventilatory support while they deal with unfinished business in their lives. In some patients an imminently terminal process is not diagnosed until they are admitted to the hospital in respiratory failure and placed on mechanical ventilation. Weaning from ventilation may not be possible for these patients, and dilemmas are faced about long-term management. The nurse must be aware of legal actions that patients can take to protect their interests in the event that they are not able to make decisions for themselves.

Recent recovery from a life-threatening exacerbation is often the stimulus for an exploration of thoughts and feelings regarding the realities of mechanical life support and can help patients decide what if any invasive interventions they want their physician to provide in the future. The nurse's role in initiating a discussion about what the patient does or does not want done has been greatly facilitated by passage of the Patient Self Determination Act of 1991. This bill mandates that patients be asked if they have prepared a living will or a durable power of attorney for health care. If they have not, the nurse must provide the patient with information on these options. Natural death acts, living wills, and other legal measures are discussed in Chapter 24.

### Funeral Arrangements

The patient and family may also be encouraged to discuss plans for the funeral and burial rites. Decisions about cremation, burial, the type of service or memorial, the eulogy, flowers, or donations are more easily made when choices are uncomplicated by time pressures and grief. This gives the patient control over the decisions and often reduces family members' apprehension. It is helpful for the family to make a list of people to be notified when death occurs.

### Legal Requirements for Anticipated Death at Home

The nurse should be familiar with the requirements of state law as they relate to anticipated death at home. Exact procedures that must be implemented in the event of an anticipated death at home vary from county to county. In most states the county medical examiner must be notified. As long as foul play is not suspected and if emergency medical services were not called, the medical examiner will simply issue a "no jurisdiction assumed" (NJA) number. Funeral homes in most areas must have an NJA number before removing the deceased from the home. In many communities the medical examiner is required by law to perform an autopsy anytime emergency medical services are involved at home, even if the death was anticipated. Prior knowledge of this requirement may help families come to a clearer decision about what

to do. If the family member is likely to be alone with the patient at the time of death, it may also help to arrange in advance for someone who could come to be with them immediately after the death.

Prior arrangements should be made with the physician about notification of death, signing the death certificate, and autopsy arrangements. Caregivers should be prepared to provide the medical examiner with the following information at the time of death:

- Name, age, and diagnosis of deceased
- Time of death
- Address
- Name of caller and relationship to the deceased
- Physician's name and telephone number
- Name and address of funeral home

### Spiritual Advisors

Individuals who are facing death often reevaluate their spiritual selves. They may question their relationship with God, have unresolved conflicts in their lives, or ponder the existence of an afterlife. The nurse or social worker can determine who has comforted the patient during times of stress in the past and whether formalized religion has been a part of the patient's support system. If the patient has roots established in a formalized religion, the nurse can contact a minister, priest, or rabbi to discuss specific religious rites that may be appropriate as the time of death nears.

### When the Dying Patient Lives Alone

One of the most difficult and challenging ethical dilemmas faced by home health care staff is that of the terminally ill patient who lives alone on a low fixed income with no identifiable support system and who is adamant about wanting to die at home. Older patients, especially, want the security of familiar surroundings and are often terrified of being sent to a nursing home to die.

Issues of safety often become a primary concern. By posing "what if" questions, the nurse can help patients consider the realities of remaining alone—for example, "What if you can't get from the bed to the commode and no one is here to help you?" and "What if you fall and are unable to reach the phone?" By discussing these possibilities, patients are helped to make informed choices about the degree of risk and potential for discomfort they are willing to take.

To maximize patient safety and comfort, the nurse must pull together a wide variety of agency and community resources, including frequent home health aide visits for personal care, homemaker services, and meal, grocery, and drug delivery services. Medicare reimbursement constraints must be considered and applications for state-funded homemaker assistance made as quickly as possible. A social work referral is usually indicated.

Because most people do not want to die alone, it is important to determine in advance whom the person most wants to have by his or her side when death comes and to facilitate this if possible. Hospice volunteers, neighbors, or church volunteers may be willing to help.

## The Dying Child and Adolescent

*Few things are more difficult than caring for a terminally ill child or adolescent. The sharp dichotomy between childhood, a time of life's beginning and becoming, and death, the ending of life, defies the natural order as we envision it. To assist these children and their families, caregivers must understand how children view themselves within their world.*

*Children and families who are coping with the final stages of a chronic illness draw from all their life experiences. The child's view of death and dying may not be communicated verbally. Thus it is important for the home health care nurse to watch for nonverbal cues and support the child in communicating concerns in whatever way he or she can. For example, young children may become preoccupied with the loss of their parents, pets, and other familiar things. They may make references to heaven or an afterlife or may focus on graves and burial rites. These are noted most often in their play or drawings. Children frequently avoid discussing matters related to dying for fear of upsetting their parents. Their ability to discuss death depends on long-standing family communi-*

*cation patterns and the degree to which parents and health care professionals support the discussion of uncomfortable subjects.*

*Worsening functional ability, frequent exacerbations and hospitalizations, and unrelieved shortness of breath or pain may become catalysts for a discussion of quality of life issues. Talking with children about what they do or do not want to happen gives them more control over their lives and may diffuse potentially maladaptive behavior. When children change the subject during discussions of emotionally charged issues, they may be signaling an unwillingness or inability to deal with the issues at that time (Larter, 1987).*

*Siblings seem to cope better if they are kept informed and, if desired, involved in the child's care. They also need an opportunity to work out feelings of guilt or anger.*

*Home intravenous therapy, oxygen, and other supportive measures permit care of the dying child in a familiar setting and with good control of symptoms. Families need to realize that a child's risk of sudden death at home is higher than in the hospital. In most cases the obvious benefits for the child of being at home outweigh this risk. Prior discussion of the risks and benefits may assuage feelings of guilt if the child does die suddenly while at home.*

## Interventions to Minimize Burnout

Spouses often greatly increase their burden of responsibility as death approaches and may manifest symptoms of burnout. The nurse must be alert for somatic symptoms such as headaches, excessive fatigue, shortness of breath, or a pounding heart. Emotional responses include feelings of loneliness and social isolation from others despite "constant togetherness" with their ill partner; depression; anger; resentment; and guilt. Guilt may be exhibited as a driving need to manage all the dying patient's care needs and reluctance to accept a home health aide or other respite services. Interventions include the following:

- Encourage spouses to spend quiet time together, uninterrupted by tasks (e.g., reading,

talking, listening to music, or holding hands).
- Explain and repeat often the importance of recuperative time away from the patient.
- Arrange respite care so that the spouse can spend a few hours away from the home at least once a week.

## Bereavement Visits After Death

One or more bereavement visits by the home health care nurse after the death of an adult or child in the home can be extremely beneficial to the grieving family. An optimal time is 6 to 8 weeks after the death when the support of other family and friends may be waning. It is also helpful to follow up with a phone call to the family at the 1-year anniversary. Many communities have support groups to help parents and family members work through the grieving process.

## TAKING CARE OF AGENCY CAREGIVERS

Caring for terminally ill patients at home often forces caregivers to look inside themselves and deal with issues of their own mortality and loss. Every day, home health care workers care for patients who may remind them of significant people in their own lives, triggering a more personal response than they might have anticipated. Such experiences are important and can lead to new areas of growth. However, they can also be exhausting and at times may be difficult to put into perspective.

Home health care agency staff are alone in the field most of their workday. This autonomy in practice is one of the more positive elements of community-based nursing. However, it must be balanced with an opportunity to share and work through intense experiences with colleagues.

A support group with a skilled facilitator is an effective vehicle by which staff (including the home health aide) can seek counsel about problems in patient care and share both successes and grief as the need arises. Home care agencies willing to make this investment of time and resources for their staff will benefit richly in the long run through reduced staff burnout and turnover.

## REFERENCES

Blues AG, Zerwekh J: *Hospice and palliative nursing care,* New York, 1984, Grune & Stratton.

Brown ML et al: Lung cancer and dyspnea: the patient's perception, *Oncol Nurs Forum* 13:19, 1986.

Foote M, Sexton DL, Pawlik L: Dyspnea: a distressing sensation in lung cancer, *Oncol Nurs Forum* 13:25, 1986.

Graffam S, Johnson A: A comparison of two relaxation strategies for the relief of pain and its distress, *J Pain Symptom Manage* 2:229, 1987.

Larter N: Patterns of impairment: cystic fibrosis. In Rose M, Thomas R, editors: *Children with chronic conditions: nursing in a family and community context,* Orlando, Fla, 1987, Grune & Stratton.

Lawrence DB: *Massage techniques,* New York, 1986, Perigee Books Putnam Publishers.

McCaffrey M: *Nursing management of the patient with pain,* Philadelphia, 1979, JB Lippincott.

McCaffrey M, Beebe A: *Pain: clinical manual for nursing practice,* St Louis, 1989, Mosby.

Schwartzstein RM et al: Cold facial stimulation reduces breathlessness induced in normal subjects, *Am Rev Respir Dis* 136:58, 1987.

White E: Home care of the patient with advanced lung cancer, *Semin Oncol Nurs* 3:216, 1987.

## SUGGESTED READINGS

Clark C et al: Hospice care: a model for caring for the person with AIDS, *Nurs Clin North Am* 23:851, 1988.

Ekberg JY, Griffith N, Foxall MJ: Spouse burnout syndrome, *J Adv Nurs* 11:161, 1986.

Hearth K: Fostering hope in terminally ill people, *J Adv Nurs* 15:1250, 1990.

Hooyman NR, Lustbader W: Taking care of your aging family members, New York, 1988, Free Press.

Lustbader W: Counting on kindness, New York, 1991, Free Press.

Marvan-Hyam J: Occupational stress of the home health nurse, *Home Healthc Nurse* 4:18, 1986.

Sexton DL: Relaxation techniques and biofeedback. In Hodgkin JE, Petty TL, editors: *COPD: current concepts,* Philadelphia, 1987, WB Saunders.

# CHAPTER 23

# ETHICAL ISSUES

MARSHA D.M. FOWLER

When patients with chronic lung disease are cared for at home, issues with legal or ethical implications inevitably arise. These situations tend to be difficult and often highly emotionally charged. They are usually situations for which the practitioner must seek peer, supervisory, or outside counsel to ensure the patient's welfare. Practitioners are encouraged to seek such counsel promptly.

Following are three care situations that illustrate scenarios commonly encountered in a respiratory home care practice. This chapter discusses the ethical ramifications of these situations and presents general information relevant to broader ethical issues that may be encountered in a community health care practice. Legal issues are discussed in Chapter 24. It is important for the home care practitioner to realize that in some instances the ethically correct course of action may be in opposition to that which is legally indicated. In such instances a sense of internal conflict is inevitable and support and counsel for the practitioner are even more important.

## CASE SITUATIONS
### Case 1

The patient is a 66-year-old male with severe emphysema, being treated by a neighborhood general practitioner. His treatments include digitalis and furosemide, supplemental potassium, multiple bronchodilators, and chest physiotherapy. He is malnourished, is barely able to get around in the home, and lives alone. Smoking seems to be one of his few pleasures. His niece comes to his apartment at least every other day to cook meals for him. The nursing care plan includes monitoring and adjusting medical treatment modalities as necessary, nutritional teaching and maintenance, chest physiotherapy, and limited breathing retraining.

The niece has expressed concern recently that her uncle is becoming forgetful and refuses to stop smoking even though it clearly makes his condition worse. Her original agreement with her uncle was that he would smoke only when she was present but that he would not smoke in her absence. She is concerned that he is not sticking to the agreement and that he has recently fallen asleep in bed while smoking. When she raised the possibility of having him move to a nursing home, he became incensed and stated, "I've lived in this apartment for 33 years, young'un, and nobody is going to move me out!" He and the niece have a basically sound relationship, although she describes him as "hard-headed and crotchety."

In addition to these concerns the patient's general practitioner persists in refusing to order oxygen for the patient, whose $P_{O_2}$ and $P_{CO_2}$ both consistently run about 50 mm Hg. The physician says that he will not order oxygen because "the patient is a $CO_2$ retainer." Even if the patient was permitted oxygen therapy, the issue of his smoking in an oxygen-enriched environment presents an additional hazard to both the patient and his neighbors.

To complicate nursing concerns, the physician frequently orders changes in respiratory medication, not necessarily relating to changes in the patient's condition and sometimes without regard for drug interactions. The nurse has informally discussed the case with a pulmonary physician, who concurs with the nurse's conclusions but says, "He's a private patient. My hands are tied."

## Case 2

The patient is a 43-year-old ventilator-dependent woman who is the mother of three school-aged children and has advanced multiple sclerosis. She is fed by nasogastric tube and occasionally receives antibiotics and other medications by intravenous infusion. Her respiratory status has limited her to bed or a chair for the past year, and her husband has struggled without assistance to keep her in the home, to keep the household going, and to maintain the family income in the face of huge medical bills.

The family is tightly knit, supportive, and almost overwhelmed in the face of the patient's now apparent decline. They have jointly decided that they will keep her at home, at almost any cost, even if she survives another year.

For the past 2 months the patient has repeatedly asked that the ventilator be withdrawn although she wishes to continue the nasogastric feedings and the intravenous fluids when necessary. The husband supports the wife in spirit; it is clear that watching her suffering is emotionally stressful for him. However, he has difficulty coping with the certainty of death if the ventilator is removed. Nonetheless, he has asked the physician to meet the wife's request to have the ventilator discontinued. The physician adamantly refuses, stating that once the ventilator has been started, it cannot be stopped because that would be "tantamount to murder."

## Case 3

The Martin family is a close-knit family of four. Both parents are teachers. The sons—Peter, who is 14 years of age, and Steven, who is 7 years of age—have cystic fibrosis. The parents are conscientious and over the years have developed a great deal of skill in caring for their children.

Peter has frequent bouts of pneumonia, chronic *Pseudomonas aeruginosa* infection, and a 40% hearing loss from antibiotic ototoxicity. He is debilitated, weak, and failing. He is now at home, receiving continuous oxygen therapy and frequent intravenous antibiotics administered through a central venous catheter. He has deteriorated to the point that hospital readmission for more aggressive bronchial hygiene and nutritional support is being considered. The possibility of evaluation for lung transplantation has also been raised with the family. Peter, however, wishes to have all treatment stopped and refuses to go to the hospital. He is aware of the consequences of that decision, but he is tired of the struggle with his disease and the social isolation it imposes on him. "Leave me alone. I don't want to be sick anymore" is his repeated statement. Nurses and family disagree over Peter's treatment. Although the nurses have become extremely attached to Peter over the years, they feel, although not uniformly, that further aggressive treatment is inappropriate. The parents are adamant that their son receive all medical treatment available and are interested in pursuing lung transplant evaluation.

Peter is subverting treatment to the limits of his energy, such as pocketing oral medications and removing the oxygen when alone. He has told his brother, "Don't ever let them do this to you!" Nursing staff and family have exhausted the approaches for securing Peter's cooperation and for swaying his opinion. The parents are at the point of issuing commands to their son and have shut off all two-way communication.

The parents are physically and emotionally exhausted. In addition to their battle with Peter, they are communicating poorly with Steven. Although they know that Peter is failing, they suppress their feelings. They are also now talking openly about having another child.

## EVOLUTION OF ETHICAL DILEMMAS FACED IN HOME CARE

Ethical dilemmas confront the home health care nurse now as in the past. What has changed, however, is the increased awareness within nursing of the prevalence of ethical issues and dilemmas, of the failure of contemporary nursing education to prepare nurses for ethical decision making, and the lack of mechanisms and processes to deal effectively with such dilemmas. Changed, too, are ethical issues that confront home health care nurses.

Earlier in the century, nursing care took place almost exclusively in the home. Such home care included public health, private duty, and visiting nurses. Regardless of their specific role, nurses had to deal with a variety of moral issues, often related to their duties in the home or responsibility to the patient, the referring physician, or the registry or agency that employed them. The questions that nurses raised regarding care in the home included the following:

- Limits of housekeeping duties
- Whether a nurse had to take care of family members, other than the designated patient, who fell ill
- Whether a nurse had to leave a patient if the referring physician were discharged by the family
- Whether a nurse should take on a patient whose physician did not have standard credentials or had not seen the patient in months
- How to handle the sexual advances of a patient's spouse
- Whether the nurse should demand to be treated as a professional or was really one of the domestics

Early ethical dilemmas in home health care also included concerns about reporting illegal procedures (e.g., criminal abortions) and diseases the physician failed to report; caring for patients of ill-prepared, incompetent, or negligent physicians; the actual role of the nurse in relation to household chores and other members of the family; and a variety of issues regarding the economic and general welfare of the nurse.

These issues were no less gripping than the issues and dilemmas nurses currently face in home health care. The specific nature of the dilemmas has shifted. There is an increased emphasis on the rights of the patient and the rights of "status individuals" such as the elderly, superimposed on a general cultural concern for individualism and freedom. Those dilemmas are even more pointed when they involve older, declining, single patients who live alone and whose condition, circumstances, or life-style poses an increased risk to themselves or others.

These are not the only new dilemmas the home health nurse encounters in respiratory care. Advancing technology in the home health environment has increased the frequency with which the nurse encounters "high-tech" patients in the home. This reality brings issues—formerly and primarily faced in intensive care units—directly into the home care realm. Increasingly patients are being treated at home with life-sustaining interventions such as ventilators. Technology has allowed patients with chronic illnesses to remain alive longer. These patients include an increasing number of children whose lives have lengthened but who remain on life-sustaining treatments in the home.

## ETHICAL PRINCIPLES: TOOLS FOR DECISION MAKING

The three case studies presented at the beginning of this chapter are examples of complex situations encountered in delivering respiratory home care nursing. Ethical decision making, for which nurses generally have little educational preparation, is not a matter of visceral or hormonal responses, personal preferences, or a vague set of subjective values. Tools for analysis and decision making are found in ethical theories, and more specifically in ethical principles and rules (Fowler, 1989). There is great agreement (more than is often acknowledged) on the ethical principles that should be applied to decision making in health care. These principles should be regarded as objectively valid and not as a matter of subjective preference.

Beauchamp and Childress (1989) identify four principles in biomedical ethics: justice, autonomy, nonmaleficence, and beneficence. The preamble to the *Code for Nurses* identifies respect for persons as the fundamental principle from which the principles of autonomy, beneficence, nonmaleficence, veracity, confidentiality, fidelity, and justice are derived (American Nurses Association, 1985). There are other lists of principles; differences between lists depend on what the ethicists consider to be root principles, rather than derived rules, and not on a disagreement over which principles are important and which are not.

Dilemmas in the clinical practice of respiratory home care frequently involve the principles of autonomy, nonmaleficence, and beneficence (Fowler, 1987). Autonomy (or more fully, respect for autonomy) deals with the freedom to choose and to act on choices. Nonmaleficence is usually understood as the noninfliction of harm. Sometimes, however, nonmaleficence is combined with beneficence to form one principle. When that is done, beneficence is held to have four aspects: the noninfliction of harm, the prevention of harm, the removal of harmful conditions, and the positive benefiting of another (Franken, 1973). These principles are discussed in relation to the previous cases.

## CASE DISCUSSIONS
### Case 1

The issues in case 1 center on the principle of respect for autonomy. Specific issues are (1) whether the pulmonary patient can give free consent, (2) whether to control the patient's smoking, (3) whether it is morally permissible to prevent a patient from smoking in an oxygen-enriched environment, and (4) how to handle moral dilemmas involving suboptimal medical practice.

Respect for autonomy means that we accord others the same right to moral decision making that we ourselves would want. It involves allowing people the freedom and information necessary to make decisions and the freedom to act on those decisions. There are, however, limits to the extent to which a person can act autonomously; the line must be drawn where the person's action will harm another (Mill, 1978).

The way in which the principle of autonomy operates in clinical practice is through the doctrine of informed consent. The two constitutive aspects of informed consent are full informedness and free consent (Fowler, 1986a, 1987a). To be fully informed, a patient must have all the information a reasonable person would need to make a decision in a similar sort of situation. This is called the reasonable person criterion or standard. Although this standard is necessary, it is not sufficient. Giving the patient all the information a reasonable person would need is not useful if the patient is unable to understand the information as given. Thus a second criterion, the individual patient standard, is necessary. The individual patient standard holds that the information must be given in a manner (e.g., method, vocabulary) that the patient will comprehend and that any additional information, made necessary by virtue of who the patient is as a person, must also be communicated (President's Commission, 1982).

The consent aspect of informed consent deals with the issue of voluntariness. For a person's consent to be free, it must not be influenced by coercion, duress, fraud, deceit, impulse, habit, or other internal or external factors that unduly influence the person or disrupt rationality.

Under the doctrine of informed consent and the principle of respect for autonomy, two major grounds exist for interfering with a patient's liberty. Those are (1) decisions in which the person's informedness or consent is impaired (i.e., decisions that are uninformed or ill informed or not freely consenting and situations where the individual is cognitively incapable of making an informed decision [e.g., advanced Alzheimer's disease]) or (2) decisions that have significant potential for harm to others. Apart from these grounds, it is ethically difficult to justify interfering with a person's (patient's) liberty.

When caregivers are tempted to intervene and to prevent a patient from acting autonomously, it is generally on the grounds of "protecting the patient from his or her own bad judgment." Such interference can be called paternalism. Paternalism falls under the principle of beneficence and is a problem because it involves the assertion that doing good for a person is more important than respecting that person's autonomy. Strong paternalism, which is overriding a patient's "bad judgment" when it is fully informed and freely consenting, is rarely if ever morally justifiable. Weak paternalism, which is overriding a patient's judgment when the patient's informedness or consent is affected, can sometimes be justified. On the whole, however, ethics requires that persons be autonomous moral agents and that their autonomy be preserved and respected.

The issue of autonomy arises in case 1 of the 66-year-old man who is living alone and being treated for emphysema. Several questions need to be addressed before the issues surrounding autonomy can be resolved. First, has the patient been informed, and second, is the patient capable of being fully informed and freely consenting?

There should be no question that the patient has been amply informed, and if the patient is informed, this issue can be dispensed with. The more crucial question is the patient's capacity to deal with the information. In any patient who has pulmonary disease and whose blood gas values document severe respiratory failure, there is no question that the thinking processes are dramatically altered. However, with a chronically ill patient who has long-standing hypoxia and some hypercapnia, it is unlikely that cognition is sufficiently impaired to disqualify consent for being involuntary. Furthermore, there is not sufficient evidence—despite the alleged "hard-headedness" and "crotchetiness" of the patient in case 1—that his cognition is affected to the point of altering his level of voluntariness. Thus it is unlikely that his ability to understand the relationship between his health and smoking or between oxygen use and smoking is impaired. It is additionally unlikely that his cognition is so burdened as to render his decisions not freely consenting.

Strong paternalism is rarely justifiable, although weak paternalism is sometimes justified. Is there an issue of paternalism in case 1? Basically, patients must be allowed to make autonomous decisions, even when they make decisions we would not make for ourselves or for them. This patient does have the right to continue to smoke, despite its effect on his health. Preventing him from smoking would be an instance of strong paternalism.

But what about the oxygen-enriched environment? Would it be permissible to deny the patient oxygen on the grounds that smoking while using oxygen poses a high degree of danger? This is not an issue of paternalism, but rather an issue of harm to others. There are two possible approaches.

First, if the risk of fire is truly great, the patient must be offered the choice of supervised smoking only (or no smoking if he chooses) when oxygen is in use or a choice between oxygen and smoking. We must accept that some patients will choose smoking over oxygen. Second, if by evaluation the risk of fire is insubstantial, the patient must be cautioned and given all the information necessary for safety, but then allowed to make his own choices.

Another choice that the patient makes is to remain in his own home. Here again, health professionals have a duty to respect patient autonomy insofar as it is fully informed, freely consenting, and does not pose a danger to others. This patient does have the right to stay in his own home, even if it leads to problems of hygiene or cleanliness, as long as others are not harmed.

The *Code for Nurses* affirms the preceding comments on patient autonomy. It maintains that "truth telling" and the process of reaching informed choice underlie the exercise of self-determination, which is basic to respect for persons (American Nurses' Association, 1985). Patients' rights to self-determination must be supported even when they make "wrong" choices.

Case 1, however, raises another issue—that of the less-than-optimal physician. Nursing declares itself to be a patient advocacy profession, with ultimate responsibility to the patient (Fowler, 1990). The *Code for Nurses* asserts that

the nurse's primary responsibility is to the health, welfare, and safety of the client. As an advocate for the client, the nurse must be alert to, and take appropriate action regarding any instances of incompetent, unethical, or illegal practice by any member of the health care team (American Nurses' Association, 1985).

The nurse is called on to act when a physician seems not to be practicing in the best interests of the patient or is simply irregular or inappropriate in issuing the medical orders. The unfortunate problem is that in many instances the home health nurse does not have agency mechanisms whereby such a situation can be easily handled, and the nurse is left either to muddle along or to attempt to bring indirect pressure. In some situations orders are simply circumvented. This puts the nurse in both moral and legal jeopardy.

Traditionally nurses have been enjoined to work "up the administrative ladder" in reporting or expressing concern about incompetent, illegal, or unethical medical practice. Ladders are usually inexorably slow, often ineffective, and even more often responsive to political rather than ethical concerns. Furthermore, this route does not effectively differentiate between problems that are questions of legality, ethics, or competence. Ideally there would be specific mechanisms for addressing each category of concern.

A more satisfactory mechanism for expressing clinical concern with moral overtones is through an intraagency or interagency ethics committee. Hospital ethics committees necessarily are somewhat different.

Ethics committees can serve a variety of functions, including educating staff, providing forums for discussion and recommendations regarding the resolution of ethical dilemmas, establishing guidelines for dealing with selected recurrent issues, and counseling patient, family, and staff. Hospital ethics committees should be constructed on the "rule of thirds"—that is, one third should be nurses, one third physicians, and one third others (clergy, lay, or community respresentatives and other health professionals). In a home health care agency it is reasonable to increase the proportion of nurses on the committee. It is customary and appropriate for ethics committees to accept referrals of dilemma or inquiry from any source—staff, patient, family, and administration.

Ethics committees generally function on an optional model, in which review of a case is optional and recommendations are optional. Decision-mak-ing authority remains with the primary caregivers. The virtue of ethics committees is that they can serve to clarify or illuminate ethical dilemmas in clinical practice (Fowler, 1986). However, and perhaps most important for respiratory home health care nursing, they can serve as authoritative bodies, representing the agency and using their power of moral suasion to safeguard patient (and nurse) well-being. This serves to ratify the nurse's moral judgment where appropriate and relieves the nurse of the burden of having to fight moral battles alone.

## Case 2

The issues in case 2 include (1) patient autonomy as expressed in the woman's desire to terminate treatment once begun, (2) the permissibility of withdrawing treatment, (3) reluctance by professionals or family members to withdraw treatment, and (4) coparticipatory decision making within the family.

Nonmaleficence and beneficence entail aspects other than paternalism. Nonmaleficence, the non-infliction of harm, requires that health professionals not engage in *vitalism*. Vitalism involves sustaining life at virtually any cost and is seen as a violation of the dignity of the patient; it is not morally defensible and is a misreading of the *sanctity of life* principle.

The sanctity of life principle asserts that life is a relative (not an absolute) value and that our duty to preserve it is a relative one (McCormick, 1981). Some lives are of such low quality that they are not worth living (Fowler, 1987b). But how is such a judgment to be made?

Nursing refuses to judge the quality of a person's life on the basis of social worth criteria—that is, the quality of a person's life does not depend on his or her contribution to society. Nursing ethics insists on making quality of life judgments based on what the patient deems to be a quality of life worth living. Thus the patient is the determiner of his or her own quality of life; it is not an external judgment based on the patient's potential for social contribution, nor is it an external judgment of what might be in the patient's "best interests."

Of course, here the presumption is that the patient can express his or her own wishes or values or that they are known through a "durable power of attorney for health care," "living will," or other advance directive or through family members, despite a patient's present inability to voice them. The *Code for Nurses* states that

clients have the moral right to determine what will be done with their own person; . . . to accept, refuse or terminate treatment without coercion; and to be given necessary emotional support (American Nurses' Association, 1985).

Nursing locates the discussion of the patient's desire to terminate treatment (i.e., the issue of patient autonomy) within the discussion of "respect for human dignity." In recent years nursing has tended to regard the observance of patient values and wishes (i.e., respect for patient self-determination or autonomy) as one aspect of the larger principle of respect for persons. To override the patient's wishes in the interest of "doing good" for the patient by continuing treatment is seen as a paternalistic violation of the patient's human rights, dignity, and worth.

In a case such as this the patient clearly is fully informed and freely consenting. Her death is inevitable and is expected by the family. Although her death would be a tragedy, it cannot be declared a "harm to others" to justify professional intervention preventing her termination of treatment.

The *Code for Nurses* is not the only document that supports this position. Additional support can be found in the report of the President's Commission (formally the President's Commission for the Study of Ethical Problems in Medicine and Biomedical and Biobehavioral Research) entitled *Deciding to Forego Life-Sustaining Treatment* (President's Commission, 1983). Both documents acknowledge that it is ethically wrong to force a patient to accept a treatment that will in essence increase or prolong the person's suffering. The President's Commission report goes further by stating that

nothing in current law precludes ethically sound decision making. Neither criminal nor civil law—if properly interpreted and applied by lawyers, judges, health care providers, and the general public—forces patients to undergo procedures that will increase their suffering when they wish to avoid this by foregoing life-sustaining treatment.

Thus a patient may refuse treatment that will prolong suffering; however, may the patient terminate treatment once started? It is often thought that it is easier to withhold treatment than to withdraw it and that withdrawal of treatment is impermissible. It is easier never to give a treatment than to take it away once begun. However, the difference between not starting and taking away a treatment is a psychologic and emotional one, albeit a powerful difference to the professional. The difference is not one of either law or ethics.

Additionally, health professionals have been and remain reluctant to withdraw life-sustaining treatment from a patient, under the mistaken belief that, while it might be morally appropriate, they will be susceptible to a charge of deliberately taking another person's life. Withdrawal of treatment at the request of the patient (or family when the patient cannot participate), particularly when treatment prolongs suffering and dying, is not legally actionable; it is neither homicide nor suicide. A lawsuit can be brought for any (even a frivolous) reason, but it will not necessarily be sustained. At some point health professionals must refuse to allow a fear of litigation to drive clinical decision making. Lawsuits are inevitable, even when nothing that warrants legal action has been done.

The distinction between failing to initiate and stopping treatment—that is, withholding versus withdrawing treatment—is not of moral importance. Adequate justification for not commencing a treatment is also sufficient for ceasing it (President's Commission, 1983).

Morally adequate justifications for withholding treatment are (1) the patient does not wish it, (2) it will harm the patient, or (3) it will not medically benefit the patient. The same reasons are sufficient to justify the withdrawal of treatment (Fowler, 1987c).

It is not unusual to find situations in which the physician or family members do not want to honor the patient's wishes. When the physician objects, it is important to ascertain the reasons. The objection may be based on a mistaken interpretation of the law, or perhaps the objection is based on a lack of understanding or misinterpretation of the patient's wishes. If communication has not been closed off, dialogue with the patient, family, or nurse might resolve this situation. However, if the physician declines to permit the withdrawal of treatment because of an emotional, psychologic, or characterologic predisposition, the assistance of an ethics committee, a medical peer review group, or another advisory body may be needed. In the end, however, if a physician persists in continuing a treatment against the patient's wishes and refuses to sanction its termination, the patient is forced to terminate the treatment himself or herself, to bring legal charges against the physician, or to seek another physician. None of these avenues enhances the patient-physician relationship at a time when a patient might most need support from the medical profession. The professional who cannot live with the autonomous decision of a competent patient (when that decision will not harm others) should make provisions for another practitioner to oversee the patient's care.

In the event that the person who objects to the discontinuation of treatment is a family member, health professionals (sometimes through a fear of a lawsuit) have tended to continue treatment, even over the patient's objections. This constitutes the infliction of harm by failing to respect autonomy and is morally inappropriate. Where there is disagreement within the family, the members should be assisted and supported in reaching a joint conclusion.

To be morally right, decisions should take place within the community of moral discourse—that is, those directly involved with the decisions should participate in formulating them. Thus decisions with respect to a family member should be made between and among spouses, children, parents, and other significant persons in the patient's life.

However, professionals should not attempt to rectify dysfunctional family dynamics, at the time

of decision making about life-sustaining treatment, unless direct harm to the patient may result. Family communication and decision-making patterns undoubtedly have been long set before the professional ever encounters the dying patient. Unilateral decision making, especially to stop treatment, is problematic from an ethical point of view; families should be assisted, insofar as is necessary, to make decisions jointly or at least to corroborate the decision made. Sometimes support for an appropriate but hard decision is all that is necessary. In instances when family members disagree, the patient's decision must ultimately prevail.

An additional issue in cases 2 and 3 is that of the provision of respite care for overburdened family members. Perhaps as a result of its early and continued practice in the home, nursing consistently identifies the patient as the person in the bed, plus his or her "relational web," usually the family. Care is not given to the patient alone, but also encompasses the family network. Respite care is a part of the nursing concern for the patient.

Unfortunately, respite care is seldom covered financially, and families are left to care for themselves. Although local solutions may be available to individual nurses or agencies, respite care is a system-wide concern that calls for nursing advocacy at the sociopolitical level.

In the current economic climate, patients are discharged from the hospital at a higher level of acuity or are left in the home when formerly they would have been hospitalized. It is appropriate for the health care system to discourage inappropriate uses of its resources, and it is appropriate for patients and families to participate in their own care. We have to question, however, whether the measures designed to reduce third-party costs actually hide costs in unreimbursed professional and quasi-professional services that are provided by a family member. Predominantly, care giving in the home by family members falls to the responsibility of one individual who is almost always a female. Thus it can be legitimately asserted that, while benefiting third-party payors, in the end cost cutting is borne on the backs of the women in society. When costs are kept low by virtue of family participation in the provision of care, it seems that a just allocation of social resources should include third-party payment or other provision for respite care.

Nursing advocacy at the sociopolitical level is accomplished only through nurses' participation in the political processes of the states or nation, whether individually or collectively (Fowler, 1989 and 1989a). Nurses who have no inclination to participate in such processes must be advocates for change by supporting the professional organizations and political action groups that can, with their collective voice, have an impact on the system.

## Case 3

The issues in case 3 include (1) autonomy of pediatric patients, (2) disagreement about treatment between parents and child, and (3) the social control of reproduction.

Family disagreement can occur not only between spouses but also between parents and child. Minor children who are not emancipated cannot legally give consent to or refuse treatment of the sort this case involves. Here, law and ethics diverge. In ethics, the right to self-determination, to expression of values, and to respect for autonomy is not limited to adults. Minors, particularly those who have entered the teenage years, have an ethical right to self-determination that may not be extended to them under the law. Whether the patient is a child or an adult, the standard of informed consent still applies. Explanations must be simplified as necessary to make them comprehensible to the individual child. In this case Peter's wishes must be taken with ultimate seriousness; he is fully informed and freely refusing treatment (Fowler, 1988).

Although it can be argued that Peter's level of physical compromise is so acute that it renders his decision involuntary, this is not a strong argument. Peter's decision appears to be based on his history of struggle, rather than on this particular crisis. His disease is such that death from the disease itself is inevitable; the question is one of the prolongation of his life. Peter apparently views his suffering as

unendurable—that is, he judges his life to be of a quality not worth living, as reflected in his comments that he does not want to be sick anymore. His refusal of rehospitalization should be taken seriously. It is both an expectation and a necessity for health professionals to

maintain a predisposition for sustaining life (while accepting that prolongation of dying may serve no worthwhile purpose for a particular patient) . . . . until it is quite clear that a patient is making an informed, deliberate, and voluntary decision to forego specific life-sustaining interventions . . . . (President's Commission, 1982).

Peter's comment to Steven—"Don't ever let them do this to you"—may indicate that his sense of human dignity or self-worth has been assaulted and that harm has been inflicted, in which case nursing must take measures to shore up his sense of worth. Nurses must take care to reinforce a dying patient's courage, self-worth, and dignity, while not pressing for life-sustaining measures or even hospitalization that will violate that dignity. This is a delicate balance, not easily achieved, but more clearly approximated when the patient's wishes are accorded great weight, even when that patient is a minor.

Unfortunately, few agencies or institutions have adequate mechanisms or processes for dealing with parent-child disagreement. Currently the best options are the involvement of parents and siblings in community support groups, conferences with the family members and additional staff, if available, and the provision of consistent staff to work with the parents. Clergy, where available, can be an invaluable resource to the home health care nurse and the family. Although counseling does not solve all problems, open communication and vigilant anticipatory discussion of potential dilemmas can prevent eventual standoffs.

Case 3 raises the additional question of the parents' indiscreet mention of having another child within Peter's and Steven's hearing. This is undoubtedly a symptom of their grief response, made worse by the fact that they will eventually face a similar situation with their second son. However, such an expression may harm the emotional well-being of the two boys. These parents need a supportive avenue for voicing their sense of loss and grief in a fashion that will not silence their expression of that grief, yet will also not harm the boys.

It is also possible that the parents have discussed the issue of having other children with Peter and Steven. The chance that a third child may also have cystic fibrosis poses some serious questions. Decisions about procreation are generally regarded as falling within a legal "sphere of privacy." Parents (even those who may produce a child with genetic defects) are permitted to regulate their procreative decisions without interference. Mill (1978) maintains that

the only part of conduct of anyone for which he is amenable to society is that which concerns others. In the part which merely concerns himself, his independence is, of right, absolute.

Reproductive decisions are generally regarded as falling outside the domain of social control.

From an ethical perspective, nursing generally affirms the rights of an individual patient over the "social good"—that is, although the social "cost" of a child with congenital defects is of broad concern to the nurse, it is overshadowed by the nurse's concern for the emotional cost to the individual couple.

## CONCLUSION

Ethical dilemmas and ethical decision making are not new to home health care nurses. However, the content of those dilemmas has shifted dramatically, partly as a result of the increased use of nurse specialists in the home, which creates an environment for more complex interventions or procedures and treatments.

This brief discussion of three cases is intended to introduce some nursing perspectives on ethical issues that the respiratory home health care nurse may encounter. We cannot provide anything more than the briefest of examinations of relevant issues here. A greater depth of learning in ethics and nursing requires an in-depth exploration of the bioethics literature.

The bioethics literature is more attentive to medical concerns than those of nursing. Nonetheless, this literature is important because it argues various positions and discusses a range of options that are considered morally right. It is not nursing specific—that is, the dilemmas often are not applied to nursing and they do not discuss nursing perspectives on the issues. Nursing perspectives and concerns may differ from those of medicine.

The function of ethics is to clarify and illuminate the moral dilemmas of clinical practice and to provide comfort by reducing moral uncertainty. It can provide insight into the values or obligations that may be in conflict and can provide guidelines for analysis and decision making. However, although ethics can help to clarify and illuminate a dilemma and thus help to increase our confidence in our moral decisions, it cannot always remove the pain or anguish of the situation. Illness and disease are human tragedies. The hope of ethics is that, in the midst of suffering, human dignity and worth will be affirmed and respect for persons will prevail against the assaults of disease, illness, and even treatment.

### REFERENCES

American Nurses' Association: *Code for nurses with interpretive statements,* Kansas City, Mo, 1985, The Association.

Beauchamp TL, Childress JF: *Principles of biomedical ethics,* ed 3, New York, 1989, Oxford University Press.

Fowler MDM: The intrainstitutional ethics committee: response to a primal scream, *Heart Lung* 15:101, 1986.

Fowler MDM: Tain't cricket: an ethical commentary on informedness, *Heart Lung* 15:414,1986a.

Fowler MDM, Levine-Ariff J, editors: *Ethics of the bedside: a sourcebook for the critical care nurse,* Philadelphia, 1987, JB Lippincott.

Fowler MDM: Voluntariness, *Heart Lung* 16:102, 1987a.

Fowler MDM: The nurse's role: rights and responsibilities. In Mapes, Zembaty, editors: *Biomedical Ethics Review,* ed 3, New York, 1990, McGraw-Hill .

Fowler MDM: Unendurable illness, *Heart Lung* 16:454, 1987b.

Fowler MDM: And the rabbi Judah the Prince died: on the withdrawal of treatment, *Heart Lung* 16:576, 1987c.

Fowler MDM: Pediatric informed consent, *Heart Lung* 17:584, 1988.

Fowler MDM: Ethical decision making in clinical practice, *Nurs Clin North Am* 24:955, 1989.

Fowler MDM: Nursing and social ethics. In Chaska NL, editor: *The nursing profession: turning points,* St Louis, 1989a, Mosby.

Franken W: *Ethics,* ed 2, Englewood Cliffs, NJ, 1973, Prentice Hall.

McCormick R: *How brave a new world?* New York, 1981, Doubleday.

Mill JS: *On liberty,* Indianapolis, 1978, Hackett.

President's Commission for the Study of Ethical Problems in Medical and Biomedical and Behavioral Research: *Deciding to forego life sustaining treatment,* Washington, DC, 1983, US Government Printing Office.

President's Commission for the Study of Ethical Problems in Medical and Biomedical and Behavioral Research: *Making health decisions: the ethical and legal implications of informed consent in the patient practitioner relationship,* Washington, DC, 1982, US Government Printing Office.

## SUGGESTED READING

Husted GL: *Ethical decision making in nursing,* St Louis, 1991, Mosby.

# CHAPTER 24

# LEGAL ISSUES

JUDY I. MASSONG

Community health professionals' practices are unique because their practice, more than any other health care practitioner, involves the enforcement of health laws and regulations at the federal, state, and local levels. In addition, a review of case law involving health care shows that the community health care professional is involved in a multitude of specific legal issues, such as guardianship matters, clients' rights with regard to termination of life support, issues of child and adult abuse, and situations involving clients' wills.

Because of the nature of their conditions, patients with chronic respiratory problems are especially likely to find themselves in situations with legal ramifications. For example, severe hypoxemia is often present in patients with chronic lung disease, and this can alter cognitive function sufficiently to impair the patient's judgment and decision-making ability. These chronic lung diseases may leave the client so physically or mentally disabled that he or she is dependent on the care of others. Occasionally these "others" prove to be neglectful or abusive.

The close and personal contact that characterizes home health care means that the home health care practitioner is often the first person approached for advice on complex legal or medical issues. Therefore the practitioner must be prepared.

In addition, medical care of many patients with chronic lung disease is provided by physicians without specialty training in pulmonary medicine,

who may not be practicing state-of-the-art pulmonary medicine. Home health care nurses who have developed expertise in the care of patients with chronic lung diseases (e.g., through advanced education or practice) may find themselves in the difficult position of knowing more about certain aspects of a patient's management than the patient's physician. When medical management poses a threat to the patient's safety, the home health care practitioner may be legally required to take action. The preceding examples are just a few of the specific ways home health care practitioners enter the legal labyrinth.

This chapter discusses the legal issues most often confronting the community health practitioner, discusses legal ramifications of cases described in Chapter 23, and ends with a brief overview of professional negligence (malpractice). The chapter is not intended to be a source of legal advice for specific situations, nor is it a substitute for legal counsel.

## LEGAL CONCEPTS

The legal issues influencing community health care practitioners and the rights of their clients are manifold. Over the years the functions of community health care practitioners have changed radically. For example, nurses used to be seen as an extension of the physician, the agency, or the hospital in which they worked. They are now seen as independent, professional practitioners. Currently, as a result of consumers' heightened awareness of health care practitioners as independent professionals with expanded roles, skills, and knowledge, practitioners are no longer able to sit back and be "protected" legally by the physician, agency, or hospital. With professional autonomy and a rise in the economic standard of the practitioner have come legal accountability and lawsuits.

## Sources of Laws Governing Professional Practice

The laws that govern practice are developed from a multitude of sources. The ultimate source is, of course, the U.S. Constitution. Other federal laws include statutes passed by Congress and regulations established by different federal agencies. A similar arrangement exists on the state level. The different state constitutions, state statutes, and agency regulations govern nursing's professional practice. The state statutes and agency regulations set forth the definition and scope of nursing's practice. A health care practitioner must act within the statute's definition and scope of practice or be subject to civil or criminal discipline by the appropriate state agency or to a civil lawsuit brought by a patient for personal injury. Information on specific state statutes relevant to the health care practitioner and health care may be obtained from local bar associations and may also be available from state nurses' associations.

## APPLICATION OF LEGAL CONCEPTS TO CASE DISCUSSIONS
### Inappropriate Medical Orders

The first case presented in Chapter 23 illustrates the legal issues involved when a home health care practitioner works with a physician whose medical orders do not reflect standard medical practice. For example, in this first case, an elevated $PaCO_2$ is not, in and of itself, sufficient reason for withholding supplemental oxygen from a hypoxemic patient. This is especially true when hypoxemia is severe enough (as in this instance) to impair the patient's judgment.

In the situation described the nurse also believed that the physician was not prescribing appropriate

medications. The nurse confirmed this belief by talking with a pulmonologist. However, this was not sufficient action. The standard of care probably requires that the nurse go further than just substantiating his or her knowledge. An expert probably would argue that the nurse must "consult with the chain of command" (i.e., talk with the supervisors and document all actions). The nurse would be expected to talk with the attending physician about the orders and their effects on the patient's condition. This discussion also needs to be charted. If the nurse does all of the preceding and the physician still does not change, he or she probably has done what could be done within the definition and scope of nursing practice and has acted as a reasonably prudent practitioner.

In such situations, it is tempting for a concerned home health care practitioner to warn the patient or family of the physician's apparently inadequate care or encourage the client to change to a different physician. However, to do so might subject the nurse to ethical criticism or legal action. If the patient or family volunteers dissatisfaction with the physician's care or specifically asks for a referral to a different physician, the home health care practitioner is free to suggest the names of other physicians.

In summary, every nurse has an independent (i.e., independent of the physician) duty to provide care within the scope and knowledge of his or her education, training, and license requirements. In a number of states, such as California, Pennsylvania, Minnesota, North Carolina, Washington, Colorado, Montana, Delaware, and Louisiana, the nurse as a condition of licensure is held directly responsible for a patient's welfare (Northrop, 1987). Therefore the nurse may be held liable for following through with an improper order given by a physician if the standard of care was such that the practitioner knew or should have known that the order was improper.

### Guardianship

Because of the nature of the practice, the home health care practitioner may be the first person to find that a patient is no longer able to cope independently at home, either because of increasing physical disability or because of mental impairment. A family member or friend may be able to step in for a time but usually cannot be responsible for all the care, daily transactions, and decisions. Therefore the practitioner may be in a position to suggest the appointment of a guardian. The intent of guardianship is to legally protect a person without the necessity for determining incompetency and without the attendant deprivation of civil and legal rights that incompetency determinations usually require (Revised Codes of Washington [RCW], 11.88.005).

Guardianships can be arranged for either minors or adults; they can be either temporary or permanent and either limited in scope or plenary. Under every state guardianship statute the laws provide procedural safeguards for the person for whom the guardianship is arranged (Logan, 1987). In case the matter is contested by someone with legal authority to object, the procedural safeguards include notice of hearing to appoint the guardian and description of the type and terms of the guardianship (Northrop, 1987).

For example, we can consider the case description of the elderly man who was living alone (case 1). From the description of his circumstances, it seems that he would be a candidate for the appointment of a guardian. However, this depends on whether the health care practitioner assessed him as "disabled/incompetent." Each state's definition of what constitutes "disabled/incompetent" differs, and practitioners are well advised to become familiar with their state's definition. For example, the State of Washington defines the "incompetent" adult as one who is incompetent—by reason of mental illness, developmental disabilities, senility, habitual drunkenness, excessive use of drugs, or other mental incapacity—in managing his property, caring for himself, or both (RCW, 11.88.010). Since the elderly man in case 1 is "forgetful" and is endangering his life by smoking while unattended, he arguably fits the description of "incompetent." However, this same behavior may be descriptive of pure stubbornness. It may

also be descriptive of a condition that is reversible with proper medication and oxygenation. The essential question for the practitioner then becomes to what degree the patient is cognitively impaired and a threat to his own safety. The practitioner needs to make a thorough assessment. If the patient is adequately treated with medication and oxygen but is still a threat to his own safety, guardianship should be considered. It would seem prudent for the practitioner to broach the subject with the man's niece.

Another frequently seen type of guardianship is one for minors or disabled adults. This type of guardianship is called guardian ad litem. A guardian ad litem is usually an attorney who has been appointed by the court to protect and advocate the interests and rights of the minor during the pendency of proceeding before court. The guardian ad litem may also have the authority to authorize or withhold emergency life-saving medical services when the individual is unable to decide because of his minority or disability.

In case 3, Peter, who is 14 years old and as such is still considered a minor, wants to have all treatment stopped and refuses to go to the hospital, even though his failing health suggests a need for more aggressive therapy, including possible evaluation for a lung transplant. Peter's parents adamantly insist that Peter be treated aggressively, despite his wishes. It would seem that in such a polarized situation the minor's right to control his destiny needs to be advocated. The nurse is in a position to suggest that a guardian ad litem be appointed by the court for the minor. It would then be the guardian's responsibility to advocate or commend to the court Peter's rights, should the situation come to that.

In summary, there are a multitude of situations for which the appointment of a guardian is appropriate. The practitioner is in a position to assess the need for a guardian and to find a guardian if others in the family are unable or unwilling to do so. The practitioner should know how to gain access to the state's guardianship system. Information about guardianships can usually be obtained from the state bar association.

## Neglect and Abuse

Because home health care practitioners are in the patient's home, they are well positioned to assess the adequacy of care a patient is receiving. In most instances family members provide the best care they can. However, neglect and abuse do occur, and their prevalence appears to be increasing rapidly (Northrop, 1987). Respiratory patients ill enough to require home care are often highly dependent on those with whom they live. Dyspnea, disability, and frailty make them particularly vulnerable. The constant care demands of these chronically ill individuals can stress a caregiver beyond tolerable limits. This may result in neglect simply because of the caregiver's fatigue and burnout.

Most states now have statutes covering abuse of dependent persons. Such statutes generally require a health practitioner to file a report with the appropriate state agency whenever there is a reasonable cause to believe that a child or developmentally disabled or incompetent adult has suffered abuse or neglect.

Some states, such as Washington, have gone further and include those elderly adults who have not yet been declared incompetent but who may be functionally disabled. The various state statutes concerning elderly abuse require the health care practitioner to make a report within a specified time after there is reasonable cause to believe that the elderly person has suffered abuse or neglect. Failure to make a report to the appropriate state agency usually exposes the health care practitioner to civil or criminal liability (RCW, 74.34.010 *et seg*).

Almost all states that have abuse statutes requiring a health care practitioner to report abuse also have clauses that protect a person who makes a report in good faith, based on a reasonable cause to believe that the abuse has occurred. However, the laws seek to discourage and prevent malicious reporting.

If a home health care practitioner is concerned that a patient may be suffering neglect or abuse, the situation should be discussed promptly with a supervisor and that discussion documented. If the supervisor concurs, the appropriate authorities should be notified promptly. If indications of ne-glect or abuse are more subtle, it may be prudent to seek legal counsel, which is available on retainer in most home health care agencies.

## Natural Death Acts and Living Wills

A significant percentage of pulmonary patients referred for home health care have diseases severe enough to be classified as end-stage. Exacerbations occur frequently and tend to be more life threatening when they do occur. A pattern of frequent intensive care hospitalizations, some involving intubation, often develops. After a few such episodes many patients decide they are no longer willing to endure this degree of episodic invasive intervention and seek assurance that they will not be subjected to such "unusual" measures in the future.

## The Patient Self-Determination Act

In response to such cases and to the much publicized Cruzan case, U.S. Senators Patrick Moynihan and John Danforth introduced federal legislation concerning patients' rights of self-determination. The Patient Self-Determination Act of 1991 is applicable to all patients who are 18 years of age or older, covered by Medicare or Medicaid, and receiving care by hospitals, nursing homes, health maintanence organizations (HMOs), and home health care agencies. The legislation requires that, on admission, patients are (1) advised of their rights to accept or refuse treatment and (2) asked if they have completed any advanced directive (e.g., living will or durable power of attorney for health care). If the answer is yes, the health care provider may ask, depending on state law, for a copy of the document. If the answer is no, the health care provider must provide the patient with written information regarding the documents, specific to the laws of each particular state. The health care provider must then document that the discussion took place and record the outcome of the discussion.

## Living Wills and Advanced Life Directives

A growing number of states have acknowledged that adults have the fundamental right to control decisions relating to their health care, including the decision to have life-sustaining procedures with-held or withdrawn. Some states have chosen to resolve the question of the termination of life support systems by enacting living will statutes and brain death statutes. However, these acts affect only a limited number of "qualified patients" because of their restrictive language.

The living will concept works relatively well when the competent adult patient has anticipated in advance and fulfilled the legislative requirements as set forth by state statute. An advanced life directive goes beyond a living will and specifies what treatment the person wishes and does not wish to have if that person becomes ill. For an example of such statutes, see Washington's Natural Death Act, (70.122.010 *et seq.*). This directive is not a legal document but rather enables a person to clearly communicate end-of-life preferences (e.g., no mechanical ventilation or tube feedings) (Fig. 24-1).

## Durable Power of Attorney for Health Care

As a direct result of the cumbersome requirements of the different state statutes, many states, such as California and Washington, have enacted a Durable Power of Attorney for Health Care (Cal. Civil Code #2410-2421, 2430-2451 [West Supp., 1986]; RCW, 11.94). Under this arrangement the patient may execute a durable power of attorney authorizing an "attorney in fact" to make health care decisions for the person (principal) executing the directive. An attorney in fact is a person designated by another to make decisions regarding health care when the patient (principal) is no longer capable of making those decisions. To be effective, the durable power of attorney must be drawn up while the principal is competent and must specifically authorize the attorney in fact to make health care decisions for him or her. In general, other requirements are as follows:

- The document must be dated and witnessed by two people who are not the attorney in fact and who are neither related to nor a beneficiary of the principal.
- The witnesses must attest that the principal (patient) is of sound mind.

- The witnesses may not be the health care provider or employees of the health care provider.

Each state's statute differs somewhat, and practitioners are encouraged to look at their state's statute for specific requirements.

Under the durable power of attorney the attorney in fact can act only when the principal is unable to give consent or make decisions. If the attorney in fact must act, he must act in a manner consistent with the desires of the principal as expressed in the durable power of attorney or through information known to him as attorney in fact. If the principal's desires are unknown, his duty is to act in the best interests of the principal. Generally speaking, however, an attorney in fact may not give consent to abortion, sterilization, psychosurgery, convulsive treatment, or commitment to a mental health facility (C. Civil Code #2434 [a] through [b]).

Health care providers are immune from civil and criminal liability as long as they follow the conditions set forth in each state's statute and the durable power of attorney. Key to the immunity is to make a good faith effort to determine whether the principal's documents comply with the state statute requirements (RCW, 70.122.010 *et seq.;* Cal. Civil Code #2438 [c]).

Looking at the facts as presented in case 2 (the ventilator-dependent mother), we can analyze how the current laws may be applied. First, because state and federal case law recognizes an adult's right to determine matters concerning one's own health care (see *Roe v. Wade,* 91 S. CT. 1610, 1973), the woman in case 2, as a competent adult, could request that the ventilator be turned off. If the physician refused to comply, the patient would be forced to go to court to seek judicial resolution of her decision.

Another way to approach this same problem is to have the woman enact a living will, if she resides in a state that has such statutes. If this woman does not reside in such a state, she might be able to appoint an attorney in fact who could advocate for her when she is no longer able. The attorney in fact could advise the physician of the woman's decision to have life support systems terminated. Even with such documents in place, if the hospital

## Natural Death
## Directive to Physicians


Directive made this _____ day of _____ 19 _____ .

I, _____ , being of sound mind, willfully, and voluntarily make known my desire that my life shall not be artificially prolonged under the circumstances set forth below, and do hereby declare that:

(a) If at any time I should have an incurable injury, disease, or illness certified to be a terminal condition by two physicians, and where the application of life-sustaining procedures would serve only to artificially prolong the moment of my death, and where my physician determines that my death is imminent whether or not life-sustaining procedures are utilized, I direct that such procedures be withheld or withdrawn and that I be permitted to die naturally.

(b) In the absence of my ability to give directions regarding the use of such life-sustaining procedures, it is my intention that this directive shall be honored by my family and physician(s) as the final expression of my legal right to refuse medical or surgical treatment and I accept the consequences from such refusal.

(c) I understand the full import of this directive and I am emotionally and mentally competent to make this directive.


Signed _____
Seattle, King County, State of Washington


The declarer has been personally known to me and I believe him or her to be of sound mind.


Witness _____

Witness _____


_____
Notary Public

Witnesses may not be related to patient by marriage or blood, may not be an heir, and may not be a care provider.

**Fig. 24-1**   Natural death directive to physicians.

or attending physician has no policy or does not recognize an adult's right to decide such matters as termination of life support systems, the person is forced to go to court to seek resolution of the matter. Currently hospitals or health care practitioners are not liable for refusing to follow an individual patient's living will (Cal. Civil Code #2438 [c]).

Although each individual's decision and reasons for withdrawing or withholding life support mechanisms are compelling, society as a whole is still not ready to allow termination in all cases. Both medicine and the law wrestle endlessly with these medicolegal ethical considerations. To date there is no remedy in sight. Each situation must be plead individually, and that may be the best solution.

## OTHER LEGAL ISSUES
### Wills

Even though the health care practitioner is not trained in the techniques or law of executing a will, there are cases of impending death when no time is available for the patient to seek counsel from an attorney. Therefore the following information is given to assist the practitioner who is faced with an emergency situation.

A will is a declaration of a person's mind about what is to be done after his or her death with his or her property. The will is operative only at death and applies only as the situation existed at death (*Restatement,* Property, 2nd ed, 1954, #8). The factors necessary for a valid will are the following:
- Sound mind
- Testamentary capacity
- Freedom from fraud and undue influence
- Legal age

For the purposes of making a will a person must be of sound mind—that is, he can understand and carry in his mind the following: the type and amount of his property, the persons who are the natural objects of his generosity and their claim on him and the disposition of his property (*Whitworth's Estate,* 110 Cal. App. 256,294 Pac. 84 [1931]). If the preceding qualifications are lacking,

he is not mentally competent to make a will (*Halbert's Will,* 15 Misc. 308, 37 N.Y.S. 757 [1895]). However, if the person's mental power is reduced below ordinary as the result of severe illness, extreme old age, or illiteracy, yet he has enough intelligence to understand the act of making a will as detailed above, there is capacity to make a will (Wood-Renton, "Testamentary Capacity in Mental Disease," 4 Law QR, 442 [1888]).

If the practitioner is assisting the patient in drafting the will, the practitioner is well advised to be aware of the following general rules:
- Ordinarily a will must be in writing. A nuncupative, or oral, will is frowned on by the courts but may be valid in some states.
- A written will must be signed by the patient and at least two competent witnesses.
- The person making the will should sign before the witnesses subscribe. In a few states the person making the will must inform the witnesses that the document being signed is a will.
- The practitioner should know that the universal requirement is for all the witnesses to be present at the same time and to sign the will in the presence of the person making the will.
- Witnesses should not be beneficiaries under the will because being a witness may affect their right to receive under the will.
- Lastly, the most important aspect for the practitioner, if present at the time of drawing up of the will, is to chart the patient's apparent mental and physical condition and the fact of his writing of the will. Such charting will be important in a will contest.

### Informed Consent

The basis for the doctrine of informed consent is the theory that an adult of sound mind has the right to determine what shall be done with his or her body. Therefore, to exercise that right, a person must be given sufficient information to make an intelligent decision (*Smith v. Shannon,* 100 Wn. 2d 26, 666 P. 2d 351 [1984]).

Most states have statutes concerning informed consent. However, even if an individual state does not have an informed consent statute, the common law doctrine on informed consent governs. The common law doctrine of informed consent requires that a health care practitioner disclose to a patient all relevant material information that a person needs to make an informed decision to accept or reject the proposed treatment. The doctrine places a heavy burden on the health care practitioner to inform the patient. Failing to so inform a patient can be the basis for a malpractice suit against the health care practitioner. Material facts that the health care practitioner must explain include the nature and character of the proposed treatment; the anticipated results, risks, and benefits of the proposed treatment; and the recognized possible alternative forms of treatment. It is not necessary, however, to explain every conceivable alternative. However, one must explain those that are generally recognized as reasonable, including the alternative of no treatment (88 ALR 3d 1008).

In deciding what is "material," the practitioner must analyze whether a reasonable person would consider the information important in deciding whether to consent. A material risk is one that occurs frequently or that is rare but serious (*Miller v. Kennedy,* 91 Wn. 2d 155, 588 P. 2d, 734 [1987]).

Under common law the informed consent doctrine applied only to physicians. Currently, in most states with informed consent statutes, the doctrine applies to all health care providers, including nurses (RCW, 7.70.020). With nurses practicing in expanded roles, informed consent is an area of increasing potential liability for nurses. Generally, the elements necessary to prove lack of informed consent are the following:

- That the health care provider failed to inform the patient of important facts relating to the proposed treatment
- That the patient consented to the treatment without being fully informed of the important facts
- That a reasonably prudent patient under similar circumstances would not have consented to the treatment if informed of such a material fact(s)

- That the treatment rendered caused the injury about which the patient complains

This places a heavy burden on the health practitioner to explain facts and determine whether the patient understands. The clearest and best way to prevent malpractice in this area is to document conversations concerning consent to treatment and to document that the client's signature was obtained. Exceptions to the general rule to disclose are the following:

- The health care provider is not liable for not disclosing risks that are not reasonably foreseeable and not inherent in the procedure.
- The health care provider is not required to disclose a risk for which full disclosure would be detrimental to the patient's best interests.
- The practitioner is not required to disclose risks commonly known (i.e., when it is reasonable to assume that the patient already knows the risk).
- The practitioner is not required to disclose risks of treatment if the patient requested that he not be told of the dangers.
- The practitioner is not required to disclose risks of treatment and alternatives in an emergency situation when the patient is not in a condition to make a determination for himself (*Holt v. Nelson,* 11 Wn. App 230, 523 P. 2d 211 [1974], 88 A.L. R. 3d 1008).

In summary, prudent and reasonable practice requires that the practitioner discuss all material risks of treatment and alternatives to treatment so that the client may give informed consent to treatment or procedures. The practitioner must then briefly document the information given and the client's responses. To do less might subject the practitioner to a suit for malpractice.

## PROFESSIONAL MALPRACTICE
### Anatomy of a Lawsuit

A civil lawsuit for professional negligence is initiated by the plaintiff (client) filing with the court a summons and complaint and delivering the summons and complaint to the defendant (health care practitioner). The complaint is a statement of facts to the court and defendant. The complaint contains the allegations of the plaintiff (patient) on which he bases his right to damages. The filing of the summons and complaint must be done by the plaintiff in a timely fashion or the plaintiff will be forever barred from bringing his action before a court. State statutes vary concerning the time in which a plaintiff must file a claim.

The summons is a paper that is directed to the named defendant and notifies the defendant that the lawsuit has commenced. The practitioner (defendant) then notifies his insurance carrier or agency who in turn notifies an attorney. The attorney for the defendant then prepares an "answer" to the complaint. The answer is the document in which the defendant admits or denies the plaintiff's allegations. In addition, the defendant asserts any defenses he might have to the plaintiff's allegations within the answer.

After the answer is filed, discovery begins by both sides. Discovery is the time period between filing the complaint and trial. Both sides must conduct discovery pursuant to the rules of court. The rules usually allow discovery by interrogatories, depositions, and requests for documents. Interrogatories are written questions from one party to the other party, whereas the deposition is a face-to-face questioning session on oath before a court reporter. The attorneys for both sides are present during the taking of a deposition. The attorney is present to protect the rights of his client by interposing appropriate objections.

During the pendency of a lawsuit, the health care practitioner may participate in the lawsuit in one of three roles—party to lawsuit (defendant or plaintiff, as explained above), fact witness, or expert witness. As a defendant, the community health care practitioner is a "party" to the lawsuit and is being sued for negligent acts or omissions. As a party defendant, the community health care practitioner will defend his or her charting, treatment, diagnoses, and judgments. The injured party (plaintiff) will charge that the community health care practitioner's acts or omissions fell below the

skill and practice of what a reasonably prudent practitioner would have done in the same or similar situations or circumstances (*Restatement [Second] of Torts* #282).

Another health care practitioner, usually with the same professional schooling and experience as the defendant practitioner, will be called on to act as an "expert witness." The expert will testify as to what should have been done—what a reasonably prudent professional would have done in the same or similar circumstances. The expert witness must be qualified as an expert to the satisfaction of the court before he or she may testify about the issues involved in the case (Federal Rules of Evidence 702, 703, and 704). The expert usually has worked, had educational experience, or has done research in the area of concern and will therefore be able to testify that the professional either acted within the standard of care or fell below the standard of care for the year the incident occurred.

The third role is that of a fact witness. A fact witness is one who neither is acting as an expert nor is a party to the lawsuit. The fact witness is merely one who describes the facts surrounding the incident as remembered. For example, in a lawsuit brought by heirs who are contesting a will, an issue might arise as to whether the patient (decedent) was under the influence of mind-altering prescription drugs and therefore not of sound mind. The practitioner, having cared for the decedent, may be called on as a fact witness to describe the medications given, times given, and their effect on the patient to the court so that the court might render a decision about whether the patient (decedent) had the mental capacity to write the will.

## Professional Negligence

Other than knowing the roles that the practitioners might be called on to play in any given lawsuit, health care practitioners should also understand, for their own protection and the safety of their clients, the necessary elements for proving professional negligence (malpractice). At common law, four elements have to be proved for the injured client to prevail in a claim of professional negligence. It was and still is necessary for the injured client to prove each and every element to be successful. The four elements are duty, breach of duty, proximate cause, and damages. Intent to cause harm is not a necessary element of professional negligence. If the client is injured by the practitioner's acts or omissions and the client is able to prove all four elements of negligence, the client will prevail even though the practitioner did not intend harm (*Restatement [Second] of Torts, #* 281-296). Most states have codified these elements within their professional negligence statutes—for example, Washington's statute provides:

*Revised Codes of Washington 7.70.040. Necessary elements of proof that injury resulted from failure to follow accepted standards of care.* The following shall be necessary elements of proof that injuries resulted from the failure of the health care provider to follow the accepted standard of care:

The health care provider failed to exercise that degree of care, skill and learning expected of a reasonably prudent health care provider in the profession or class to which he belongs, in the State of Washington, acting in the same or similar circumstances. Such failure was a proximate cause of the injury complained of.

## Duty

The first element of negligence is duty. The professional's duty is to comply with the applicable standard of care (i.e., to act as a reasonably prudent professional would in similar circumstances). The standard of care is the yardstick with which to measure performance of a health care provider. A community health nurse who renders professional services to an ill or injured client is under a legal duty to that client to exercise due care in the performance of such services (*Ybarra v. Spangard*, 25 Cal. 2d 486, 154 P. 2d 687 [1944]).

## Breach of Duty

The second element that must be present is a breach of duty. Because the duty is to conform to the applicable standard of care, breach of duty is a failure to conform to the standard of care applicable to the situation. When a professional fails to act as a reasonably prudent health care professional, he or she breaches his or her legal duty to the client. The way this is demonstrated at trial is through the testimony of an expert witness who describes what the standard of care is in a particular set of circumstances. The expert witness opines whether the health care practitioner acted within the applicable standard of care for the year in which the incident occurred. After hearing all the evidence at trial, including expert witnesses from both sides, the judge or jury decides whether the health care practitioner acted within the standard of care.

## Proximate Cause

The third element of negligence is proximate or direct cause. The term "proximate cause" means a cause that, in a direct sequence, unbroken by any new independent cause, produces the injury complained of without which such injury would not have happened (*Restatement [Second] of Torts,* #281.) This element requires proof of a reasonably clear connection between the defendant's act or omission and the resultant harm or injury. Therefore merely proving that the professional fell below the applicable standard of care does not entitle the patient to recover damages. The plaintiff must prove that *but for* the professional's negligent action, the patient would not have suffered harm.

## Damages

The fourth and last element that must be present is actual damage. The patient must show that the health care practitioner's negligence damaged the patient in some way—for example, damage may be proved at trial by an accounting of the time that the patient was off work, which would be in the form of lost wages. If permanently injured, the patient may recover for loss of future earning capacity. The patient may recover for past and future medical expenses attributable to the injury and past and future pain and suffering.

## Most Common Areas of Liability

The following discussion is not an exhaustive list of all areas of recurring professional liability but may heighten the awareness of problem areas so that the practitioner can avoid liability by being more cautious.

The most common allegation of negligence against practitioners is medication errors (Northrop, 1987). These errors include administering the wrong medication, wrong dosage and concentration, and using the wrong route. The cases involving drug errors are multitudinous and expensive. For example, in *Wagner v. Kaiser Foundation Hospitals* (285 OR 81, 589 P. 2d 1106 [1979]), a nurse anesthetist gave an overdose of narcotics during surgery. The plaintiff (patient) sustained permanent brain damage, and the jury awarded him $750,000. Home care nurses routinely teach patients and families how to administer prescribed medications and frequently administer medications directly. Legal responsibility is the same whether a nurse directly administers the medication or teaches the patient or caregiver to administer it. Responsibility with regard to teaching, however, ends with the dissemination of correct information and the assurance that the patient or caregiver has understood the instruction (i.e., a nurse cannot be held liable when a patient takes medications in contradiction to how he or she was instructed).

Another common allegation against the practitioner is liability for burns. Cases involving vaporizers, douches, enemas, sitz baths, showers, heating pads, and lamps are numerous. In *Bowers v. Olch* (120 Cal. App. 2d 108, 260 P.2d 997 [Cal. 1953]) the nurse attending a paraplegic was held liable when the patient suffered serious burns from a pipe that started his bedclothes on fire. The nurse had given the patient the lit pipe and left the room. The pipe fell from the patient's mouth, and because of his paraplegic condition he was unable to put out the fire. The court held that the nurse had a duty to ensure the safety of the patient, especially from known hazards.

A third concern is reporting changes in patients' conditions. In an Ohio case the court held that a nurse was liable for not observing and reporting changes in her patient's condition (*Richardson v. Doe,* 176 Ohio 371 [1964]). Failure to observe and report changes that result in harm to the patient can result in negligence.

## Importance of Charting

Charting is the linchpin of most malpractice suits and as such is an important area of concern. The chart is the patient's legal record. Therefore the practitioner must use due care when writing in it. In addition, good, concise charting can be the practitioner's best defense in the event of a malpractice suit. The old phrase, "Everything was normal or I would have charted it," never repeats well before a jury 3 or more years after the fact. The best course is to write legibly and chart all actions taken—that is, everything that was done for the patient and all pertinent information and follow-up instructions. The usual excuse that the practitioner does not have enough time will not hold up under cross-examination at trial (Creighton, 1981). The jury usually requires proof of actions taken by the professional when faced with a devastation allegedly caused by health care professionals.

In summary, people are more apt to believe something if it is in writing. Besides, good charting not only prevents lawsuits, it facilitates patient care.

## Malpractice Risks Associated with Improper Medical Orders

Nurses are under a legal duty to follow physicians' orders (*Abille v. U.S.A.,* 482 F. Supp. 703 [1980]). However, this holds only if the order is a proper one. If a nurse carries out an improper order, the nurse *and* the physician are held liable if the other side is able to prove that the nurse fell below the standard of care by carrying out the improper order. Therefore, before carrying out any prescribed treatment plan, the practitioner's duty is to understand the treatment, to understand its effects, and to know whether it is appropriate for the patient.

Because of the type of patient and the home-based nature of the practice, the home health care practitioner is faced with legal or ethical quandaries on an almost daily basis. The preceding pages highlight only a few areas of concern, give an overview of the law as it might relate to various situations, and discuss ways the practitioner can manage his or her job in a legally safe manner for both the patient and the practitioner. If unsure about a legal issue, the practitioner should always consult an attorney.

**REFERENCES**

Creighton H: *Law every nurse should know,* ed 4, Philadelphia, 1981, WB Saunders.

Logan B, Dawkins D: *Family centered nursing in the community,* Reading, Mass, 1987, Addison-Wesley.

Northrop C, Kelly M: *Legal issues in nursing,* St Louis, 1987, Mosby.

# INDEX

*t* indicates a table; number in italics indicates a figure.

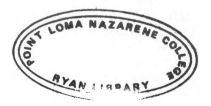

POINT LOMA NAZARENE COLLEGE
RYAN LIBRARY